Population and Community Biology

POPULATION DYNAMI
INFECTIOUS DISEASES
THEORY AND APPLIC.

Population and Community Biology

Series Editors

M. B. Usher, Senior Lecturer, University of York, UK

M. L. Rosenzweig, Professor, Department of Ecology and Evolutionary Biology, University of Arizona, USA

The study of both populations and communities is central to the science of ecology. This series of books will explore many facets of population biology and the processes that determine the structure and dynamics of communities. Although individual authors and editors have freedom to develop their subjects in their own way, these books will all be scientifically rigorous and often utilize a quantitative approach to analysing population and community phenomena.

THE POPULATION DYNAMICS OF INFECTIOUS DISEASES: THEORY AND APPLICATIONS

Edited by

Roy M. Anderson

Reader in Parasite Ecology
Imperial College, London University

Springer-Science+Business Media, B.V.

British Library Cataloguing in Publication Data

The population dynamics of infectious diseases.
1. Communicable diseases.
I. Anderson, Roy M.
614.4   RA651

ISBN 978-0-412-21610-7   ISBN 978-1-4899-2901-3 (eBook)
DOI 10.1007/978-1-4899-2901-3

Contents

Contributors

Roy M. Anderson Department of Pure and Applied Biology, Imperial College, London University, London SW7 2BB, England.

Joan L. Aron Laboratory of Mathematical Biology, National Institutes of Health, Building 10, Room 4B-56, Bethseda, Maryland 20205, USA

Andrew D. Barbour Statistical Laboratory, University of Cambridge, 16 Mill Lane, Cambridge CB2 15B, England.

David J. Bradley Ross Institute of Tropical Hygiene, London School of Hygiene and Tropical Medicine, Keppel Street, London WC1E 7HT, England.

B. Cvjetanović Institute of Immunology, Rockefeller Street 10, 4100 Zagreb, Yugoslavia.

Klaus Dietz Institute for Medical Statistics, Tübingen University, Hallstattstrabe 6, D-7400 Tübingen 1, West Germany.

Anne Keymer Molteno Institute, University of Cambridge, Downing Street, Cambridge, England.

Robert M. May Biology Department, Princeton University, Princeton, NJ 08544, USA.

Gary Smith Department of Pure and Applied Biology, Imperial College, London University, London SW7 2BB, England.

Mervyn Thomas Research Support Unit, Faculty of Arts and Social Studies, University of Sussex, Brighton, Sussex, England.

Alan Wilson Department of Biology, University of York, Heslington, York YO1 5DD, England.

Preface

Since the beginning of this century there has been a growing interest in the study of the epidemiology and population dynamics of infectious disease agents. Mathematical and statistical methods have played an important role in the development of this field and a large, and sophisticated, literature exists which is concerned with the theory of epidemiological processes in populations and the dynamics of epidemic and endemic disease phenomena.

Much of this literature is, however, rather formal and abstract in character, and the field has tended to become rather detached from its empirical base. Relatively little of the literature, for example, deals with the practical issues which are of major concern to public health workers.

Encouragingly, in recent years there are signs of an increased awareness amongst theoreticians of the need to confront predictions with observed epidemiological trends, and to pay close attention to the biological details of the interaction between host and disease agent. This trend has in part been stimulated by the early work of Ross and Macdonald, on the transmission dynamics of tropical parasitic infections, but a further impetus has been the recent advances made by ecologists in blending theory and observation in the study of plant and animal populations.

The present book aims to review and draw together recent work on the population dynamics of infectious disease agents (including viruses, bacteria, protozoa and helminths), to show how mathematical models can shed light on empirical epidemiological observations. The chapters focus attention on the population biology of the disease agent, and on the biological assumptions which underlie the various models. Some of these models describe the dynamics of specific infections in a very detailed way, while others discuss the general properties that emerge from a broad theoretical framework. The approach is in the main descriptive, with emphasis on the biological detail that must be included in mathematical models, on the epidemiological concepts and principles that emerge from theoretical work and on the role theory can play in the design of disease control programmes. A special feature of the chapters is their attempts to summarize and distil the available empirical evidence and to incorporate this epidemiological information into the body of theory.

The book therefore seeks to fill a useful niche intermediate between mathematical texts on disease dynamics and texts on practical epidemiology. Mathematical details are kept to a minimum and the book is directed towards epidemiologists, public health workers, parasitologists and ecologists. It is hoped, however, that sufficient details of the models are included to stimulate interest amongst mathematicians and statisticians. Although primarily aimed at review and synthesis, the book does contain much new material. As indicated by the chapter headings, the book is mainly concerned with infections of man but two chapters deal with diseases of veterinary importance.

Chapter 1 describes the dynamics of directly transmitted viral and bacterial infections of man, and focuses on the concept of herd immunity and its significance in the design of vaccination programmes. It introduces the notion of the basic reproductive rate of an infection, and shows how this parameter plays a central role both in determining observed epidemiological patterns and in the design of policies for disease control. This theme is further developed and refined in the other contributions.

Chapter 2 deals with the dynamics of acute bacterial infections and emphasizes the role complex simulation models can play in the design of optimal control policies. This chapter also underlines the important contribution played by inapparent infections in the persistence and stability of bacterial disease agents in human communities.

Chapter 3 gives a brief survey of the basic dynamical features of geohelminth infections of man and discusses the impact of chemotherapy on observed population behaviour. The concepts of transmission thresholds and breakpoints are discussed in relation to two of the most prevalent human diseases; namely, hookworm and roundworm infections. Similar themes are discussed in Chapter 4 in the context of human tapeworms, some of which have very complex life cycles involving one or more intermediate host species. These complex life cycles create many problems in model development and analysis, and in the acquisition of quantitative epidemiological data.

Chapter 5 gives an in depth treatment of the dynamics of one of the most important human infections in the world today; namely, malaria. This particular group of parasites stimulated some of the earliest attempts to use models to investigate disease dynamics. The chapter focuses on the complications introduced by vector transmission and examines the important topic of acquired immunity to reinfection. For malaria the degree of immunological protection acquired by the human host appears to depend on the frequency of exposure to infection.

The dynamical properties of another important group of parasites, the schistosomes (which also triggered early developments in mathematical epidemiology), are examined in Chapter 6. These parasites are transmitted indirectly via a molluscan intermediate host and the pathology of the infection to man is dependent on the burden of worms harboured. The chapter explores the significance of various biological complications to the dynamics of helminth infections such as transmission via a molluscan host, sexual mating behaviour of the adult worms, acquired immunity and heterogeneity introduced by spatial effects and human behaviour patterns.

Chapter 7 presents a detailed analysis of the epidemiology of onchocerciasis which is one of the most important diseases caused by the human filarial nematodes. Special attention is given to the density-dependent factors which regulate parasite population growth of this vector-transmitted infection and to the significance of transmission rates dependent on the age and sex of the human host. Theoretical models are used to examine the impact of vector control on the dynamics of the disease.

The next two of the remaining three chapters discuss the dynamics of disease agents within animal populations. In Chapter 8 an analysis is presented of the population biology of the rabies virus in European fox populations and models are described which help to assess the impact of various control options. The fox host in Europe is an important reservoir of infection, transmitting this highly pathogenic virus to domestic animals with the associated risk of frequent human contact. Chapter 9 gives a survey of fascioliasis in cattle and sheep, a disease caused by a helminth parasite which is transmitted indirectly via a molluscan host. The chapter places special emphasis on the significance of climatic and spatial factors in determining observed fluctuations in disease prevalence, and describes the use of simulation models to assess the effectiveness of various control options.

The final chapter, Chapter 10, presents a suitably cautionary tale for a book of this nature. It draws attention to the dangers inherent in using oversimplified models to explain epidemiological phenomena and argues that theoretical studies in epidemiology have had, up to now, little impact on public health policy. The book therefore ends with a challenge to future workers in this field.

I hope that the selection of chapter topics has provided a representative picture of recent and past developments in the population study of disease dynamics. The chapters may serve to indicate unanswered questions, areas in which our biological knowledge is inadequate and directions for future research. I further hope that the contributions convey the feeling that this relatively new field of scientific study is an exciting one in which much remains to be done.

The number of people whose influence has helped to form this multi-authored volume is too large to list but I wish in particular to thank M. J. Anderson, M. S. Bartlett, N. A. Croll, A. Crowden, R. M. May and T. R. E. Southwood.

1 Directly transmitted viral and bacterial infections of man

Roy M. Anderson

1.1 INTRODUCTION

The origins of contemporary epidemiological theory can be traced back to the early part of the 20th century. Just prior to this period the mechanisms by which infectious disease agents spread within populations had been revealed by microbiological research, notably that of Pasteur and Koch, and this, together with a statistical familiarity with epidemiological data (particularly the geometry of the epidemic curve (Farr, 1840; Brownlee, 1906)), laid the groundwork for future developments.

The first major theoretical contribution was that of Hamer (1906) who postulated that the course of an epidemic depends on the contact rate between susceptible and infectious individuals. This notion has become one of the most important concepts in mathematical epidemiology; it is the so-called 'mass action principle' in which the rate of disease spread is assumed to be proportional to the product of the density of susceptibles times the density of infectious individuals. This simple assumption is central to most deterministic and stochastic theories of disease dynamics.

Hammer formulated the mass action principle in a discrete time model but in 1908 Ronald Ross (celebrated as the discoverer of malarial transmission by mosquitoes) translated the problem into a continuous-time model in his pioneering work on the dynamics of malaria (Ross, 1911, 1915, 1916, 1917). The structured form of Ross's model meant that, for the first time, it was possible to use a clearly defined mathematical theory as a genuine research tool in epidemiology.

The ideas of Hamer and Ross were extended, and explored in more detail, by Soper (1929), who deduced the underlying mechanisms responsible for the often observed periodicity of epidemic outbreaks of disease, and by Kermack and McKendrick (1927) who established the celebrated threshold theorem. This theorem, according to which the introduction of infectious individuals into a community of susceptibles will not give rise to an epidemic outbreak unless the density of susceptibles is above a certain critical value, is, in conjunction with the mass action principle, a cornerstone of modern theoretical epidemiology.

Since this early beginning the growth in the literature concerned with mathematical epidemiology has been very rapid indeed. Recent reviews of this literature have been published by Bailey (1975) and Becker (1979). From an early stage it became apparent that the elements of chance and variation were important determinants of disease spread and this led to the development of stochastic theories. Much of the literature over the past three decades has been concerned with probabilistic models (see for example Bartlett, 1955, 1960; Bailey, 1975).

In recent work there has been an emphasis on the application of control theory to epidemic models (Wickwire, 1977), the spatial spread of diseases (Mollison, 1977) and the extension of the threshold theorem to encompass more complex deterministic and stochastic models (Whittle, 1955; Becker, 1977a). Despite the current sophistication of the mathematical literature dealing with epidemic phenomena, the insights gained from theoretical work have in general had little impact on public health policy. This may be due, in part, to the abstractly mathematical nature of much of this research. Becker (1979), for example, notes that of 75 papers on epidemiological models published since 1974, only five contained any data. If theoretical work is to make a contribution to the solution of practical problems in disease control, there clearly is a need for more data-oriented studies.

Some progress in this direction has been made, particularly with respect to the estimation from epidemiological data of parameters such as the incubation period and the duration of infectiousness (see Bailey, 1975, for a review of this work). More recently, attention has begun to be focused on the estimation of the rate of disease reproduction within human communities (the basic reproductive rate of infection, R) and on the use of this measure to determine immunization levels for disease control or eradication (MacDonald, 1957; Dietz, 1974, 1976; Yorke, Hethcote and Nold, 1978; Yorke *et al.*, 1979; Anderson and May, 1982a, b).

This chapter attempts to summarize the main trends in the more data-oriented sections of the literature. The emphasis is placed on recurrent epidemic behaviour and on the manner in which simple models can provide broad insights into the factors controlling the persistence and stability of directly transmitted viral and bacterial infections within large human communities (large-scale epidemic phenomena, Anderson and May, 1979a; May and Anderson, 1979). Of all disease agents, these directly transmitted infections have attracted the greatest attention from theoreticians. This is due, in part, to the relative simplicity of their life cycles but is also a consequence of the availability of long-term records of the population behaviour of such infections in Britain and North America.

1.2 HISTORICAL PERSPECTIVE

The observed improvement in human mortality rates within Europe and North America over the past three centuries, with life expectancy increasing from around 25–30 years in 1700 to around 70–75 years in 1970, comes mainly from a decline in deaths from directly transmitted infectious diseases. A combination of nature and nurture is implicated: higher standards of hygiene and nutrition have combined with probable changes in the genetic structure of human and parasite populations to decrease the pathogenicity of many common childhood infections (McNeill, 1976; McKeown, 1979). An illustration of this trend is displayed in Fig. 1.1 where the number of deaths in England and Wales attributed to measles is recorded for the period 1897 to 1939.

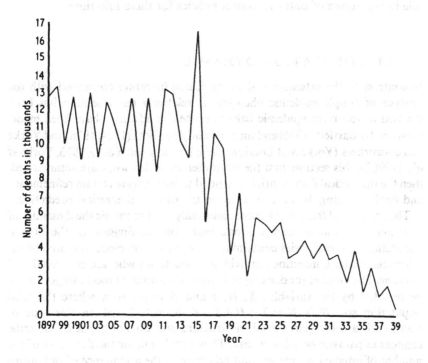

Figure 1.1 Yearly number of deaths attributed to measles in England and Wales over the period 1897 to 1939. (based on information from the Registrar General's statistical review of England and Wales).

In parallel with this decline in mortality, the frequency and magnitude of disease epidemics increased during the 18th and 19th centuries as a result of changing social patterns and the growth of large centres of population in increasingly industrialized societies. The reversal of this trend during the present century is largely due to the development and widespread use of vaccines to immunize susceptible populations against a variety of directly transmitted viral and bacterial diseases. The world-wide eradication of smallpox and the decline in the incidence of diptheria and paralytic poliomyelitis in Europe are testimony to the effectiveness of this method of disease control.

In many regions of the world, however, many viral and bacterial infections remain endemic, despite the widespread use of vaccines. On the continents of Africa and Asia certain common childhood infections such as measles and whooping cough still remain a significant threat to life. The effective control of these infections will, in part, be dependent on an improved understanding of the population biology of the disease agents. Mathematical studies, combined with detailed statistical analysis of epidemiological data, can play an important role in the design of optimal control policies for these infections.

1.3 POPULATION DYNAMICS

In contrast to the extensive and sophisticated literature concerned with the analysis of simple epidemic phenomena, relatively less attention has been devoted to recurrent epidemic behaviour. Major advances have been made, however, by Bartlett (1956) and more recently by Dietz (1974, 1976) and Yorke and co-workers (Yorke and London, 1973; London and Yorke, 1973; Yorke *et al.*, 1979). In this section, first the main themes of this work are summarized, then the theoretical framework is extended to incorporate certain refinements, and finally existing data are analysed in the light of theoretical predictions.

The theoretical framework most commonly used to mimic the dynamics of viral and bacterial infections is one based on the division of the human population into categories containing susceptibles, infecteds who are not yet infectious (latent), infectious individuals, and those who are recovered and immune. The number (or density) of individuals in each of these categories will be denoted by the variables X, H, Y and Z respectively where the total population size N is $N = X + H + Y + Z$. Models based on this type of framework are compartmental in structure and do not explicitly describe changes in parasite population size. They simply mirror the dynamics of the number of infected people without reference to the abundance of organisms within each individual. Broadly speaking, they seek to answer such questions as: can the infection be stably maintained within the population? Is the disease endemic or epidemic in character? Does the infection exhibit recurrent epidemic behaviour? How do the proportions of susceptibles, infecteds and immunes change through time after the infection is introduced into a susceptible population? What is the critical density of susceptibles necessary to maintain the infection?

It is conventional to assume that the size (or density) of the human population, N, remains roughly constant, or at least changes on a time scale that is long compared to all other time scales of interest in an epidemiological context. This assumption is reasonable for most populations in western societies. The assumption corresponds to the net input of susceptibles into the population (by births) being roughly equal to the net mortality μN (where μ is the per capita death rate and $1/\mu$ denotes life expectancy).

In accord with the 'mass action' transmission principle of Hamer (1906), we initially assume that the net rate at which infections are acquired is proportional to the number of encounters between susceptible and infectious individuals, βxy, where β is a transmission coefficient. Individuals pass from the latent state to the infectious stage at a per capita rate σ (such that the average latent period is $1/\sigma$), and recover to join the immune class at a per capita rate γ (where $1/\gamma$ represents the average infectious period).

Acquired immunity is taken to be lifelong, as it appears to be for most common childhood viral and bacterial diseases. This assumption, however, is easily modified in the model defined below. The assumption that all the rate parameters, β, σ, γ and μ, are simple constants is clearly artificial, but the resulting model provides a convenient point of departure for subsequent elaborations.

Under the above assumptions, a set of four first-order differential equations describe the dynamics of the infection within the human population (Dietz, 1974, 1976; Anderson and May, 1982a) and may be expressed as follows:

$$dX/dt = \mu N - \mu X - \beta X Y \tag{1.1}$$

$$dH/dt = \beta X Y - (\mu + \sigma)H \tag{1.2}$$

$$dY/dt = \sigma H - (\mu + \gamma)Y \tag{1.3}$$

$$dZ/dt = \gamma Y - \mu Z \tag{1.4}$$

Adding all four equations gives $dN/dt = 0$, corresponding to the original assumption that human population size, N, is constant.

The model defined by Equations (1.1) to (1.4) has two broad patterns of behaviour. The disease will be maintained within the population provided the 'basic reproductive rate', R, of the infection is greater than, or equal to, unity. The quantity R is of central importance to the dynamics of infectious disease agents and represents the expected number of secondary cases produced by an infectious individual in a defined population of X susceptibles (Dietz, 1974; Anderson and May, 1980). For the system defined above,

$$R = \frac{\sigma \beta X}{(\sigma + \mu)(\gamma + \mu)} \tag{1.5}$$

In more biological terms, secondary infections are produced at a rate βX throughout the expected lifespan, $1/(\gamma + \mu)$ of an infectious individual. Of these a fraction $\sigma/(\sigma + \mu)$ will survive the latent period to become the second generation of infectious individuals. Note the similarity of R to Fisher's net reproductive rate, R_0, a quantity widely used in the disciplines of ecology, population genetics and demography (Fisher, 1930). Also note that, although called a rate, R is in reality a dimensionless quantity. If $R < 1$, the disease cannot establish within the host population.

The criterion $R > 1$ for the establishment of the disease can equivalently be expressed as the requirement that the population of susceptibles exceed a critical 'threshold density', $X > N_T$, with the definition,

$$N_T = (\gamma + \mu)(\sigma + \mu)/\beta\sigma \qquad (1.6)$$

This is the celebrated threshold theorem of Kermack and McKendrick (1927). More generally, therefore we may express R as

$$R = X/N_T \qquad (1.7)$$

namely, the ratio of the number of susceptibles in the population divided by the threshold density necessary for disease persistence. In the absence of a continual inflow of susceptibles (when $\mu N = 0$), the criterion $R > 1$ represents the condition which must be satisfied for an epidemic to occur. Under such circumstances the disease will eventually die out once the supply of susceptibles drops below N_T.

For most of the common childhood viral and bacterial diseases, such as measles, whooping cough and chicken pox, the durations of the latent and infectious periods, $1/\sigma$ and $1/\gamma$, are of the order of a few days to a few weeks, while $1/\mu$ is of the order of 70 years or more. Under these circumstances ($\sigma \gg \mu$ and $\gamma \gg \mu$), Equations (1.5) and (1.6) may be accurately approximated as $R = \beta X/\gamma$ and $N_T = \gamma/\beta$.

Of the parameters determining the value of R, some are specific to the disease agents; examples are the parameters σ and γ, and that component of β which reflects the transmissibility of the disease. Other components of R, such as the density of susceptibles, X, and that component of β which reflects the average frequency of contact between individuals, vary greatly from one locality to the next depending on the prevailing environmental and social conditions. Even the value of $1/\gamma$ may be influenced by such conditions, since the isolation of infected children can substantially reduce the effective infectious period. The density of susceptibles depends mainly on the net birth rate in the community, which itself depends on the total population density, N. This observation underlies the observed correlation between endemic maintenance of disease without periodic fade out and community size. For measles in Britain and North America, the critical community size appears to be around 200 000–300 000 people (Table 1.1a) (Bartlett, 1957, 1960; Yorke et al., 1979), although from an analysis of epidemiological data for relatively isolated island communities Black (1966) suggests a figure in the region of 500 000 (Table 1.1b). On a more local scale, in low-density rural communities (where $X < N_T$) epidemics will be unable to develop and the disease will not persist in the absence of a continual inflow of infecteds.

The model defined by Equations (1.1) to (1.4) predicts that provided $R > 1$, the system will exhibit damped oscillations to a stable state (Dietz, 1974). At equilibrium the proportions of susceptibles, infected but not infectious,

infectious and immune individuals, namely, x^*, h^*, y^* and z^* respectively are given by:

$$x^* = 1/R \tag{1.8}$$

$$h^* = (1 - 1/R)(\gamma + \mu)/(\sigma C) \tag{1.9}$$

$$y^* = (1 - 1/R)/C \tag{1.10}$$

$$z^* = \gamma(1 - 1/R)/(\mu C) \tag{1.11}$$

where R is as defined in Equation (1.5) and

$$C = 1 + \gamma/\mu + (\gamma + \mu)/\sigma$$

The damped oscillatory behaviour of the model is clearly at odds with observed patterns of disease behaviour such as the regular 2-year cycle in measles epidemics in Britain and North America. This issue will be discussed more fully in a later section of this chapter.

Table 1.1a Reported cases of measles in cities of North America, 1921–1940 (adapted from Bartlett (1960) and Yorke et al. (1979)).

City	Population size (units of 100 000)	Years with a month in which no cases were reported
New York	75	0
Chicago	34	0
Philadelphia	19	0
Detroit	16	0
Los Angeles	15	0
Montreal	10	0
Cleveland	9	1
Baltimore	9	0
Boston	8	0
Toronto	7	0
Washington	7	0
Pittsburgh	7	0
Milwaukee	6	0
Buffalo	6	0
Minneapolis	5	0
Vancouver	3	20
Rochester	3	3
Dallas	3	18
Akron	2	8
Winnipeg	2	7

Table 1.1b   The persistence of measles within 19 island communities (adapted from Black (1966)).

Island	Population size (units of 100 000)	Percentage of months in which no cases were reported
Hawaii	5.50	0
Fiji	3.46	36
Iceland	1.60	39
Samoa	1.18	72
Solomon	1.10	68
Fr. Polynesia	0.75	92
New Caledonia	0.68	68
Guam	0.63	20
Tonga	0.57	88
New Hebrides	0.52	70
Gilbert and Ellice	0.40	85
Greenland	0.28	76
Bermuda	0.41	49
Faroe	0.34	68
Cook	0.16	94
Niue	0.05	95
Nauru	0.03	95
St. Helena	0.05	96
Falkland	0.02	100

1.4   PARAMETER ESTIMATION

The values of certain parameters of the model, such as the expectation of life, $1/\mu$, and the annual input of susceptibles, μN (the annual birth rate), can be obtained from published demographic statistics. Other parameters such as the average latent and infectious periods are more difficult to estimate and clearly vary for each disease agent.

To estimate these rate parameters it is necessary to turn to data reflecting transmission within family groups. The classic data on measles, collected by Hope Simpson in the Cirencester area of England during the years 1946–1952 (see Bailey, 1975), record the distribution of the observed time interval between two cases of measles in 219 families with two children under the age of 15 as listed in Table 1.2. The bulk of these observations represent case-to-case transmission within a family. However, in a small number of families, where the observed interval is only a few days it may be assumed that these cases are double primaries, both children having been simultaneously infected from some outside source. Early work on the estimation of latent periods was based on chain binomial models where it is assumed there is a constant incubation period which is terminated by a very short interval of high infectiousness since,

Table 1.2 Observed time interval distribution between two cases of measles in families of two (adapted from Bailey (1973); Hope Simpson's data from Cirencester, England 1946–1952)).

Time interval between the two cases (days)	Total number of families observed	Presumed double primaries	Presumed case-to-case transmission
0	5	5	.
1	13	13	.
2	5	5	.
3	4	4	.
4	3	2	1
5	2		2
6	4		4
7	11		11
8	5		5
9	25		25
10	37		37
11	38		38
12	26		26
13	12		12
14	15		15
15	6		6
16	3		3
17	1		1
18	3		3
19	.		.
20	.		.
21	1		1

once symptoms appear, the case is promptly removed from circulation. Susceptibles in contact with the case at the time of infectiouness have a certain probability of themselves becoming infected and this leads to successive crops of cases in a group of susceptibles (i.e. a family or school), the crops being separated in time by the incubation period (the time to appearance of symptoms). The variable number of cases actually observed at any given stage can be shown to have a binomial distribution (Wilson and Burke, 1942; Greenwood, 1931). Recently, more sophisticated models have been developed which assume that the latent period is variable, with say a normal distribution, and that it is followed by an extended but constant period of infectiousness (see Bailey, 1975, chapters 14 and 15; Becker, 1976, 1977b; and Gough, 1977). A rough guide to the latent, incubation and infectious periods of certain common viral and bacterial infections is recorded in Table 1.3. Some of these estimates are based on the detailed statistical analyses of household data while others are more speculative.

Table 1.3 Epidemiological parameters (information compiled from Fenner and White (1970); Christie (1974) and Benenson (1975)).

Infectious disease	Latent period, $1/\sigma$ (days)	Infectious period, $1/\gamma$ (days)	Incubation period (time to appearance of symptoms; days)
Measles	6–9	6–7	11–14
Chicken pox	8–12	10–11	13–17
Rubella	7–14	11–12	16–20
Infectious hepatitis	13–17	19–22	30–37
Mumps	12–18	4–8	12–26
Polio	1–3	14–20	7–12
Smallpox	8–11	2–3	10–12
Influenza	1–3	2–3	1–3
Scarlet fever	1–2	14–21	2–3
Whooping cough	6–7	21–23	7–10
Diphtheria	2–5	14–21	2–5

A direct estimate of the basic reproductive rate, R, from Equation (1.5) (or equivalently, of N_T from Equation (1.6)) is usually impossible, because of the difficulties inherent in obtaining any direct estimate of the transmission parameter, β. Dietz (1974, 1976) has, however, shown that R can be estimated from the relation

$$R = 1 + L/A \qquad (1.12)$$

Here L is the human life expectancy ($L = 1/\mu$), and A is the average age at which individuals acquire the infection. Dietz's derivation assumes all the rate parameters ($\sigma, \gamma, \mu, \beta$) are constants, independent of the age of the host. A more general expression for R has been derived by Anderson and May (1982a) and is discussed below, but Equation (1.12) remains a useful approximation even when the rate processes are age-dependent.

The average age at infection, A, can be estimated from data recording the proportion in each age class who have experienced the infection. The most accurate data of this form are provided by serological surveys but other, less accurate methods, are often employed, such as questionnaire surveys, or estimates can be obtained from age-classified notification records (Muench, 1959; Griffiths, 1974; Dietz, 1974). If the transmission parameter, β, of Equations (1.1) to (1.4) is age-independent, then $A = 1/\lambda$ where λ is the 'force of infection' of simple catalytic models (Muench, 1959). Under equilibrium conditions for example, in the context of Equations (1.1) to (1.4), $\lambda = \beta y^* N$. Typical data recording the proportion in each age class who have experienced the infection are displayed in Fig. 1.2. A more extensive collection of estimates of A for various diseases in various localities and times are presented in Table

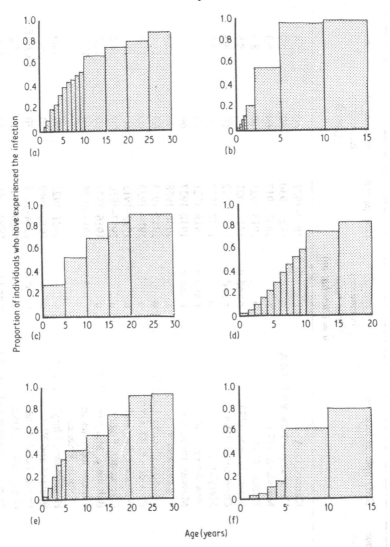

Figure 1.2 Examples of age-prevalence curves, based on either serological surveys or case notifications. (a) Poliomyelitis in the USA 1955 (serology) (b) Pertussis in England and Wales 1970 (case notifications) (c) Rubella in West Germany 1977 (serology) (d) Diphtheria in New York State 1915–1924 (case notifications) (e) Epstein–Barr virus in England and Wales 1970 (serology) (f) Mumps in Baltimore USA 1943 (case notifications).

1.4. Knowledge of A and L leads, via Equation (1.12), to an estimate of R as also catalogued in Table 1.4.

Most commonly the transmission parameter, β, and hence the force of infection λ, are age-dependent; this complication will be treated in a later section (Anderson and May, 1982a; Griffiths, 1974).

Table 1.4 The average age, A, at which various infections are acquired (see Anderson and May (1982a) for data sources).

Infectious disease	Average age at infection, A (years)	Geographical location	Type of community (r = rural, u = conurbation)	Time period	Assumed life expectancy (years)	R
Measles	11.7	Kansas, USA	r	1918–1921	60	5.4
	10.5	Cattaraugus, New York, USA	r	1920–1930	60	6.0
	10.0	Maryland, USA	r	1907–1917	60	6.3
	7.7	Kansas, USA	u	1918–1921	60	8.3
	7.3	Massachusetts, USA	r and u	1918–1921	60	8.8
	7.3	Connecticut, USA	r and u	1921–1922	60	8.8
	6.9	Maryland, USA	u	1907–1917	60	9.4
	6.7	New Jersey, USA	r and u	1918–1921	60	9.7
	6.7	Massachusetts, USA	r and u	1932–1937	60	9.7
	6.1	England and Wales	r	1956–1968	70	12.5
	5.9	London, Ontario, Canada	u	1912–1913	60	11.1
	5.8	Providence, RI, USA	u	1919–1935	60	11.3
	5.6	Willesden, England	u	1912–1913	60	11.7
	5.5	Cirencester, England	u	1947–1950	70	14.0
	5.4	Baltimore, Maryland, USA	u	1916–1927	60	12.2
	5.3	Various localities in North America	r and u	1912–1928	60	12.5
	5.1	Hagerstown, Maryland, USA	u	1921–1923	60	13.0
	4.8	England and Wales	u	1956–1969	70	16.3
	4.4–5.6	England and Wales	r and u	1944–1979	70	13.7–18.0
	4.2	Gary, Indiana, USA	u	1920–1922	60	16.2
	3.5	Zambia, Rhodesia and S. Africa	r and u	1960–1968	40	11.4

Disease		Location		Period		
	2.9	Ghana	r and u	1960–1968	40	13.8
	2.5	Eastern Nigeria	r and u	1960–1968	40	16.0
Whooping cough	9.4	Cattaraugus, New York, USA	r	1920–1930	60	6.4
	6.5	Various localities in North America	r and u	1912–1928	60	9.2
	6.5	Maryland, USA	r	1908–1917	60	9.2
	5.9	Hagerstown, Maryland, USA	u	1921–1923	60	10.2
	5.7	London, Ontario, Canada	u	1912–1913	60	10.6
	5.6	Connecticut, USA	r and u	1921–1922	60	10.7
	5.4	New Jersey, USA	r and u	1918–1921	60	11.1
	5.3	Massachusetts, USA	r and u	1918–1921	60	11.3
	4.9	Maryland, USA	u	1908–1917	60	12.2
	4.3	Baltimore, Maryland, USA	u	1943	70	16.23
	4.1–4.9	England and Wales	r and u	1944–1978	70	14.3–17.1
Chicken Pox	8.6	Maryland, USA	u	1913–1917	60	7.0
	8.5	Various localities in North America	r and u	1912–1928	60	7.1
	7.6	New Jersey, USA	r and u	1917–1921	60	7.9
	7.1	Massachusetts, USA	r and u	1918–1921	60	8.5
	6.8	Baltimore, Maryland, USA	u	1943	70	10.2
	6.7	Maryland, USA	u	1913–1917	60	9.0
Diphtheria	19.1	Pennsylvania, USA	r	1910–1916	60	3.1
	14.2	New York, USA	r	1918–1919	60	4.2
	12.8	Kansas, USA	r	1918–1921	60	4.7
	12.6	Maryland, USA	r	1908–1917	60	4.8
	11.6	Kansas, USA	u	1918–1921	60	5.2

Table 1.4 (continued)

Infectious disease	Average age at infection, A (years)	Geographical location	Type of community (r = rural, u = conurbation)	Time period	Assumed life expectancy (years)	R
	11.2	New York, USA	u	1918–1919	60	5.4
	11.0	Virginia and New York, USA	r and u	1934–1947	70	6.4
	10.4	Various localities in North America	r and u	1912–1928	60	5.8
Scarlet fever	14.9	Various localities in North America	r and u	1912–1928	60	4.0
	12.3	New York, USA	r	1918–1919	60	4.9
	10.8	Kansas, USA	r	1918–1921	60	5.5
	10.1	Maryland, USA	r	1908–1917	60	5.9
	10.0	Kansas, USA	u	1918–1921	60	6.0
	9.8	Pennsylvania, USA	r	1910–1916	60	6.1
	9.0	Pennsylvania, USA	u	1910–1916	60	6.7
	8.0	Maryland, USA	u	1908–1917	60	7.5
Mumps	13.9	Various localities in North America	r and u	1912–1916	60	4.3
	9.9	Baltimore, Maryland, USA	u	1943	70	7.1
Rubella	11.6	England and Wales	r and u	1979	70	6.0
	10.5	West Germany	r and u	1972	70	6.7
Poliomyelitis	17.9	USA	r and u	1955	70	5.9
	11.2	Netherlands	r and u	1960	70	6.2

1.5 THE INTER-EPIDEMIC PERIOD

Long-term records reveal that many common childhood diseases exhibit marked variations in incidence from year to year. These fluctuations are often of a regular nature, tending to arise as a broad consequence of the depletion and renewal of the supply of susceptibles. The 2–3-year cycles of measles, a typical example of which is shown in Fig. 1.3, is particularly remarkable. In general, the interval between major epidemics is termed the inter-epidemic period and values of this parameter, for a variety of childhood diseases, are recorded in Table 1.5.

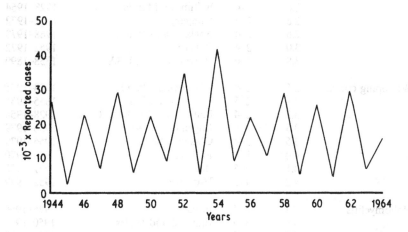

Figure 1.3 Measles in New York City from 1944 to 1964 (data from Yorke and London, 1973).

The deterministic model of Equations (1.1)–(1.4) exhibits damped oscillations, where, for diseases which are of short duration relative to the host lifespan ($\sigma \gg \mu$, $\gamma \gg \mu$), the period, T, of the oscillations is approximately (Anderson and May, 1982a):

$$T = 2\pi[LD/(R-1)]^{1/2} = 2\pi(AD)^{1/2} \qquad (1.13)$$

Here D is the sum of the lengths of the latent and infectious periods (i.e. $D = 1/\sigma + 1/\gamma$), and R, L and A are as defined previously. The tendency of these oscillations to damp out is clearly at odds with the patterns of persistent oscillations shown in Fig. 1.3 and documented in the studies listed in Table 1.5. The damping rate, however, is small and hence the stability of the system is 'weak' (Grossman, 1980). It is therefore to be expected that relatively small destabilizing effects, due to either external excitation or structural changes in the model, could neutralize the damping and bring about undamped oscillatory behaviour.

Stochastic effects and seasonality in transmission can perpetuate the

Table 1.5 The average inter-epidemic period, *T*, for various diseases (see Anderson and May (1982a) for data sources).

Infectious disease	Inter-epidemic period (years)		Geographical location	Time period
	Average	Range		
Measles	2.2	2–4	England and Wales	1855–1968
	2.2	2–3	New York City, USA	1928–1964
	2.3	2–4	Glasgow, Scotland	1929–1968
	2.3	2–3	Providence, RI, USA	1900–1923
	2.6	2–4	Baltimore, Maryland, USA	1928–1964
	2.6	2–5	Hungary	1952–1972
	2.6	2–4	England and Wales	1968–1979
	3.0	2–4	Bulgaria	1952–1972
	3.8	2–6	Providence, RI, USA	1858–1899
Whooping cough	2.5	2–4	Glasgow, Scotland	1928–1955
	2.8	2–5	England and Wales	1855–1955
	3.2	2–4	Baltimore, Maryland, USA	1928–1954
	3.5	2–5	England and Wales	1956–1979
	3.5	3–4	Glasgow, Scotland	1956–1979
	4.0	3–4	Finland	1940–1970
	4.1	2–5	Bulgaria	1921–1972
	4.2	4–5	Hungary	1952–1972
Poliomyelitis	2.8	2–4	Bulgaria	1926–1956
	4.0	3–5	England and Wales	1950–1965
	4.2	2–5	Finland	1940–1972
	4.6	4–5	Netherlands	1950–1965
Chicken pox	2.5	2–4	New York City, USA	1928–1972
	2.8	2–4	Baltimore, Maryland, USA	1929–1973
	3.0	2–4	Glasgow, Scotland	1929–1972
Rubella	3.3	2–5	Glasgow, Scotland	1929–1964
	3.4	2–7	Baltimore, Maryland, USA	1928–1974
	3.7	2–6	New York City, USA	1933–1972
Mumps	3.0	2–4	Baltimore, Maryland, USA	1928–1973
	3.0	2–6	New York City, USA	1928–1967
Diphtheria	5.1	4–6	England and Wales	1897–1979
Scarlet fever	4.4	3–6	England and Wales	1897–1978

oscillations of the system indefinitely. Bartlett (1956), for example, demonstrated that a full stochastic model of an epidemic process, with renewal of susceptibles plus an immigration rate of new infectives, generates an undamped succession of outbreaks. These outbreaks will not follow a strict cycle but will tend to be rather irregular in their occurrence.

More recently, a series of studies have shown that the inclusion of seasonal periodicity in the transmission parameter β of Equations (1.1) to (1.4) can 'pump' the otherwise-damped deterministic oscillations, locking the system into sustained cycles whose periods are an integral number of years (London and Yorke, 1973; Yorke and London, 1973; Dietz, 1976; Grossman, Gumowski and Dietz, 1977; Yorke et al., 1979; Grossman, 1980). This mechanism has been succinctly described by Yorke et al. (1979) in the following manner. 'We may think of the level of susceptibles as similar to a pendulum swinging back and forth past equilibrium. Seasonal variation gives the pendulum a shove every year and these regular shoves are required to keep the pendulum in motion'.

The precise conditions under which this mechanism generates subharmonic resonance (imposed over the regular seasonal cycles in prevalence) depend, in a complicated manner, on the amplitude of the seasonal cycles and on the magnitude of the basic reproductive rate R (Dietz, 1976; Grossman, 1980). Broadly speaking, to induce 2- or more-year cycles both the amplitude of the seasonal transmission and the magnitude of R must be relatively large. These conditions are satisfied, for example, by measles which has very marked seasonality in transmission and hence exhibits the most regular and clearly defined inter-epidemic period (Fig. 1.3). Seasonality in transmission is a common feature of many common childhood infections, some examples of which are shown in Fig. 1.4, but the mechanisms which generate such patterns are poorly understood at present. The main causes are probably climatic effects such as temperature and humidity influencing the survival and dispersal of transmission stages, and seasonal changes in social behaviour such as children returning to school after vacation periods.

Irrespective of the mechanisms which perpetuate the oscillations, the resulting inter-epidemic period is approximately determined by the period T defined in Equation (1.13) which depends on the biological parameters $1/\sigma$, $1/\gamma$, R and L. These relations between D $(1/\sigma + 1/\gamma)$, R(or A) and T are illustrated in Fig. 1.5.

Anderson and May (1982a) have pointed out that there is striking agreement between the simple theoretical insights embodied in Fig. 1.5 and observed values of the epidemiological parameters T, D and A or R (catalogued in Tables 1.5, 1.4 and 1.3). For measles in Britain, the average value of D is around 10 to 16 days (Table 1.3) noting that D is the sum of the latent period plus the effective infectious period, allowing for the fact that children are usually withdrawn from circulation once symptoms appear. The average value of R is about 14 to 18 (Table 1.4), and life expectancy is approximately 70 years. With these figures, Equation (1.13) predicts a value of T between 2 and 3 years, in agreement with the observed inter-epidemic period (Table 1.5). In the case of whooping cough in Britain and North America, the value of D is around 20 to 30 days (Table 1.3) and R is about 14 to 17 (Table 1.4), leading to the prediction

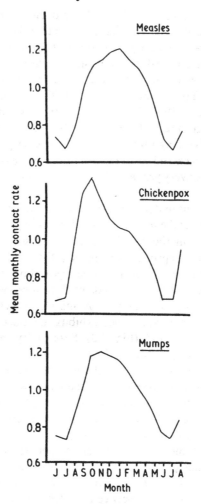

Figure 1.4 Examples of seasonal trends in the mean monthly contact rates (finite transmission rates for measles, chicken pox and mumps in New York City, USA (modified from London and Yorke, 1973)).

that the inter-epidemic period T is around 3 to 4 years. This again is in general agreement with the observations (Table 1.5).

It is important to note that the foregoing analysis pertains to macro-epidemiological patterns in large communities, and substantial variations from the predictions are to be expected in small subpopulations. In addition, within those developing countries where birth rates are high and life expectancy short, Equation (1.13) suggests a pronounced reduction in the inter-epidemic period compared with the corresponding period in a developed country (small L values and high R values in developing countries).

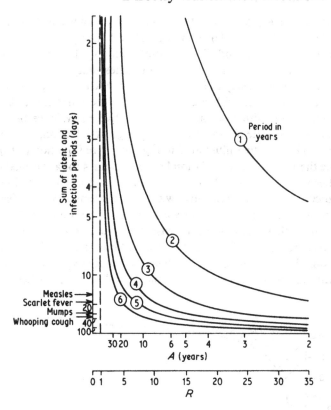

Figure 1.5 This figure shows the inter-epidemic period, T, as a function of the sum of the latent and infectious periods, D, where $D = 1/\sigma + 1/\gamma$, and the basic reproductive rate of the disease, R, for $L = 70$ years. (the approximate relationship defined in Equation (1.13)). Equivalently, as shown in Equation (1.12) T may be expressed as a function of D and A, the average age at which infection is acquired. The contour lines are for specified values of T, labelled according to the period in years. The values of D for some particular diseases are indicated on the y-axis (see Table 1.3) (after Anderson and May, 1982a).

1.6 CONTROL BY IMMUNIZATION

The concept of the basic reproductive rate, R, is central to an understanding both of the population behaviour of infectious diseases and of the impact of control policies (Anderson, 1982b). To eradicate an infection, it is necessary to reduce R below unity. This may be achieved by immunizing a proportion, p, of the population soon after birth, provided

$$p > [1 - 1/R] \tag{1.14}$$

This expression follows from the observation that, in such a population, the number of susceptibles is at most $N' = N(1 - p)$, such that the effective

reproductive rate R', is $R' = R(1 - p)$ with R as defined in Equation (1.7) (Dietz, 1974; Smith, 1970). The condition $R' < 1$ then gives Equation (1.14). The relation between p and R is illustrated in Fig. 1.6. If R is large, the proportion that must be immunized approaches unity. If other things are equal (such as the efficiency of a vaccine, or the ease of its application within the population) diseases with high R values will be much more difficult to control than those with low values. The effective equivalence between the basic reproductive rate R and the average age at infection, A, defined in Equation (1.12), is further illustrated in Fig. 1.6 where Equation (1.12) is used to re-scale the x-axis to give a relation between p and A for a specified value of L. In other words diseases which have a low average age at infection will be more difficult to control than those with a high average age at infection.

Immunization programmes clearly act to reduce the value of R and hence theory predicts they will tend to increase, both the inter-epidemic period, T, and the average age at infection, A (see Equations (1.12) and (1.13)).

For example, in England and Wales, as a consequence of widescale immunization, the average inter-epidemic period for measles has increased

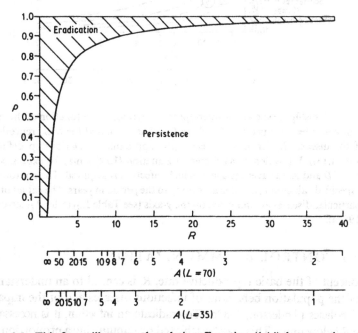

Figure 1.6 This figure illustrates the relation, Equation (1.14), between the proportion, p, of a community that must be immunized (at or near birth) to eradicate an infection, and the basic reproductive rate R. Alternatively p may be expressed as a function of A (using Equation (1.12)); this relationship is shown for $L = 70$ and $L = 35$ years. The infection is eradicated for values of p in the shaded area and it persists otherwise (Anderson and May, 1982a).

from 2.2 to 2.6 years, and for whooping cough it has increased from 2.8 to 3.5 years (Anderson and May, 1982a). The frequency distributions of inter-epidemic periods for both diseases, before and after the introduction of immunization, are displayed in Fig. 1.7. The epidemiology of rubella in the United States is a good example of the impact of immunization on the average age at which individuals acquire infection. As documented in Table 1.6, the introduction of

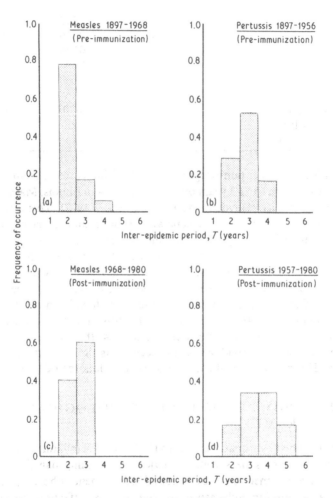

Figure 1.7 This figure shows the frequency distributions of the inter-epidemic period, T, for measles and whooping cough in England and Wales. (a) Measles prior to the introduction of immunization; 1897–1968. (b) Pertussis prior to the introduction of immunization; 1897–1956. (c) Measles after the introduction of immunization; 1968–1980. (d) Pertussis after the advent of immunization, 1957–1980. The mean periods for graphs (a), (b), (c) and (d) are 2.2, 2.8, 2.6 and 3.5 years respectively. Data from the Registrar General's statistical review of England and Wales.

Table 1.6 Cumulative proportion of reported cases of rubella in Illinois, Massachusetts and New York City, USA, by age group for three different periods. A nationwide immunization programme was introduced in the United States in 1969 (data from Hayden, Modlin and Witte, 1977).

	1966–1968	1969–1971	1972–1974
Age (years)			
0–4	0.216	0.215	0.132
5–9	0.601	0.566	0.345
10–14	0.771	0.726	0.555
15–19	0.898	0.897	0.870
20+	1.000	1.000	1.000
Total number of cases	17 960	10 709	6512
Average age A (years)	9.6	9.9	13.3
R	8.3	7.1	5.3

a nationwide immunization programme in 1969 increased A from 9.6 years prior to vaccination to 13.3 years by the end of 1974 in Illinois, Massachusetts and New York City (Hayden, Modlin and Witte, 1977). This attribute of immunization programmes has generated wide comment, since the risks associated with infection by certain common viral diseases such as measles and rubella increase with age. In the case of rubella, the infection is of major significance to pregnant women since the virus has a capacity to produce congenital abnormalities (Greenberg *et al.*, 1957), while, for measles, the likelihood of neurological complications (encephalitis) is known to increase with age (Miller, 1964). It is important to note, however, that although immunization will tend to increase the value of A, the *total number* of cases occurring in older individuals may decline as immunization coverage increases. This point is well illustrated by rubella data recorded in Table 1.6.

1.7 AGE-DEPENDENT EPIDEMIOLOGICAL PARAMETERS

The model defined by Equations (1.1) to (1.4) is helpful in illuminating certain basic principles but it suffers from one major short-coming, namely all the rate parameters are assumed to be constant and independent of host age. This is a reasonable assumption with respect to the latent and infectious periods, $1/\sigma$ and $1/\gamma$. Other parameters, however, such as the transmission rate, β, and the mortality rate, μ, are functions of host age. Furthermore, in the context of control, immunization programmes are often highly age-specific. To illustrate this point, Fig. 1.8 records a series of examples of transmission, mortality and vaccination rates at various ages for measles and pertussis in England and Wales.

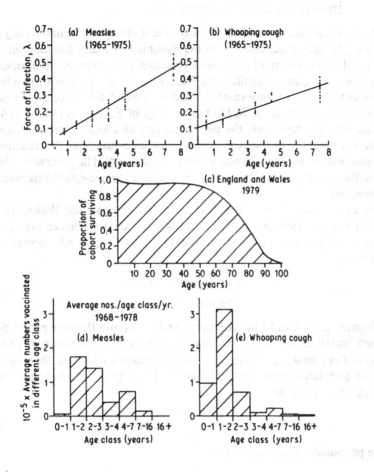

Figure 1.8(a) The 'force', or instantaneous rate, of infection, λ, is shown as a function of age, a, for measles in England and Wales between 1965 and 1975. This rate λ is estimated from case notifications presented in the Registrar General's Statistical Reviews, by methods described by Griffiths (1974); λ is defined per annum per susceptible. The dots represent yearly estimates of the age-dependent rates, while the solid line is the best-fit linear model. Up to the age of 10 years, the relation between λ and age, a, is well described by the linear expression $\lambda(a) = \alpha + \delta a$, where α and δ are constants: $\alpha = 0.030, \delta = 0.057$ ($r^2 = 0.99$). (b) As for Fig. 1.8(a), except that the data are for whooping cough. The linear relation between λ and a has coefficients $\alpha = 0.109$, $\delta = 0.033$ ($r^2 = 0.95$). (c) This figure shows the age-dependent survival curve for the population of England and Wales in 1977 (data from the Registrar General's Statistical Review, 1977). The age-specific mortality rate, $\mu(a)$, is the logarithmic derivative of this curve with respect to age, a. (d) The average number of individuals, in various age classes, who were vaccinated against measles in England and Wales between 1968 and 1978 (data supplied by the Department of Health and Social Security, UK). (e) As for Fig. 1.8(d), except the data are for whooping cough from 1965 to 1978.

In developed countries the mortality rate, μ, changes little in the early years of life (the ones most relevant to the dynamics of many common viral and bacterial infections) and hence age-dependency in the transmission parameter is the factor of greatest significance. The estimation of age-dependent infection is usually based on simple catalytic models in which the 'force of infection' is denoted by $\lambda(a)$ at age a. In the terminology of Equations (1.1) to (1.4), the parameter $\lambda(a)$ represents the per capita rate at which susceptibles acquire infection when the disease is at its endemic equilibrium (with the total number of infectious individuals having a constant value Y^*). The parameter $\lambda(a)$ can be written as $\lambda(a) = \beta(a)Y^*$, with $\beta(a)$ denoting the age-specific transmission parameter.

In an analysis of measles-incidence data in England and Wales, Griffiths (1974) suggests that the function $\lambda(a)$ is approximately linear over the age range 0–10 years of age (and this includes over 95% of all reported cases) where

$$\lambda(a) = \alpha + \delta a, \quad t > \tau,$$
$$\lambda(a) = 0, \quad t \leqslant \tau \tag{1.15}$$

The parameters α and δ are constants while τ denotes the time period during which maternal antibodies provide protection from infection in newborn infants. For measles the value of τ is roughly 6 months. If $\bar{x}(a)$ is the proportion of the population that remains uninfected by age a, then the mean age at attack, A, is given by

$$A = \int_0^\infty \bar{x}(a)\,\mathrm{d}a \tag{1.16}$$

The proportion $\bar{x}(a)$ is defined as

$$\bar{x}(a) = \exp\left[-\int_0^\infty \lambda(a)\,\mathrm{d}a \right] \tag{1.17}$$

Griffiths discusses the estimation of the parameters of the function $\lambda(a)$ from case notification records for a series of age classes and describes a maximum-likelihood estimation procedure. Ideally serological data would be the best information on which to base such estimation procedures, but in the case of measles, for example, case notifications provide a reasonable data base since over 95% of all cases occur in the young age classes of the population.

Catalytic models take no account of the recurrent epidemic cycles of infections but since the epidemic process is being averaged over a number of years, including several cycles, the fluctuations in incidence can be effectively ignored. Estimates of the age-dependent force of infection $\lambda(a)$ for measles in England and Wales are displayed in Fig. 1.8(a) and the fit of a simple catalytic model of the form defined in Equation (1.17), to case notification records is shown in Fig. 1.9

Dietz (1974, 1976) and more recently Anderson and May (1982a) have

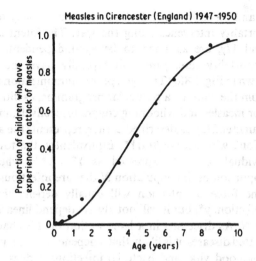

Measles in Cirencester (England) 1947-1950

Figure 1.9 The fit of the 'catalytic' model defined in Equation (1.17) in the main text to the proportion of children who experienced an attack of measles at various ages in the Cirencester region of England during 1947–1950. This proportion, $y(a)$, is given by $1 - \bar{x}(a)$ where $\bar{x}(a)$ is as defined in Equation (1.17). The dots are observed points while the solid line is the best-fit 'catalytic' model (data from Griffiths, 1974).

generalized the model described in Equations (1.1) to (1.4) to form a set of partial differential equations describing the change in, for example, the number of susceptibles as a function of time and age, $X(a, t)$. The analysis of such models may be simplified by following the dynamics of a cohort of $\bar{N}$ newly born susceptibles, within a community where the population has a constant size and a stable age distribution, and where the disease is at its endemic equilibrium, Y^*. In order to increase the generality of the following model we assume that disease control is being attempted by an immunization schedule in which susceptibles are vaccinated at an age-dependent rate $c(a)$ and that vaccinated individuals join the immune class and remain protected for life.

The numbers of susceptibles, latent, infectious and immune individuals as functions of age a (denoted by $X(a)$, $H(a)$, $Y(a)$ and $Z(a)$, respectively) in the cohort of size $\bar{N}$ can now be represented by the following differential equations:

$$dX/da = -[\lambda(a) + \mu(a) + c(a)] X(a) \qquad (1.18)$$

$$dH/da = \lambda(a)X(a) - [\sigma + \mu(a)]H(a) \qquad (1.19)$$

$$d Y/da = \sigma H(a) - [\gamma + \mu(a)] Y(a) \qquad (1.20)$$

$$dZ/da = \gamma Y(a) + c(a)X(a) - \mu(a)Z(a) \qquad (1.21)$$

Individuals leave the susceptible class as a result of natural mortality, vaccination (passing directly to the immune class), and infection passing into the latent class and thence to the infectious class, and finally to the immune state unless mortality intervenes along the way. The latent and infectious periods, $1/\sigma$ and $1/\gamma$, are assumed to be age-independent. In developed countries the mortality rate, $\mu(a)$, will typically have the type of age-dependence shown in Fig. 1.8(c). The age-specific immunization rates, $c(a)$, can be estimated from the data for a particular programme, as illustrated in Figs 1.8(d) and (e) for measles and whooping cough, respectively, in England and Wales. The parameter $\lambda(a)$, as described earlier, represents the age-dependent 'force of infection', with $\lambda(a) = \beta(a)Y^*$. Equivalently, the total number of infectious individuals can be expressed as $Y^* = y^*N$ where y^* is the equilibrium proportion of the population N that are infectious, whence $\lambda(a) = \beta(a)y^*N$. The force of infection will usually depend linearly on the prevalence of infection, y^*, but it will not always depend linearly on the total population size N. As discussed in a later section of this chapter, for most sexually transmitted diseases, it is likely that λ depends only on y and not on N.

For most childhood viral and bacterial infections λ does depend on N, although, as noted by Anderson and May (1982a), the dependence is often less strong than the conventionally assumed linear dependence of Equations 1.1–1.4. Some evidence presented by these authors is documented in Tables 1.7 and 1.8 which show the mean age at first infection, A, as a function of community size (Table 1.7) and of the degree to which the population is an urban rather than a rural one (Table 1.8) for several diseases. The data are for unvaccinated populations and A is thus inversely proportional to λ. As expected, A tends to increase with decreasing N or decreasing urbanization but the effects are weaker than linear. These complications, however, can be avoided by using Equations (1.18) to (1.21) and simply determining $\lambda(a)$ from empirical data.

From the definition and discussion given earlier (see Equation (1.7)) the basic reproductive rate R for a disease in a given population is, in general, equal to the number of susceptibles there would be in the absence of the disease,

Table 1.7 Average age at first infection, A, as a function of community size, for various childhood diseases (data for New York state in the years 1918–19, see Anderson and May, 1982a).

Community size	Mean age A (years)			
	Measles	Whooping cough	Scarlet fever	Diphtheria
200 000–50 000	9.0	6.3	10.5	10.6
50 000–10 000	9.0	5.7	10.2	11.5
10 000–2 500	10.7	6.9	11.2	12.5
under 2 500	12.9	8.2	12.3	14.2

Table 1.8 Average age at first infection, A, in relation to the degree of urbanization for various childhood diseases (data for different states in the USA in the years 1910–22, from reference (data for different states in the USA in the years 1910–22, see Anderson and May, 1982a):

State	Percentage of population living in urban, rather than rural, communities	Mean age A (years)				
		Measles	Whooping cough	Chicken pox	Scarlet fever	Diphtheria
Mass.	94.8	7.3	5.4	–	9.5	9.7
N.J.	78.4	6.7	5.4	7.1	9.7	9.0
Conn.	67.8	7.3	5.6	7.6	10.4	10.5
Penn.	64.3	–	–	–	9.2	9.6
Maryland	60.0	8.4	5.7	7.6	8.9	10.4
N.Y.	57.6	–	–	–	11.1	11.6
Kansas	24.9	10.8	–	–	10.7	12.7

divided by the number of susceptibles when the disease is established at an endemic equilibrium. From Equations (1.18)–(1.21) we therefore obtain (Anderson and May, 1982a)

$$R = \frac{\int_0^\infty \exp\{-\int_0^a [\mu(v)+c(v)]dv\}da}{\int_0^\infty \exp\{-\int_0^a [\lambda(v)+\mu(v)+c(v)]dv\}da} \quad (1.22)$$

In the simplest limiting case when all the rate parameters (λ,c,μ) are constants, and in the absence of vaccination $(c = 0)$ Equation (1.22) reduces to $R = 1+(\lambda/\mu)$ where the average age at first infection $A = 1/\lambda$. This gives Equation (1.12) (where $L = 1/\mu$) as discussed earlier. If a proportion p of the population is immunized at the constant rate c, the effective reproductive rate R' under the pressure of vaccination is

$$R' = R[1-cp/(c+\mu)] \quad (1.23)$$

Here R is the basic reproductive rate before the implementation of immunization.

To eradicate the infection we require $R' < 1$ and from Equations (1.12) and (1.23) the fraction of the population to be protected must satisfy

$$p > \frac{1+V/L}{1+A/L} \quad (1.24)$$

where V is the average age at which individuals are immunized $(V = 1/c)$ and A remains the average age at first infection prior to control. Since p cannot exceed unity, it is clear that $V < A$ is a necessary condition for eradication to be achieved.

Provided R is estimated from the age-dependent rates $\lambda(a), \mu(a)$ and $c(a)$ (Equation 1.22) then Equation (1.24) remains a very good approximation for determining the proportion p where A, V and L are the reciprocals of the appropriately average values of the age-dependent rates. The conclusion that eradication is impossible if $V > A$ is of practical importance. In the case of rubella (German measles) in Britain, for example, evidence suggests the value of A is roughly 10–12 years (Knox, 1980). The adopted control policy is to vaccinate girls, and only girls, between 11 and 15 years of age, combined with selective post-partum vaccination in women found not to have antibodies during antenatal care. This clearly protects the individuals most at risk but Equation (1.24) suggests it will have little impact on the overall incidence of rubella in Britain. This prediction is in agreement with available evidence and with experience in the United States where a greater reduction in rubella prevalence has been achieved by vaccinating boys and girls at a pre-school age (see Table 1.6). A detailed appraisal of which of the two policies is the 'better' depends on other factors such as cost–benefit considerations.

The main conclusion to be drawn from the age-structured model defined by Equations (1.19)–(1.21) is that the optimum vaccination policy (optimum in the sense of either eradication or the degree of reduction in disease prevalence) will maintain the value of V as low as possible. It is important to note, however, that the duration of protection provided by maternal antibodies (τ, see Equation (1.15)) must be taken into account in the design of immunization programmes for children.

1.8   MEASLES AND WHOOPING COUGH IN ENGLAND AND WALES

A detailed examination of the impact of immunization programmes on the epidemiology of a disease agent is, of course, dependent on the availability of long-term records of both incidence and numbers vaccinated. Such data are available for both measles and pertussis in England and Wales (Anderson and May, 1982a; Griffiths, 1973).

1.8.1   Measles

The epidemiological trends for measles in England and Wales since 1940 are recorded in Fig. 1.10. Measles is a highly infectious disease with the average age of acquisition, A, being between 4 and 6 years in developed countries. In certain regions of Africa and Asia with high birth rates the value of A is much lower (Table 1.4). Significant differences also exist in the value of A between rural and urban communities (see Tables 1.7 and 1.8) with the average age being higher in smaller and less densely populated areas.

In England and Wales, A decreased from 5.5 years to 4.4 years between 1944 and the introduction of widescale immunization in 1968 (Fig. 1.11a), a trend

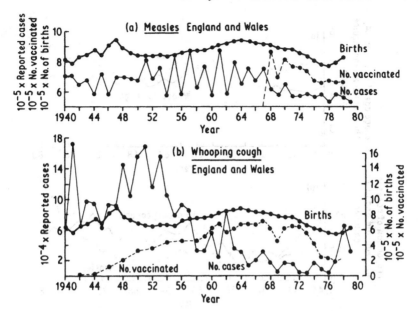

Figure 1.10   Reported cases of (a) measles and (b) whooping cough in England and Wales are shown, from 1940 to 1979. The figures show the total number of births (thick line), the total number of reported cases (thin line) and the total number of people vaccinated (dashed line) each year (Anderson and May, 1982a).

thought to be due to greater intermixing within the population and increased population density. Since the introduction of immunization, the trend has been reversed and both the inter-epidemic period, T (Fig. 1.7), and the average age at infection, A (Fig. 1.11a), have increased. Throughout the span of 1944 to 1979, 90–98 % of reported cases have been in children less than 10 years old (Fig. 1.11b). By following specific cohorts through time to monitor the decline in the proportion that are susceptible, these data have been used to estimate that the degree of under-reporting of cases, on a national scale, lies between 40 and 45 % (Anderson and May, 1982a). Similar estimates have been made in North America (Yorke *et al.*, 1979).

Vaccination coverage in England and Wales has been relatively low. As recorded in Fig. 1.12(b), of each yearly cohort, 15–35 % have been vaccinated by an average age at vaccination, V, of between 2.0 and 2.6 years. In total, roughly 46–57 % of each cohort has been vaccinated since 1968. This level of immunization has had relatively little impact on the reproductive rate R. For example, Fig. 1.13(a) records the decline in the susceptible population over time for the 1956 cohort (pre-vaccination) and for the 1970 cohort (post-vaccination). Anderson and May (1982a) estimated the value of R (using Equation (1.22)) to be in the range 14 to 18 pre-vaccination and in the range 12 to 13 post-vaccination. Thus the vaccination of a total of the order of 50 % of

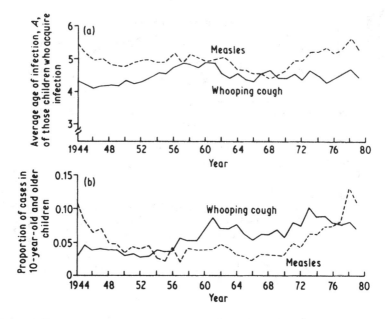

Figure 1.11 (a)   This figure shows the average age, A, at which children experienced an attack of measles (dashed line) or pertussis (solid line) in England and Wales over the years 1944 to 1979. The values of A were estimated by numerical integration of the expression

$$A = \int_{\tau}^{t} \exp\left[-\int_{\tau}^{a} \lambda(v)dv \right]da$$

where the age-dependent infection rate, $\lambda(v)$, for each specific year is as defined in the text. The limits of the integral are τ, defined to be the interval of time after birth during which maternal antibodies protect a newborn child against infection (assumed to be 0.5 years for measles, and negligible for pertussis), and t, an arbitrarily determined upper limit (which is set at 10 years since 90–98 % of cases occur in children less than this age). In calculating A, the death rate is taken to be negligible during the first 10 years of life (Anderson and May, 1982a). (b) This figure shows the proportion of reported cases of measles (dashed line) and whooping cough (solid line) that were from individuals past the age of 10 years, in England and Wales from 1944 to 1979.

whom roughly 30% are vaccinated by the average age of vaccination at roughly 2–2.2 years reduced the value of R by about 20%.

On the basis of Equation (1.24), with average A and V values of 4.6 and 2.2 years respectively, it appears as though approximately 96% of each cohort would have to be immunized for measles to be eradicated in Britain. Figure 1.14 depicts the relations between p, V and A as predicted by Equation (1.24). Even if the average age at vaccination was reduced to close to, or less than, 1 year, to eradicate the disease would require an immunization coverage of close to 94%.

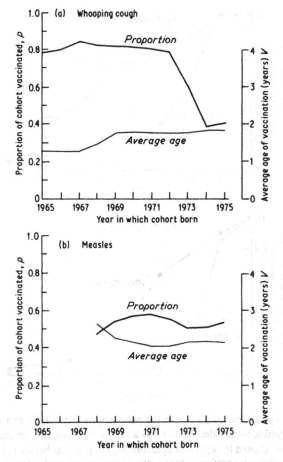

Figure 1.12(a)   The thick line (corresponding to the vertical axis to the left) shows the proportion of the cohorts born in England and Wales during the years 1965 to 1975 who were vaccinated against whooping cough. The thin line (corresponding to the vertical axis to the right) represents the average age, *V*, at which vaccination was received by the individuals in these cohorts who were vaccinated (data from the Department of Health and Social Security, UK). (b) As for (a), except that the data are for vaccination against measles in cohorts born in the years 1968 to 1975.

This figure is an average value for England and Wales and higher levels of coverage would be required in densely populated cities and lower levels in rural communities. Stochastic effects, accentuated by seasonality in disease transmission, would probably result in the fade out of infection at marginally lower levels of protection than those predicted by deterministic models. The magnitude of the predicted level of immunization required to eradicate measles is a direct consequence of the high infectiousness of this disease (high *R* values and low *A* values).

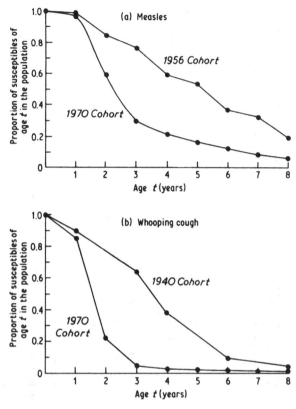

Figure 1.13(a) The estimated decline in the proportions of the 1956 and 1970 cohorts that were susceptible to measles is shown as a function of age, in England and Wales. The cohorts were chosen to represent epidemiological patterns before (1956) and after (1970) the introduction of immunization programmes for measles (see Anderson and May (1982a) for further details). The basic reproductive rate, R, for measles within these cohorts was estimated by numerical integration of Equation (1.22): for the 1956 cohort, $R = 16.0$; and for the 1970 cohort, $R = 12.8$. Of the 1970 cohort, a total of 57% were vaccinated at an average age, V, of 2.3 years. (b) As for (a) except this figure shows the decline in the proportions of the 1940 and 1970 cohorts susceptible to whooping cough as a function of age, in England and Wales. The cohorts were again chosen to show patterns before (1940) and after (1970) the introduction of immunization programmes. Values for R were estimated as $R = 16.3$ and 6.3 for the 1940 and 1970 cohorts respectively (see Anderson and May, 1982a). Of the 1970 cohort a total of 81% were vaccinated at an average age, V, of 1.7 years.

1.8.2   Whooping cough

Anderson and May (1982a) have also analysed, along the lines outlined above, the available data for pertussis in England and Wales between 1940 and 1979 (Fig. 1.10). Their analysis, based on the decline in the proportion of

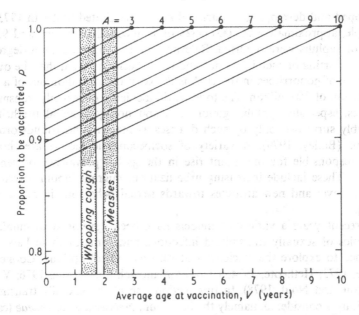

Figure 1.14 This figure shows the approximate relationship, Equation (1.24), between the proportion, *p*, of each cohort that must be vaccinated, and the average age at vaccination, *V*, for eradication of an infection. The solid lines represent the boundaries between eradication (above the line) and persistence (below the line) for various values of the average age at first infection, *A*, in the population before the introduction of immunization. The average life expectancy is taken to be 70 years. The shaded vertical bands depict the ranges of values of *V* for immunization against whooping cough and against measles, in England and Wales, during the periods 1965–1975 and 1968–1975 respectively (Anderson and May, 1982a).

susceptibles pre-vaccination and post-vaccination, gave values of *R* of roughly 16 and 6 respectively (Fig. 1.13(b)). In the 1970 cohort, for example, a vaccination coverage of 81% in total and 42% by the average age of vaccination at 1.7 years produced a 61% decline in the value of *R* and a very low overall incidence of the disease during the early 1970s. Since this time, however, public concern about the dangers of vaccination for whooping cough has led to a substantial decline in the level of vaccination and concomitantly the incidence of the disease has increased (Fig. 1.10). Anderson and May (1982a) suggest, on the basis of Equation (1.24), that with an average age of vaccination around 1.7 years (see Fig. 1.12(a)), a coverage of about 96% would be necessary to eradicate whooping cough in Britain.

1.9 SEXUALLY TRANSMITTED INFECTIONS

The widespread occurrence and increasing incidence of venereal disease, or sexually transmitted infections, is today a major public health problem in developed and developing countries alike. In the United States in 1973, for example, approximately 767 000 cases of gonococcal infections and 91 000 cases of syphilis were reported. Relevant surveys suggest a high degree of under-reporting of such infections and it has been estimated that the overall incidence of gonorrhoea in the USA is in excess of 2.5 million out of a total population of 250 million. The total world incidence of sexually transmitted diseases, especially syphilis, gonorrhoea and non-gonococcal urethritis is probably surpassed only by such diseases as malaria and roundworm infections (Bailey, 1979). A variety of socioeconomic factors are thought to be responsible for the recent rise in the global prevalence of venereal disease. These include increasing urbanization, migrant labour, expanding tourist travel and new attitudes towards sexual behaviour in modern societies.

In recent years a variety of models have been developed to mimic the dynamics of sexually transmitted infections and some of these have been designed to explore the efficiencies of various control options (Cooke and Yorke, 1973; Hethcote, 1974, 1976; Lajmanovich and Yorke, 1976; Yorke, Hethcote and Nold, 1978). In this section one of the sexually transmitted infections is considered, namely the bacterium *Neisseria gonorrhaeae* (causal agent of gonorrhoea).

Gonorrhoea has distinctive epidemiological characteristics when compared with the viral and bacterial infections discussed in the preceding sections of this chapter. First, the disease occurs only within the sexually active portion of a community. Second, the duration of infectiousness is long and differs substantially between male and female individuals. Third, and finally, acquired immunity to reinfection is virtually non-existent and hence recovered individuals pass directly back to the susceptible pool.

Models of the dynamics of gonorrhoea conventionally consider a freely mixing community which consists of sexually active males and females of densities N_1 and N_2 respectively. In the following model we assume that in a short interval of time, X_2 susceptible females have sexual contact with $S_2 X_2$ males of whom $S_2 X_2 Y_1/N_1$ are infected. The parameter S_2 represents the average number of partners that a female has sexual contact with in a defined unit of time. We further assume that the probability of infection passing from an infected male to a susceptible female during a single 'partner contact' is q_2. The net rate at which new female infections arise is therefore $S_2 q_2 X_2 Y_1/N_1$. For convenience we define $\hat{\beta}_1 = S_2 q_2/N_1$. In a similar manner the net rate at which male infections arise is $S_1 q_1 X_1 Y_2/N_2$ and we define $\hat{\beta}_2 = S_1 q_1/N_2$. The parameter S_1 denotes the average number of partners that a male has sexual contact with per unit of time and q_1 is the probability of infection passing from an infected female to a susceptible male during a single 'partner contact'. The average duration of male and female infectiousness is denoted by $1/\gamma_1$ and $1/\gamma_2$ respectively. If the populations of sexually active males and females are constant, then the above assumption gives rise to the following differential Equations:

$$dX_1/dt = -\hat{\beta}_2 X_1 Y_2 + \gamma_1 Y_1 \qquad (1.25)$$

$$dY_1/dt = \hat{\beta}_2 X_1 Y_2 - \gamma_1 Y_1 \qquad (1.26)$$

$$dX_2/dt = -\hat{\beta}_1 X_2 Y_1 + \gamma_2 Y_2 \qquad (1.27)$$

$$dY_2/dt = \hat{\beta}_1 X_2 Y_1 - \gamma_2 Y_2 \qquad (1.28)$$

This model predicts that the infection will be maintained within the population provided the basic reproductive rate, R, is greater than, or equal to, unity. For the system defined in Equations (1.25)–(1.28)

$$R = (S_1 S_2 q_1 q_2)/(\gamma_1 \gamma_2) \qquad (1.29)$$

Note that in contrast to the basic reproductive rate of the viral and bacterial infections discussed in earlier sections of this chapter (see Equation (1.5)), the expression defined in Equation (1.29) is independent of host population size. In other words there is no critical threshold density for disease persistence. The maintenance of gonorrhoea is thus simply dependent on the prevailing degree of sexual promiscuity within the community (i.e. the magnitudes of the parameters S_1 and S_2).

The estimation of the parameter R from empirical data is fraught with problems since it is dependent on the availability of accurate information on sexual habits. These clearly vary greatly both within different sections of a given community and between communities. With respect to the infectious periods, $1/\gamma_1$ and $1/\gamma_2$, the most widely quoted values are 10 days for men and 100 days for women (Constable, 1975; Reynolds and Chan, 1975). These values, however, are fairly crude and based on limited evidence (Yorke et al., 1978). Some attempts have been made to estimate average values for S_1 and S_2 on the basis of interviews, but such information is known to be highly unreliable. In a study by Darrow (1975), for example, of a large city in North America, the average patient with gonococcal infection reported 1.46 partners during the preceding 30 days. This figure is too low since at endemic equilibrium ($R = 1$) theory suggests that on average each infective person must have two effective contacts during the course of an infection, namely, a contact with an infector (the source of the infection) and a contact with a person to whom the infection is transmitted. An infective person, may of course have additional sex partners to whom the infection is not transmitted (the probabilities q_1 and q_2).

The discrepancy between theory and data may be due to several factors not least of which is the honesty of the individuals interviewed. Other factors, however, may also play an important role. The model defined in Equations (1.25) to (1.28) is based on the assumption that the sexually active proportion of the community mixes in a homogeneous manner. This is clearly far from the truth, some individuals have many more sex partners than others. In fact, many epidemiologists believe that in most communities the frequency distribution of sexual partners per unit of time is highly skewed (the variance being much greater than the mean) with the majority of individuals having one or no contacts (in a unit time interval) and a few individuals having very many contacts. The sexually active individuals in the tail of this distribution in effect form a 'core' population which is, by itself, almost entirely responsible for the maintenance of gonorrhoea in the community as a whole. In the 'non-core' segment of the population the value of R is probably much less than unity so that the activities of the core maintain the infection by continually reintroducing it into the remainder of the population.

The core is thought to consist primarily of women, whose infections would often be asymptomatic for long periods. It will also contain some asymptomatic men and people who continue sexual intercourse in spite of symptoms. Control programmes (based on screening and drug treatment) aimed at this core segment of the population are potentially highly effective (Yorke et al., 1978).

One final point to note concerning the epidemiology of sexually transmitted infections relates to the concept of an endemic disease equilibrium. As illustrated in Fig. 1.15 the incidence of infections such as gonorrhoea has increased substantially in many regions of the world over the past two decades. This implies that the parameters which control the dynamics of such infections are not in reality constants (as defined in Equations (1.25)–(1.28)) but are in fact changing with time. We therefore have a situation in which the equilibrium predicted by simple deterministic models is moving in time as the parameters which determine this state change. For sexually transmitted infections, it is highly probable that changes in the contact rates S_1 and S_2 are responsible for the observed epidemiological trends.

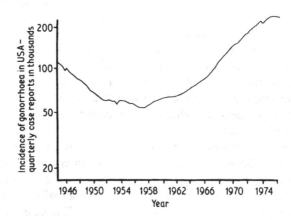

Figure 1.15   This figure shows the quarter-yearly case reports of gonorrhoea in the United States between the years 1944 and 1976 (data from Yorke et al., 1978).

1.10 CONCLUSIONS

The development of safe, effective and cheap vaccines which provide lasting (ideally lifelong) protection is clearly a first step for the successful control of many common viral and bacterial infections. Once these aims have been achieved, however, as they have for diseases such as measles, polio and rubella, important epidemiological questions remain to be resolved. Careful thought, for example, must be given to such issues as the level of artificially induced herd immunity required to eradicate an infection, the degree of reduction in case notifications to be expected from a given immunization policy and the influence of vaccination upon the average age at first infection and upon the time period between major epidemics. In certain cases, the failure to tackle these issues has led to some degree of confusion concerning the type of immunization policy to be adopted (Sutherland and Fayers, 1971; Roden and Heath, 1977; Galbraith, Forbes and Mayon–White, 1980).

Any attempt to answer these questions involves a knowledge both of the typical course of infection within an individual (e.g. the latent period and the duration of infectiousness) and of the overall population biology of the disease agent and its host. Theoretical studies of the population dynamics of infectious diseases can play a central role in the acquisition of both types of information. In the case of parameters which determine the course of an infection within an individual, mathematical models provide a framework for parameter estimation from empirical data. With respect to population behaviour, theory can help to create a basic understanding of the factors controlling dynamical behaviour. In this latter context, the concept of a basic reproductive rate, and its definition in terms of a few simple biological properties of the disease agent and its host population, are of central importance. Theory suggests that the design and implementation of immunization programmes should ideally be based on quantitative assessments of their overall impact on the quantity R, the aim being to reduce the basic reproductive rate to a level, close to, or below, unity.

Assessments of the extent to which specific infections may be controlled by immunization requires serological surveys to measure the average age at which infection is acquired and thence to estimate typical values of R (at local, regional and national scales). For those infections for which vaccines are, or soon will be, available (such as cytomegalovirus and hepatitis B virus), it would appear prudent to acquire this information before immunization schedules are introduced. Once the level of protection necessary for eradication, or a defined reduction in incidence, has been determined, other issues which influence public health policy, such as social and cost–benefit considerations, may be examined in much more rigorous terms. Further research of a statistical and mathematical nature could be of great value to such deliberations particularly if it is based on the analysis of data. There is a need, for example, for more sophisticated statistical methods to aid in the estimation of R from serological data or case notification records, and for a better understanding of the significance of non-homogeneous mixing to disease dynamics.

2 The dynamics of bacterial infections

B. Cvjetanović

2.1 INTRODUCTION

Many researchers studying infectious diseases have come to the conclusion that infections due to bacteria, as well as other pathogenic agents, can usefully be viewed as a biological process which consists of the interaction between two populations, namely, the parasite population and the host population. During an epidemic or endemic period these two populations undergo fluctuations in size which are interrelated in a dynamic manner. Some researchers have attempted to explain these fluctuations on intuitive grounds, while others have based their analyses on a mathematical framework describing the dynamics of the interaction between the two populations. We shall briefly refer to some of these latter types of studies, which are of direct relevance to the dynamics of bacterial infections.

Half a century ago Kermack and McKendrick formulated a mathematical theory of epidemic processes which was based on a simple deterministic model (Kermack and McKendrick, 1927, 1932, 1933). This model essentially describes the transmission of a disease agent within the host population and the resulting increase in the level of immunity within the community (herd immunity). Their model is relevant to bacterial diseases, since such infections typically induce a degree of acquired immunity in those hosts that recover from infection. As described in Chapter 1, Kermack and McKendrick developed the celebrated threshold theorem which simply states that an epidemic will not occur unless the density of susceptible hosts is above a critical level (Kermack and McKendrick, 1927). In 1959, Muench published an account of the use of 'catalytic models' to describe trends in disease prevalence within different age classes of a host population. Muench (1959) used his catalytic models with some success to describe the age-specific dynamics of certain bacterial infections.

Further developments in the mathematical theory of infectious diseases have been made by Bailey (1957) and others who developed stochastic models of epidemic processes. More recently, Bailey (1975) has published an extensive review of these theoretical studies of disease dynamics.

The work mentioned above deals more with the general theory of infectious disease dynamics and less with specific bacterial infections. In the last two decades, with the advent of modern computing facilities, work on the dynamics of bacterial infections has gained momentum. Much of this work is based on complex multi-state models which describe the flow of hosts between various compartments which designate a series of states of infection (i.e. latent, infectious etc.). A review of the early work on tuberculosis and chronic bacterial infections has been published by Waaler, Gesser and Anderson (1962) and a more extensive treatment of the dynamics of tuberculosis was published in 1968 (Waaler, 1968). Shortly after this, Lechat and co-workers developed a model to describe the dynamics of leprosy (Lechat, 1971).

The first model of the dynamics of acute bacterial diseases was described by Cvjetanović et al. (1971) and this work was shortly followed by specific studies of typhoid, tetanus and other major acute infections (Cvjetanović et al., 1971, 1972, 1978). This work was based on quantitative models of the dynamics of these infections and has proved useful, both in generating an understanding of epidemiological processes, and in the design and planning of practical and cost-effective control strategies.

2.2 BIOLOGICAL BASIS OF THE DYNAMICS OF BACTERIAL DISEASES

The biology and natural history of a disease agent creates the framework for the development of quantitative models of the dynamics of bacterial infections. A qualitative biological understanding of disease natural history is translated into quantitative, time-related changes within a model framework. There are some biological characteristics which are common to all bacterial diseases, but there are also many other characteristics which are specific to each disease agent.

The central characteristic of the population dynamics of bacterial diseases is the transmission of the infection from infecteds to susceptibles. The number of newly infected individuals during a unit of time depends on the number of infectious persons, the number of susceptibles in the population and the rate of effective contact between these two categories of the population. The effective contact between infectious and susceptible persons depends on a number of epidemiological factors, such as population density, environmental factors like climate, and many others. All these factors together represent a 'force of infection' which determines disease incidence and can be expressed in quantitative terms (Cvjetanović et al., 1978). However, it is at present extremely difficult to account exactly for all components of the 'force of infection', and for the interrelationships between the numerous factors which are involved.

The number of new infections in a unit of time can be expressed in a simple way as follows:

| number of infectious individuals in the population | × | force of infection | × | proportion of susceptible individuals in the population | = | number of newly infected individuals |

The number of infectious persons and the degree and the duration of their infectiousness, differ both in qualitative and quantitative terms for different diseases. Infectious persons with some bacterial diseases are clinical cases with overt disease symptoms; in others there are either many subclinical infections or many healthy carriers. The duration of infectiousness differs from one class of infectious individuals to another. In some bacterial diseases the carriers of bacteria may at one time be dangerous spreaders of infection, while at other times they may be non-infectious. The existence of dangerous (nasal) spreaders of streptococci is well known, as is the existence of intermittent spreaders of enteric infections. It is therefore essential to clearly define, in qualitative and quantitative terms, on the one hand the different classes of the infectious population and on the other hand the classes of the susceptible population. The degree of susceptibility depends on the immune status of the individual. This is governed by the level of specific antibodies, cell-mediated immunity and various factors of the general state of resistance (such as the presence or absence of gastric acidity in the case of cholera). There are many complex host-associated factors involved in the dynamics of such infections.

The dynamics of bacterial diseases also depend on parasite factors such as the number of pathogenic bacteria and their characteristics, the virulence, toxigenicity, survival in the environment and the ability to attach to the intestinal mucosa (in enteric infections) or to penetrate the meningeal barrier (in cerebrospinal meningitis). The effects of pathogenic bacteria also depend on the host's reaction, a point which underlines the interactive nature of the association between host and parasite. Present knowledge of human biology and immunity points to the existence of a great deal of variability in the susceptibility of individuals to infection. There is also similar genetic variability within bacterial populations. Accordingly, in the study of the dynamics of bacterial diseases, such variability within host and parasite populations must be taken into account and expressed, as far as possible, in quantitative terms.

While it is obvious that an over-simplification of the dynamics of bacterial diseases leads to meaningless generalities, it is also obvious that there is no need to include in quantitative models all possible factors and sources of variability. Many of these factors may play only minor, or quite unimportant, roles. It is therefore essential to distinguish the factors which are important in the dynamics of an infection in order to formulate realistic but manageable models. In other words, the biological basis of the models should ideally comprise a limited number of essential variables and parameters which permit the formulation of an epidemiological model sufficiently accurate but simple enough to be applicable.

In the formulation of a model of disease dynamics it is clearly necessary to pay attention to the biological phenomena, before considering mathematical and computational aspects. It is important to strike a balance between scientific precision and practical needs. Bailey (1975), expressed his view on this point as follows: 'there are intellectual and aesthetic satisfactions in understanding the mechanism and processes underlying the natural world: but in the face of misery and suffering on a monumental scale, epidemic theory for its own sake is a luxury mankind can ill afford. The world must not only be interpreted: it must be changed.' It is to be hoped that most studies of the dynamics of bacterial diseases are based on this philosophy.

Public health workers are obviously interested in understanding both the dynamics of bacterial diseases and the methods by which this knowledge can be used in the effective control of such infections.

2.3   GENERAL CONSIDERATIONS OF THE DYNAMICS OF THE MAJOR BACTERIAL INFECTIONS

In the construction of models of bacterial disease, which encompass a description of public health intervention (such as the effects of immunization, chemoprophylaxis or sanitation) certain difficulties have been encountered as a consequence of the large number of factors and parameters involved. It has proved possible, in certain cases, to define flow charts which describe the way in which individuals pass from one epidemiological category to another. These flow charts have been translated into difference or differential equation models, but because of their complexity, the analysis of disease dynamics has to a large extent been based on numerical studies of model behaviour. The large capacity and speed of modern computers, however, enables the behaviour of very complex systems of equations to be rapidly explored.

In the analysis of model behaviour, simulations are run until the disease reaches its stable endemic state. The impact of various control options is assessed by their influence on this stable level of disease prevalence. In a similar manner it is also possible to analyse the impact of changes in the demography of the human population on the dynamics of the disease. In the following sections, the manner in which specific diseases are modelled is described more fully but for a general treatment of the structure of models of bacterial infections the reader is referred to Bailey (1975) and Cvjetanović *et al.* (1978).

Before proceeding to describe the dynamics of certain specific infections it is important to note a few further complications of a general nature. Clearly, before attempting to formulate a model it is first necessary to understand thoroughly the biology of the causative agent of disease. In some cases more than one causative agent may be responsible for a specific disease, as in the case of the 'diarrhoeal diseases'. This sort of problem is very difficult to treat in a quantitative manner. Other problems arise as a consequence of the existence of different bacterial serogroups for which specific polysaccharide vaccines are required in order to immunize susceptible individuals. This situation arises in the case of meningococcal meningitis. A model of this disease must take into account the different serogroups within the population particularly if model construction is aimed at assessing the impact of immunization programmes. In certain cases the same causative agent may give rise to more than one type of disease. For example, tetanus bacteria give rise to neonatal tetanus and the more general tetanus disease observed in older age groups. Such age-related changes in the pattern of infection are often of importance and should ideally be incorporated in the model structure.

For diseases which are endemic in character, where the incidence of infection changes little from year to year, deterministic models will normally be appropriate to describe the dynamics. If, however, the prevalence changes dramatically through time, exhibiting sudden epidemic changes, then stochastic formulations may be more appropriate. On a national or regional scale stochastic effects will be less marked since the overall incidence levels for large populations reflects the summation of many small outbreaks of infection. In these cases deterministic models may suffice. These themes are stressed in many of the chapters in this book.

At a fundamental level there are two different types of bacterial infections, namely, the acute ones of short duration of illness (with or without a carrier state) and the chronic diseases in which individuals may be infected and infectious for long periods of time. This chapter is primarily concerned with the dynamics of acute bacterial infections, chronic diseases are only briefly discussed.

2.4 ACUTE BACTERIAL DISEASES

Acute bacterial diseases have relatively short infectious and latent periods; a short illness is followed by either transient or lasting immunity. Some diseases are characterized by having a carrier state and prolonged infectivity, while in others this state is absent.

Typical parameters which have to be taken into account in the dynamics of bacterial infections are as follows:

1. Susceptibility;
2. Infectious period; period of incubation and illness;
3. Immunity after infection (and after immunization);
4. Carrier state and its duration;
5. Death rates.

Some diseases, because of their particular natural history, involve parameters which are not mentioned above. Aside from the characteristics of infection other factors such as the birth and death rates of the host population must also be taken into account.

For the study of public health interventions it is necessary to know the effectiveness of control measures and their cost-effectiveness. Ideally cost–benefit analyses should be carried out on the cost of control, the cost of treatment and the social cost of illness.

The 'force of infection' is one of the most important parameters in the dynamics of any infectious disease. This parameter and its components will therefore be discussed in detail with respect to each specific disease.

2.5 TETANUS–INFECTION WITHOUT INTER-HUMAN TRANSMISSION

The natural history of tetanus differs substantially from that of other bacterial diseases. First, this infection is not transmitted from man to man. Second, the disease produced by the toxin of *Clostridium tetani* does not lead to acquired immunity, although immunization with tetanus toxoid does induce the production of protective antibodies. Tetanus is more an environmental hazard than a communicable disease, an issue clearly reflected in the dynamics of the infection. The number of new infections in other bacterial diseases depends on the number of infectious persons, the force of infection and the proportion of susceptibles in the population. In the case of tetanus, the number of new infections depends only on the force of infection and the number of susceptibles. The construction of an epidemiological model of tetanus has therefore proved to be somewhat simpler than is the case for other infections (Cvjetanović *et al.*, 1972, 1978).

It is relatively easy to determine the proportion of susceptibles in the population, since only those who have been adequately immunized are in fact resistant. The determination of the force of infection is also simple, since for practical purposes the force of infection is defined by the incidence rate. In the dynamics of tetanus the force of infection is the most important single factor and therefore much is to be gained by defining its components in detail. This gives greater insight into the biological and other aspects of disease dynamics. Data from various countries have been analysed and disease incidence appears to be correlated with the following factors:

1. Climate;
2. Soil (content of spores of *C. tetani*);
3. Type of agriculture and animal husbandry;
4. Profession (related to agriculture);
5. Level of economic development;
6. Level of health services;
7. Probability of wounding and soiling the wound with *C. tetani*.

These factors differ in neonatal tetanus when compared with tetanus within the general population.

It is clear that in a primitive community, where animal manure and simple non-mechanized agricultural techniques are used, health services are poor and the level of the socio-economic development low, the chances of wounds becoming infected with *C. tetani* are higher than in industrialized communities.

It has proved possible to develop methods to predict the magnitude of the force of infection in relation to climate, state of socio-economic development and the level of health services. Nevertheless, it is still not precisely clear how the numerous factors influencing the force of infection (as listed above) are interrelated and the relative role played by each factor. More studies on this subject are clearly needed. Nevertheless, it has proved possible to identify the principle factors which generate high levels of tetanus incidence (Bytchenko *et al.*, 1975) and to assess the effectiveness of various forms of control.

Another special feature of tetanus mentioned in an earlier section is the existence of two distinct epidemiological patterns: tetanus of the newborn and tetanus of all other ages. The first is the result of unhygienic delivery practices and the absence of maternal antibodies from the newborn. The second is due to soiled wounds, the failure to sterilize wounds properly and the absence of a programme of active immunization. While tetanus is a single disease entity the above two distinct epidemiological categories have different dynamic patterns which require separate treatment in the mathematical models (Bytchenko, 1966, 1967).

Models of tetanus dynamics have been constructed to assist in the planning and evaluation of public health interventions (immunization in particular). Because such models were conceived to deal with problems concerning large centres of population they are deterministic in nature. A flow chart of the structure of the tetanus model is presented in Fig. 2.1.

The flow chart begins with the class of newborn infants (of density x_1) who pass either to class x_2 (susceptible population) or, if the mother received a preventive vaccination, to class x_8 (short-lasting immunity). The susceptible population (class x_2) can pass to class x_7 (long-lasting immunity) as a result of vaccination. When infected, both the susceptible newborn and the susceptible general population will pass through their corresponding incubation and sickness classes, namely, to classes x_3 and x_5 for the newborn and to classes x_4 and x_6 for the general population. A certain fraction of sick adults and infants will die (passing to class x_9) and the remainder will return to class x_2 (susceptible population) with the exception of sick individuals, who have been vaccinated after treatment, who pass to class x_7 (long-lasting immunity). The newborn, as a consequence of the short duration of passive immunity, pass into class x_8 (passive immunity of 6 months duration) before passing back to the susceptible pool.

Quantitative estimates of the epidemiological parameters controlling the

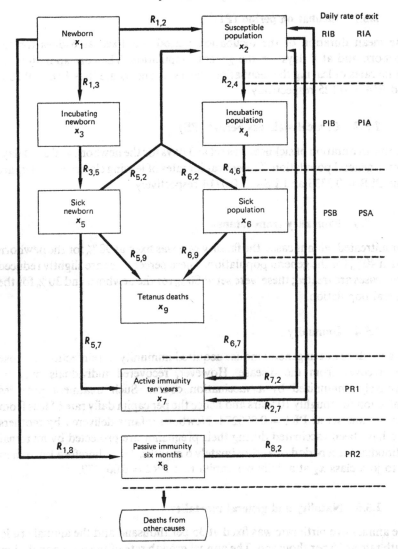

Figure 2.1 A diagrammatic flow chart of the dynamics of tetanus. The variables x_1–x_9 represent population numbers (or densities) in each of the epidemiological states, while the parameters $R_{1,3}$–$R_{8,2}$ denote the proportional transfer from one state to another (see text) (from Cvjetanović *et al.*, 1978).

flow of individuals between the various classes portrayed in Fig. 2.1 were obtained from published data and health statistics (Bytchenko, 1966; Eckmann, 1967). The basic unit of time for the estimation of the discrete quantitative changes in the disease dynamics was taken to be 1 day.

2.5.1 Incubation period (PI)

The mean duration of the incubation period was fixed at 6 days for the newborn and at 8 days for the general population. The corresponding per capita rates of leaving the incubation classes x_3 and x_4 are thus PIB = 0.1667 and PIA = 0.125 respectively.

2.5.2 Clinical sickness period (PS)

The mean duration of sickness was set at 3 days for the newborn and at 14 days for the general population. The per capita rates of leaving classes x_5 and x_6 are thus PSB = 0.3333 and PSA = 0.0714 respectively.

2.5.3 Mortality from tetanus

For untreated tetanus cases, the fatality rate was fixed at 90% for the newborn and at 40% for the general population. These percentages are slightly reduced when cases are treated; these were set at 80% for the newborn and 30% for the general population.

2.5.4 Immunity

Tetanus does not in general induce acquired immunity to reinfection in those that recover from the disease. However, recovered individuals may be effectively immunized by a vaccination course. Such treatment provides protection for roughly 10 years and hence the per capita daily rate of loss from class x_7 was set at PR1 = 0.000274. Newborn infants delivered by mothers who have been vaccinated during their pregnancy are protected by maternal antibodies for a period of approximately 6 months. They therefore leave class x_8 to join class x_2 at a daily per capita rate PR2 = 0.005479.

2.5.5 Natality and general mortality

The annual live birth rate was fixed at 35 per thousand and the annual crude death rate at 15 per thousand. The annual growth rate of the total population is thus around 2%, a level appropriate for many developing countries. The per capita input and output rates (birth and death rates) of the population were therefore set at PB = 0.0000959 and PD = 0.0000411 respectively.

2.5.6 Force of infection

In order to describe a range of common epidemiological situations in developing countries, the forces of infection acting on the susceptible newborn (RIB) and on the susceptible general population (RIA) were set at three different levels in order to mimic the following stable annual incidence rates of tetanus cases: (a) for the newborn, 200 cases, 400 cases and 600 cases per 100 000 new born; (b) for the general population, 9 cases, 18 cases and 27 cases per 100 000 population (see Bytchenko *et al.* (1975) for a more detailed account of the estimation of rates of infection).

2.5.7 Coefficients of transfer

In the flow chart (Fig. 2.1) the fraction of individuals leaving one epidemiological class to join another class is represented by a coefficient $R_{i,j}$ where i is the class of origin and j the class of destination. For any class i the sum of the coefficients $R_{i,j}$ is equal to 1 (see Cvjetanović *et al.*, 1978).

2.5.8 Mathematical model

The dynamics of the disease within a population, as described in the flow chart of Fig. 2.1, may be expressed in terms of a set of difference equations which denote daily changes, Δx_i, in the various epidemiological classes (the x_i's). These equations are as follows:

$$\Delta x_1 = x_T \text{PB} \tag{2.1}$$

$$\Delta x_2 = (x_T - x_7)\,(1 - \text{RIB})\,\text{PB} + x_7\,\text{PR1} + x_8\,\text{PR2}$$
$$+ x_5 R_{5,2}\,\text{PSB} + x_6 R_{6,2}\,\text{PSA} - x_2\,(\text{RIA}$$
$$+ \text{PD} - \Delta x_9/x_T) \tag{2.2}$$

$$\Delta x_3 = (x_T - x_7)\,\text{RIB}.\text{PB} - x_3\,(\text{PIB} + \text{PD} - \Delta x_9/x_T) \tag{2.3}$$

$$\Delta x_4 = x_2\,\text{RIA} - x_4\,(\text{PIA} + \text{PD} - \Delta x_9/x_T) \tag{2.4}$$

$$\Delta x_5 = x_3\,\text{PIB} - x_5\,(\text{PSB} + \text{PD} - \Delta x_9/x_T) \tag{2.5}$$

$$\Delta x_6 = x_4\,\text{PIA} - x_6\,(\text{PSA} + \text{PD} - \Delta x_9/x_T) \tag{2.6}$$

$$\Delta x_7 = x_5 R_{5,7}\,\text{PSB} + x_6 R_{6,7}\,\text{PSA} - x_7\,(\text{PR1} + \text{PD} - \Delta x_9/x_T) \tag{2.7}$$

$$\Delta x_8 = x_7\,\text{PB} - x_8\,(\text{PR2} + \text{PD} - \Delta x_9/x_T) \tag{2.8}$$

$$\Delta x_9 = x_5 R_{5,9}\,\text{PSB} + x_6 R_{6,9}\,\text{PSA} \tag{2.9}$$

$$\text{where } x_T = x_2 + x_3 + \ldots x_8$$

The parameters PR1 and PR2 denote the mean duration of acquired immunity in the classes x_7 and x_8 respectively (see Fig. 2.1).

The annual number of tetanus cases is given by the formulae:

$$\Sigma x_3\,\text{PIB} \quad \text{and} \quad \Sigma x_4\,\text{PIB}$$

for the newborn and the general population respectively, the summation Σ being carried out over 365 days. The total annual number of deaths from tetanus is similarly obtained by summing Δx_9 over 365 days. The size of the total population is regulated by the birth and death rates (PB and PD).

The effect of control intervention by immunization may be simulated by transferring susceptibles (x_2) to the immune class (x_7) for the average period of post-vaccinal immunity (roughly 10 years). When pregnant women are immunized, given that the efficacy of immunization is defined by the parameter E_2 (the product of the effectiveness of the vaccine times the coverage of pregnant mothers by the immunization programme), the above system of equations (Equations (2.1)–(2.9)) must be replaced by the following equations for Δx_2 to Δx_8:

$$\Delta x_2 = (1 - E_2)(x_T - x_7)(1 - RIB)\,PB + x_7\,PR1 + x_8\,PR2 + x_5 R_{5,2}\,PSB$$
$$+ x_6 R_{6,2}\,PSA - x_2(RIA + PD - \Delta x_9/x_T) - E_2(x_T - x_7)\,PB \qquad (2.10)$$

$$\Delta x_3 = (1 - E_2)(x_T - x_7)\,RIB.\,PB - x_3(PIB + PB - \Delta x_9/x_T) \qquad (2.11)$$

$$\Delta x_7 = x_5 R_{5,7}\,PSB + x_6 R_{6,7}\,PSA - x_7(PR1 + PD - \Delta x_9/x_T)$$
$$+ E_2(x_T - x_7)\,PB \qquad (2.12)$$

$$\Delta x_8 = x_7\,PB - x_8(PR2 + PD - \Delta x_9/x_T) + E_2(x_T - x_7)\,PB \qquad (2.13)$$

Computer programmes were developed to simulate the dynamics of these systems of equations and various control programmes were analysed by the exploration of the computer model's behaviour.

One problem analysed in detail was a comparison of the effects of the following immunization schemes on tetanus among the newborn segment of the population. It was assumed that the endemic incidence level of the disease prior to immunization was 400 per 100 000 newborns, a level widely observed in developing countries. The vaccine was taken to be 95% effective. Given these assumptions, and the parameter values described above, four schemes were considered: (A) single mass vaccination of the general population with a 50% coverage; (B) three mass vaccinations at 10-year intervals with 50% coverage; (C) continuous immunization of pregnant women with a 90% coverage; and (D) a combined programme of (B) and (C). The predicted outcomes of these programmes are shown in Fig. 2.2, where the numerical results produced by the model are recorded. It is clear from this figure that the continuous immunization of pregnant women has the greatest effect, effectively reducing the incidence of tetanus in newborn infants to very low levels.

The same model can also be used to study the cost-effectiveness and cost–benefit aspects of various anti-tetanus immunization programmes (Cvjetanović, 1974). The programme of continuous immunization of pregnant mothers appears to be the optimum approach to control both with respect to cost–benefit considerations and the reduction in disease incidence (Cvjetanović et al., 1978).

2.6 TYPHOID – INFECTION WITH INTER-HUMAN TRANSMISSION

Typhoid has a relatively simple natural history and its causative agent, *Salmonella typhi*, has stable characteristics. It might therefore be expected that

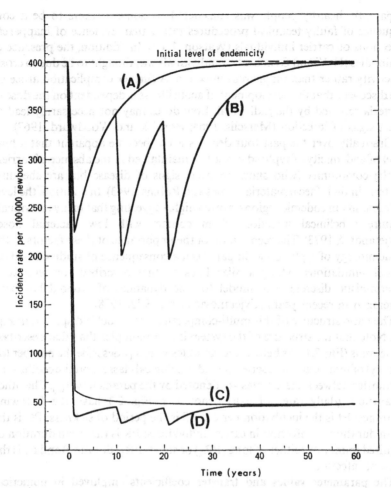

Figure 2.2 Effect of various immunization programmes on the incidence of tetanus cases in newborn infants (cases are treated and then immunized). (A) one mass programme of vaccination. (B) three mass programmes of vaccination at intervals of 10 years. (C) continuous vaccination of pregnant women. (D) combination of (B) and (C) (from Cvjetanović *et al.*, 1978).

the development of a mathematical model of the disease dynamics would be relatively straightforward given the quantity of available epidemiological information. This, however, has not proved to be the case since certain widely accepted epidemiological concepts concerning this infection appear to be inaccurate.

In the past it was believed that typhoid was an overt clinical disease with typical symptoms. As such, it was thought that the number of clinical cases notified reflected the actual incidence of the disease. The isolation of *S. typhi* in apparently healthy people was considered by some workers to be a consequence of faulty technical procedures rather than evidence of inapparent infections or carrier individuals (Watson, 1967). In addition, the presence of antibodies (H, Vi and O) in healthy individuals was thought to be due to cross-reactivity rather than inapparent infection. A further complication arose on the discovery that the development of acute illness is dependent on the dose of bacteria received by the individual. Low doses may not necessarily lead to overt signs of infection (Merselis, 1964; Hornick and Woodward, 1967).

Gradually over the past four decades it has become apparent that a high level of endemicity of typhoid cannot be maintained in the absence of carriers in the community (who show no overt signs of disease but are shedding bacteria in their faecal material; Ames and Robins, 1943). In addition, the level of immunity in endemic regions is often high, suggesting that many individuals acquire subclinical infections from contact with low bacterial doses (Cvjetanović, 1973). The recognition of the importance of these factors to the epidemiology of typhoid has in part been a consequence of studies based on model simulations. Along similar lines to that described for tetanus, a deterministic discrete time model for the dynamics of typhoid has been developed in recent years (Cvjetanović et al., 1972, 1978).

The basic structure of this multi-compartmental model is displayed in Fig. 2.3. Note that the structure of the system is more complex than that described for tetanus (Fig. 2.1). As before, the variables x_1 to x_{10} describe the number (or density) of individuals in a series of epidemiological classes and the coefficients of transfer between these states are denoted by the parameters $R_{i,j}$. The other parameters (daily rates of exit) denoted in Fig. 2.3 have the following meanings: PI is the incubation period; PS is the period of sickness; PC is the mean duration of infection in carrier individuals; PR is the mean duration of acquired immunity (either of long (PR$_2$) or short (PR$_1$) duration) and RI is the force of infection.

The parameter values and transfer coefficients employed in numerical simulations are listed in Tables 2.1 and 2.2 respectively.

Table 2.1 Typical values for the epidemiological parameters of typhoid.

Incubation period: range, 7–21 days; mean, 14 days
Duration of sickness: range, 14–35 days; mean, 28 days
Duration of relapse: range, 7–28 days; mean, 18 days
Frequency of relapses: 5% of cases
Proportion of cases: symptomatic (typical, febrile):
    20%; asymptomatic (and mild): 80%
Case fatality rate: 1–10%; average 3%
Carrier rate: chronic range, 2–5%; average 3%; temporary
    (mean duration, 90 days) range, 7–20%; average, 10%
Incidence in endemic areas per 10 000 population: 10–150

The equations to describe the daily rate of change in each of the classes are defined as follows:

$$\Delta x_1 = -(x_3 + x_4 + x_6 + x_7)(x_1/x_T)RI + (x_4 R_{4,1} + x_5 R_{5,1})PS$$
$$+ x_6 R_{6,1} PC + x_8 R_{8,1} PR_1 + x_9 R_{9,1} PR_2$$
$$+ x_T PB - x_1 (PD - \Delta x_{10}/x_T) \tag{2.14}$$

$$\Delta x_2 = R_{1,2}(x_3 + x_4 + x_6 + x_7)(x_1/x_T)RI$$
$$+ x_3 R_{3,2} PI - x_2 (PI + PD - \Delta x_{10}/x_T) \tag{2.15}$$

$$\Delta x_3 = R_{1,3}(x_3 + x_4 + x_6 + x_7)(x_1/x_T)RI$$
$$+ x_2 R_{2,3} PI - x_3 (PI + PD - \Delta x_{10}/x_T) \tag{2.16}$$

$$\Delta x_4 = (x_2 R_{2,4} + x_3 R_{3,4})PI + x_5 R_{5,4} PS - x_4 (PS + PD - \Delta x_{10}/x_T) \tag{2.17}$$

$$\Delta x_5 = (x_2 R_{2,5} + x_3 R_{3,5})PI + x_4 R_{4,5} PS - x_5 (PS + PD - \Delta x_{10}/x_T) \tag{2.18}$$

$$\Delta x_6 = x_4 R_{4,6} PS - x_6 (PC + PD - \Delta x_{10} x_T) \tag{2.19}$$

$$\Delta x_7 = x_6 R_{6,7} PC - x_7 (PD - \Delta x_{10} x_T) \tag{2.20}$$

$$\Delta x_8 = (x_4 R_{4,8} + x_5 R_{5,8})PS + x_6 R_{6,8} PC - x_8 (PR_1 + PD - \Delta x_{10}/x_T) \tag{2.21}$$

$$\Delta x_9 = x_8 R_{8,9} PR_1 - x_9 (PR_2 + PD - \Delta x_{10}/x_T) \tag{2.22}$$

$$\Delta x_{10} = (x_4 R_{4,10} + x_5 R_{5,10})PS \tag{2.23}$$

where $x_T = \sum_1^9 x_i$

Table 2.2 Typhoid fever: matrix of coefficients of transfer $R_{i,j}$.

Class of origin, i	Coefficient of transfer to class of destination, j:										Total
	1	2	3	4	5	6	7	8	9	10	
1	–	0.990	0.010	–	–	–	–	–	–	–	1.000
2	–	–	0.040	0.950	0.010	–	–	–	–	–	1.000
3	–	0.010	–	0.900	0.090	–	–	–	–	–	1.000
4	0.100	–	–	–	0.100	0.100	–	0.694	–	0.006*	1.000
5	0.100	–	–	0.200	–	–	–	0.694	–	0.006*	1.000
6	0.100	–	–	–	–	–	0.300	0.600	–	–	1.000
7	–	–	–	–	–	–	–	–	–	–	0.000
8	0.100	–	–	–	–	–	–	–	0.900	–	1.000
9	1.000	–	–	–	–	–	–	–	–	–	1.000
10	–	–	–	–	–	–	–	–	–	–	0.000

* The fatality rate is 0.03 of clinical cases. Assuming that 0.20 of classes x_4 and x_5 develop clinical symptoms, 0.006 of these classes are transferred to class x_{10}.

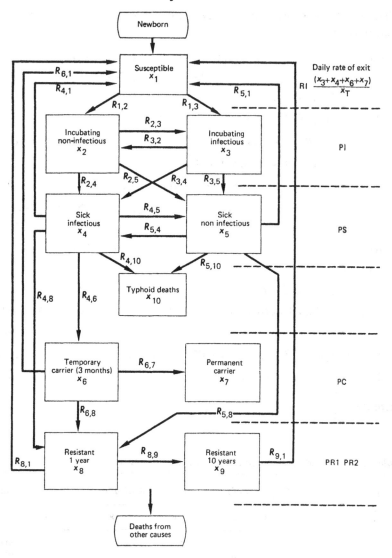

Figure 2.3   A diagrammatic flow chart of the dynamics of typhoid (from Cvjetanović *et al.*, 1978).

A computer programme was written to simulate the behaviour of these equations and to mimic the impact of various control options (Cvjetanović *et al.*, 1978).

The dynamics of the disease and its long-term stability are critically dependent on the proportion of infectious individuals within a community. For typhoid a high percentage of these infectious cases may be chronic carriers with no overt signs of disease. This point is illustrated in Table 2.3 which lists the percentage of the population in the various epidemiological classes for a

Table 2.3 Typhoid: model predictions of the percentage of individuals in the various epidemiological states at equilibrium (force of infection set at 0.002/day).

Susceptible (x_1)	84.9%
Incubating, infectious (x_3)	0.003%
Sick, infectious (x_4)	0.139%
Temporary carriers (x_6)	0.043%
Permanent carriers (x_7)	2.62%
Resistant for short period (x_8)	1.43%
Resistant for long period (x_9)	10.7%

situation in which the population is stable and endemic incidence level is stable at 348 cases per 100 000 (a daily per capita force of infection of roughly 0.002). The proportions of susceptibles and immunes within the population clearly changes for different forces of infection (which determines the overall incidence level) but the relative distribution of cases among the various infected classes $(x_3, x_4, x_6$ and $x_7)$ remains approximately stable. This point underlines the major role played by chronic carriers of the disease in the maintenance of endemic typhoid (Table 2.3).

With the development of improved environmental sanitation and rising standards of personal hygiene, the force of infection is declining steadily in many countries. The older age cohorts, with high proportions of carriers, are slowly removed by natural mortality and hence the overall number of carriers within many populations is falling rapidly. In many countries, such as England and Wales, there has been a steady decline in the incidence of typhoid which corresponds roughly to a 50% decrease every 10 years (Fig. 2.4). Once the force of infection drops below a critical level (as a consequence of improved sanitation and hygiene) where the basic reproductive rate of infection, R, is less than unity (see Chapter 1), the disease will slowly die out. However, as illustrated by the trends in England and Wales (Fig. 2.4) the constant reintroduction of infection from outside by immigrants or travellers can maintain the disease indefinitely within a country.

In regions where typhoid is endemic, the model can be used to assess the effectiveness of various control measures. These are basically of two types, immunization and improved sanitation. The effect of immunization is immediate but because of the short duration of protection provided by the available vaccines and the continual inflow of susceptibles into a community by new births, immunization coverage must be maintained at a high level and carried out on a continual basis to control the infection. In contrast, improvements in sanitation and hygiene act in a cumulative manner and, if maintained, have a long-lasting impact on disease prevalence (Cvjetanović and Uemura, 1965). An extensive discussion of the practical use of the typhoid model in the design of control measures for the disease is described in Cvjetanović *et al.* (1978).

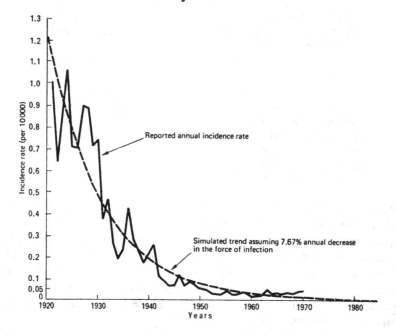

Figue 2.4   Incidence of typhoid cases in England and Wales from 1921 to 1970.

2.7   CHOLERA–AN ENDEMIC AND EPIDEMIC DISEASE

Cholera is an enteric infection with an anal–oral route of transmission but, in contrast to typhoid, carrier individuals with no overt signs of infection are not typically infectious for long periods of time. In some countries cholera is endemic in character while in others it is epidemic. Even in those countries where it is endemic there are typically seasons of high and low incidence. Extended endemic and epidemic waves in large populations are the result of many small outbreaks of infection.

As for typhoid, our understanding of the natural history of the disease has changed substantially over the past few decades since the last pandemic which began in 1961 (Barua and Burrows, 1974). In particular, it was realized that cholera is a very common infection in which only a small fraction of those who acquire infection develop clinical symptoms (WHO, 1970). Individuals who are infected but do not show symptoms of disease have been termed 'contact carriers' (Cvjetanović *et al.*, 1978; Barua and Burrows, 1974). Serological studies in endemic regions have shown that a high proportion of the population has high antibody titres as a result of frequent subclinical infection with cholera (*Vibrio cholerae*). Certain strains of cholera are more likely to produce such inapparent infections (e.g. *V. cholerae* biotype El Tor).

Taking these and other epidemiological factors into account, a model for the

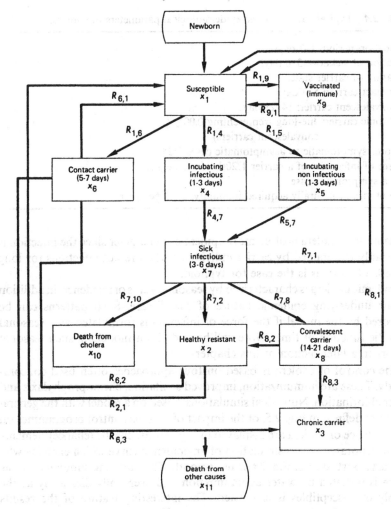

Figure 2.5 A diagrammatic flow chart of the dynamics of cholera (from Cvjetanovic *et al.*, 1978).

dynamics of the disease can be formulated along similar lines to those described for tetanus and typhoid. A flow chart of the basic structure of such a model is displayed in Fig. 2.5, while a list of typical values for certain epidemiological parameters of cholera is documented in Table 2.4.

In a population with crude birth and death rates of 40 and 20 per 1000 respectively, and with an endemic incidence of 133 per 100 000 individuals, the model predicts that roughly 95% of the population will be in the susceptible class and roughly 4% will be in the immune (or resistant) state. The incidence of carriers will typically be much lower than that for typhoid. This in part

Table 2.4 Typical values for the epidemiological parameters of cholera.

Incubation period: 1–3 days
Duration of sickness: 3–6 days
Duration of carrier state:
   Contact carrier: 5–7 days
   Convalescent carrier: 14–21 days
   Chronic carrier: life-long (representing 0.001 %
                       convalescent carriers)
Ratio of symptomatic to asymptomatic cases 1:24
Degree of infectivity of a carrier 1/20th of the degree
  of a symptomatic case
Rate of loss of naturally acquired immunity: 50 % per year

explains why cholera is often more epidemic in character since the infection is not stably maintained by carrier individuals who are not infectious for long periods of time, as is the case for typhoid.

Endemic cholera is characterized by seasonal waves of incidence, in addition to the underlying epidemic nature of the disease. Such patterns can be mirrored by the model if the force of infection is formulated as a seasonal periodic function of time. More will be said about modelling such seasonal factors in a later section of this chapter.

The control of cholera is based on four approaches often used concomitantly. These are immunization, improved sanitation, chemoprophylaxis and water chlorination. Numerical simulations, based on a model with the general structure defined in Fig. 2.5, of the impact of various control programmes on the incidence of cholera are displayed in Fig. 2.6. Stochastic (chance) elements are incorporated in this simulation of an epidemic curve which explains why the curve portrayed in Fig. 2.6 is not smooth. The outbreak simulated in this figure is initiated by water contamination and eventually dies away as the supply of susceptibles is exhausted. The interesting feature of the results portrayed in Fig. 2.6 concerns the relative efficiencies of vaccination versus water chlorination. These results suggest that the latter form of control is by far the most effective, an observation supported by practical experience (Azurin and Alvero, 1974). After the chlorination of the water supplies, water-borne transmission virtually ceases and the tail of the epidemic is the result of 'contact carriers' with inapparent infections of short duration.

The simulation of an endemic situation is more complex and a variety of control options exist with very different costs. The simulation model of cholera dynamics has proved particularly useful in examining these various options (Cvjetanović *et al.*, 1978). An example of the model's predictions of the impact of a variety of control options is displayed in Fig. 2.7. As for typhoid, improvements in sanitation have the most impact of all the control methods. Such an approach may be made more effective if used in conjunction with

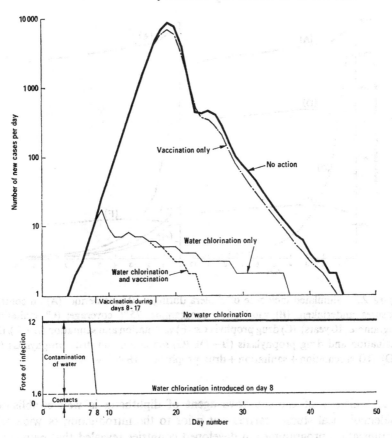

Figure 2.6 Numerical simulation of an explosive, water-borne epidemic pattern of cholera in a population of 1 million individuals. The force of infection was set at 12 in the absence of water chlorination and at 1.6 with water chlorination. It was assumed that 15 contact carriers arrived on day 0 and introduced the infection into the water supply. At the beginning of the epidemic the population consisted of 95.8 % of susceptibles. Vaccine efficacy and coverage were taken to be 70 % and 75 % respectively (for further details see Cvjetanovic *et al.*, 1978).

vaccination and drug prophylaxis (Fig. 2.7). If relevant data on the costs of the various options are available a model of the structure depicted in Fig. 2.6 may be used to design the most cost-effective form of control.

2.8 DIPHTHERIA

Diphtheria is a typical disease of childhood and one in which the force of infection changes with host age. Dynamic models of such infections must therefore take into account the age structure of the human population. The

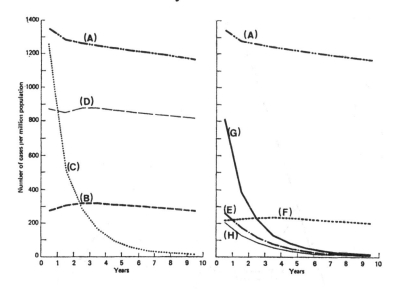

Figure 2.7 Simulated incidence of cholera during a 10-year period. (A) no control measures undertaken; (B) vaccination programme, 75% coverage; (C) sanitation programme (10 years); (C) drug prophylaxis; (E) vaccination and sanitation (B + C); (F) vaccination and drug prophylaxis (B + D); (G) sanitation and drug prophylaxis (C + D); (H) vaccination + sanitation + drug prophylaxis (B + C + D).

natural history of the causative agent of diphtheria is well established. Epidemiological studies carried out prior to the introduction of widescale immunization programmes in developed countries revealed that between 6 and 40% of children are infected each year and that 2–7% of school children were carriers of the disease. By the age of 5 years roughly 75% of children have been infected and by the age of 15 years the infection rate is close to 100%. It is thought that children, in their first 10 years of life, each experience roughly 2.5 infections. The clinical patterns of the disease differ somewhat in tropical regions but the duration of infectiousness and acquisition of immunity is essentially the same in temperate and tropical areas.

The dynamics of the disease is characterized by a high incidence of carriers and a rather low incidence of clinical cases. It is estimated that the ratio of carriers to clinical cases is roughly 19:1. This results in the acquisition of immunity by the majority of children by the age of 15, either by an inapparent infection, or an infection which results in clinical symptoms. The flow of individuals between the various epidemiological classes of the disease may be summarized as displayed in Fig. 2.8. In this flow chart, provision is made for simulating the effects of immunization programmes, since susceptibles can be transferred to a vaccinated class (x_9). Simulation studies of a model based on the structures displayed in Fig. 2.8 focused on the experiences of a cohort of

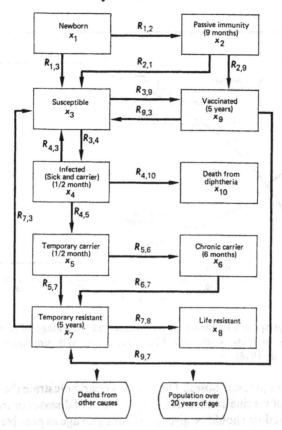

Figure 2.8 A diagrammatic flow chart of the dynamics of diphtheria (see Cvjetanović *et al.*, 1978).

newborn infants as they progressed through a series of age classes. The resultant output, of the proportion of immunes at each age through a time span of 30 years, is portrayed in Fig. 2.9. It can be seen from this figure that model predictions can be made to closely minor observed trends in the age prevalence of infection. The average age at which the infection was acquired in New York in the period 1920–1924 was approximately 11–12 years. The basic reproductive rate, R, of diphtheria in this community was therefore approximately 5–6 (see Chapter 1) (Cvjetanović *et al.*, 1978).

Vaccination against diphtheria in developed countries is often combined with immunization programmes for pertussis (whooping cough) and tetanus. A combined DPT vaccine is given to children in the first 4 or 5 years of their life. The simulated effects of various schemes of immunization on the incidence of diphtheria are recorded in Table 2.5. The schemes vary according to the age at which the vaccine is administered and the number of vaccine

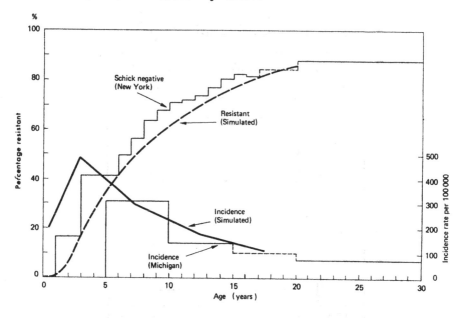

Figure 2.9 Age-specific incidence of diphtheria and percentage of people immune (observed data in New York and Michigan, USA, and simulated results; see Cvjetanović *et al.*, 1978).

administrations (booster doses). These results clearly illustrate the importance of the timing of vaccine administration to the level of disease control achieved. Ideally the first dose should be given at as young an age as possible but it must be followed by booster doses in the latter part of the pre-school period of a child's life. These predictions are substantially supported by the observed trends in European countries with different vaccination schemes. The comparative success (in contrast to cholera and typhoid) of immunization as a means of the control of diphtheria and pertussis is a consequence of the long-lasting protection that can be induced by toxoid administration (Gottlieb, 1967).

2.9 SEASONAL FACTORS

In the section concerned with the dynamics of cholera it was noted that disease prevalence often fluctuates markedly from season to season in any given year. Such patterns are a consequence of seasonal changes in the force of infection, due either to a change in host habits or changes in the infectivity of transmission stages as a consequence of climatic trends. Seasonal patterns may be easily simulated by formulating the force of infection as a periodic function of time.

In the case of certain diseases, such as cerebrospinal meningitis, seasonal

Table 2.5 Simulated effects of different immunization schemes, with 90% population coverage, on diphtheria incidence rates per 100 000 people in the age groups 0–19 years (from Cvjetanović et al., 1978).

No. of vaccine administrations	Scheme	Age at vaccination (years): ½	1	1½	3	5½	6	11	Initial rate	Incidence rate of diphtheria, Duration of programme (years): 2	5	10	20	30
1	1	DPT‡							252.7	180.2	37.6	12.2	89.0	26.8
	2		DPT‡						252.7	167.5	36.6	13.5	94.3	28.9
	3			DPT‡					252.7	172.1	41.3	16.2	100.5	34.7
1*–2†	4		DPT‡			DT			252.7	129.5	7.16	0.17	0.005	0.001
2	5	DPT‡		DPT					252.7	127.6	12.8	0.79	0.022	0.000
	6	DPT‡			DPT				252.7	139.8	7.53	0.05	0.000	0.006
	7			DPT‡		DPT			252.7	133.2	8.66	0.33	0.020	0.006
	8	DPT‡				DPT			252.7	127.0	7.12	0.28	0.006	0.000
2*–3†	9	DPT‡		DPT		DT			252.7	97.3	1.90	0.003	0.000	0.000
3	10	DPT‡		DPT		DPT			252.7	97.3	1.90	0.003	0.000	0.000
	11	DPT‡			DPT		DPT		252.7	98.4	1.36	0.002	0.000	0.000
3*–4†	12	DPT‡			DPT		DPT	DT	252.7	83.9	0.34	0.000	0.000	0.000

* Pertussis vaccine.
† Diphtheria toxoid.
‡ Primary immunization (three doses).

outbreaks are of paramount importance to the dynamics of infection (Fig. 2.10). The high incidence of this disease at certain times of the year is inversely correlated with the relative humidity of the atmosphere (Fig. 2.11), although the precise reasons for such patterns are as yet unclear (Cvjetanović et al., 1978). Such changes in the force of infection induce complex seasonal changes in the proportion of susceptibles, infecteds and immunes within the population (Fig. 2.12). The interaction of seasonal oscillations superimposed on the systems' intrinsic tendency to oscillate (induced by the exhaustion and renewal of the supply of susceptibles) can produce very complicated patterns of disease incidence. In addition, control intervention (say by immunization or mass chemoprophylaxis) can induce very bizarre patterns of oscillation in the incidence of the infection (see Cvjetanović et al., 1978). At present very little is understood concerning the generative processes of seasonal trends in the

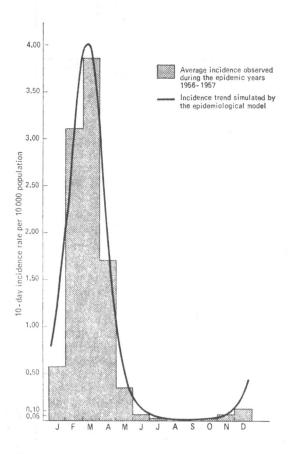

Figure 2.10 Seasonal variation in the incidence of cerebrospinal meningitis in the Upper Volta (1956–1957) by 10-day periods (from Cvjetanovic *et al.*, 1978).

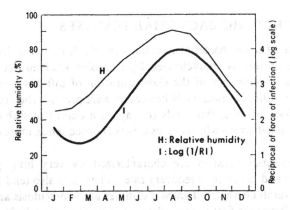

Figure 2.11 Seasonal variation in relative humidity at Bobo Dloulasso, Upper Volta, and the inverse of the force of infection of cerebrosinal meningitis (plotted on a logarithmic scale) (from Cvjetanović *et al.*, 1978).

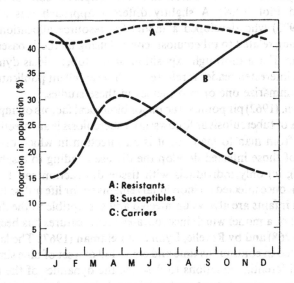

Figure 2.12 Simulated changes in the proportion of the population in different epidemiological classes for cerebrospinal meningitis infection in the Upper Volta during the epidemic year 1956–1957 (from Cvjetanović *et al.*, 1978).

incidence of many bacterial infections. It must be recognized, however, that such trends are of some importance to the interpretation of long-term oscillations (over many years) in the dynamics of such diseases (see also Chapter 1 with respect to the influence of seasonal factors on the epidemiology of measles).

2.10 CHRONIC BACTERIAL DISEASES

The dynamics of acute bacterial infections in which carrier individuals are either absent or rare is characterized by explosive epidemic outbreaks of infection as a consequence of the short duration of infectiousness and the transience of acquired immunity. When carriers are present who are infectious for long periods of time, this tends to impose a degree of stability on the dynamics of such diseases which are, as a direct consequence, more endemic in character.

Chronic bacterial diseases are characterized by very long periods of infectiousness and hence slow recovery rates. They thus also tend to be more endemic in overall character. Typical examples are tuberculosis and leprosy.

Frost (1937) was the first to formulate a quantitative model of tuberculosis and this work was later extended by Feldman (1957). A summary of early work on the dynamics of tuberculosis has been published by Waaler, Gesser and Anderson (1962). This work was further developed by Waaler and Piot in a study of an epidemiological model to mimic the impact of control intervention (Waaler and Piot, 1969). A slightly different approach was adopted by Feldman (1973) who developed a model for resource allocation in public health planning related to tuberculosis control using methods based on linear programming. For a thorough exposition of the tuberculosis dynamics and controls, the interested reader is referred to these excellent publications. Here, we briefly summarize one or two themes in these studies.

Waaler et al. (1962) pinpointed the major biological factors of importance to the dynamics of tuberculosis as follows: (a) tuberculosis is an infection directly transmitted from man to man; (b) it is an infection in which only a minor proportion of those infected develop the disease (leading to disabling tissue destructions); (c) only individuals with tissue destruction can transmit the infection; (d) once infected an individual remains so for life unless treated; and (e) newborn infants are always uninfected and susceptible to the disease. The development of a model which incorporates these features has been achieved by Waaler (1968) and by Revelle, Lynn and Feldman (1967). The latter model was formulated in continuous time and consisted of a set of nine simultaneous non-linear differential equations to describe the dynamics of the number of people in each of nine distinct epidemiological classes. Many of these classes were created by control procedures such as prophylaxis and vaccination (see Bailey (1975) for further discussion of these models).

Leprosy like tuberculosis is a chronic disease of some importance in the world today. Lechat and co-workers have made some preliminary attempts to construct models to describe the dynamics of leprosy and the impact of public health policies (Lechat, 1971). This work is to a large extent in its infancy since many factors concerning this disease are ill understood at present. The main biological features may be summarized as follows: (a) leprosy is a disease which results from the contact of a leprous patient with a susceptible individual; (b) leprosy develops into either lepromatous open leprosy or close leprosy in tuberculoid form; (c) close leprosy may develop to open leprosy but the reverse is not thought to be possible; (d) susceptibility to the disease is thought to be uniformly high in most populations and infants are susceptible when born; (e) spontaneous recovery is not possible, and (f) treated and cured patients can relapse. These ideas have enabled simple flow charts to be constructed of the disease's dynamics but as yet little progress has been made in the formal mathematical description of the rates of flow between the various epidemiological classes. There is clearly much scope for further mathematical work on the dynamics of chronic bacterial infections and on the impact of control measures on these diseases.

2.11 CONCLUDING REMARKS

It is clear from the brief discussion of acute bacterial infections presented in this chapter that a great deal of further study of the dynamics of these infections is required. Many bacterial infections exhibit features which make formal descriptions of their dynamics much more complex than is usually the case for directly transmitted viral, helminth or protozoan infections. The existence of carrier individuals, for example, who are infectious but show no overt signs of disease, raises special complications. These individuals, however, are clearly of major importance to the persistence of such bacterial infections within human communities. The duration of infectiousness of these carrier individuals is an important determinant of observed patterns of disease behaviour (i.e. whether it is endemic or epidemic in character).

One immediate consequence of the complexity of the natural history of such diseases in man is the necessity to recognize many distinct epidemiological groups within a population (for example, susceptibles, infecteds who are not infectious, infectious individuals, immunes and carrier individuals). Mathematical models must therefore consist of large numbers of equations and contain many rate parameters.

Such models, whether formulated as difference or differential equations, are difficult to analyse. Analytical solutions are rarely, if ever, possible and the derivation of equilibrium states and their associated stability properties will usually be difficult. For practical purposes, we can of course (as illustrated in this chapter) use computer methods for the exploration of model behaviour and to make time projections of the likely outcome of different forms of control intervention. Studies of this form are of obvious value in public health planning.

In order to obtain guidance for the control of say, tetanus or cholera, in any given community, we need estimates of all the model parameters for that specific community. Initially, it may not be necessary to have highly accurate estimates. Subsequent computation may be able to demonstrate whether important results are sensitive to changes in certain parameters. When this occurs, special steps may have to be taken to obtain more accurate information.

As noted by Bailey (1975) some parameters, such as birth and death rates, or relapse and recovery rates (see Tables 2.1 and 2.4), may be directly derivable from appropriate demographic and epidemiological data. Others, like the force of infection, may have to be based initially on a certain amount of guesswork. These aspects of parameter estimation have so far received insufficient attention. One major role of model construction, however, is to identify areas in which our knowledge is inadequate and hence mathematical work can help to guide the design of epidemiological surveys.

In conjunction with research aimed at improving the available epidemiological data base there is also a need for further refinements in the methods used to construct models of bacterial diseases. Complex sets of difference or differential equations can often be greatly simplified, without loss of realism, by taking note of the relative time scales over which the dynamics of the various variables defined in the model operate (Anderson and May, 1979a; May and Anderson, 1979). In certain of the diseases discussed in this chapter, it is clear that the time spent by an individual in any one epidemiological state (i.e. immune, infectious or carrier state) vary greatly. In such cases further work may be able to simplify greatly the basic model structure and hence reduce the number of parameters for which estimates are required. However, in other instances simplifications may neither be possible nor desirable.

3 The population dynamics and control of hookworm and roundworm infections

Roy M. Anderson

3.1 INTRODUCTION

More than thirty years ago Stoll (1947) noted that helminth parasites were amongst the most prevalent of all human infections within many tropical, subtropical and temperate regions of the world. Today the global pattern of infection has changed little. World Health Organization statistics, for example, suggest that approximately one billion people are currently infected with the directly transmitted nematode *Ascaris lumbricoides* (roundworms). The picture is similar for other nematode parasites such as *Trichuris trichiura* (whipworms), *Enterobius vermicularis* (pinworms) and the hookworms *Ancylostoma duodenale* and *Necator americanus* (Table 3.1).

In contrast to the viral and bacterial diseases discussed in the first two

Table 3.1 Estimates of the number of people infected with various nematode parasites in different regions of the world in 1975 (data source Peters (1978); world population size in 1975 was approximately 3967 million).

Parasite	Number of people infected (millions)					
	Africa	Asia (excluding USSR)	N., C. and S. America	Europe (excluding USSR)	USSR	World total
Ascaris lumbricoides (roundworm)	159	931	109	39	30	1269
Hookworm (two species)	132	685	106	2	4	932
Enterobius vermicularis (pinworm)	24	136	115	75	48	353
Trichuris trichiura (whipworm)	76	433	135	41	41	687

chapters, helminths are macroparasites which give rise to persistent infections with hosts being continually reinfected. In areas with endemic ascariasis and hookworm disease, for example, a newborn child can expect to harbour worms for the majority of his or her life. Direct multiplication within the host is either absent or occurs at a low rate and the immune responses elicited by these metazoans generally depend on the number of parasites present in a given host. Such responses do not tend to provide complete protection to reinfection; they simply act to increase the rate of parasite mortality and decrease worm fecundity and establishment.

Infection with helminth parasites is not necessarily synonomous with disease. Many people invaded by *Ascaris* and hookworms do not exhibit overt signs or symptoms of disease. Manifestations, such as intestinal obstruction or anaemia, are usually associated with heavy worm burdens. The frequency of appearance of disease symptoms is directly proportional to the worm burden harboured by an individual, although the impact of infection is more severe in regions where malnourishment is prevalent. Indeed, the parasites themselves may be an important contributory factor in the occurrence of malnutrition (Scrimshaw, Taylor and Gordon, 1968; Rowland, Cole and Whitehead, 1977; Whitehead, 1977).

Very few attempts have been made to study the population dynamics of direct life-cycle helminths despite their prevalence and medical significance in the world today (Leyton, 1968; Talis and Leyton, 1969; Hoagland and Schad, 1978; Nawalinski, Schad and Chowdhury, 1978a, b; Anderson, 1980, 1981b; Croll *et al.*, 1982a). An understanding of the population biology of these parasites is of obvious significance to the design and implementation of control programmes. This chapter describes some preliminary attempts to explore the dynamics of directly transmitted nematode infections of man. Attention is specifically focused on the population biologies of human hookworms and the roundworm *A. lumbricoides* since relatively good data bases exist in the epidemiological literature for these two types of parasitic infection.

3.2 LIFE CYCLES

The life cycles of directly transmitted nematodes consist of many distinct developmental stages which are identified by their morphological features and by their respective habitats (either in the host or in the external environment).

The developmental cycle of human hookworms, for example, begins with the production of eggs by mature female worms in the small intestine of the host. These pass to the exterior in the faeces and hatch to release a first stage, or L_1 larva, which feed on bacteria and organic debris in the soil. After a short period of growth they moult once to produce the second stage, or L_2 larva, and then again to produce the third stage or L_3 infective larva. The L_3 stage is responsible for host location and infection, gaining entry either by direct penetration of the epithelial layers (*Necator americanus*) or by ingestion

(*Ancylostoma duodenale*). Once inside the host a phase of migration occurs, the larvae passing via the circulatory system to the lungs and then in swallowed secretions to their final habitat in the small intestine. The larvae undergo two further moults in the intestine before sexual maturity is attained. Broadly speaking, the stages within the human host can be divided into two types: namely, immature and mature worms. The complete life cycle of hookworm parasites involves six distinct developmental stages; the egg, the L_1, L_2 and L_3 larvae and the immature and mature parasitic worms (Muller, 1975).

The net reproductive success of the parasite during development through the life cycle will depend on the rates of mortality and reproduction associated with these various stages and the average time spent in each developmental state. The ability to reproduce is invariably restricted to the sexually mature parasitic stages, although exceptions arise such as the nematode *Strongyloides stercoralis* which may undergo a phase of reproduction within the host and in the external habitat (Pampiglione and Ricciardi, 1972). Without exception, however, reproduction by the parasitic stages does not *directly* increase parasite population size within the host, but involves the production of transmission stages such as eggs or larvae which pass into the external habitat.

The life cycles of all directly transmitted nematodes are basically of similar structure, involving two principal populations: the *sexually mature parasitic worms* and the *free-living infective stages*. The infective stage is not always a motile larva (as in the hookworm life cycle), but may, as in the case of *A. lumbricoides*, be a resistant egg which hatches to release a larval parasite on ingestion by a suitable host species. The two principal populations play a central role in determining the overall transmission success of the parasite and to a large extent control parasite population growth and stability throughout the entire life cycle. The sexually mature worms are responsible for reproduction while the infective stages determine both the rate at which new hosts are 'colonized' and the rate of recruitment to established parasite populations. Infection is essentially a form of reproduction since it is the means by which a parasite gains access to a habitat in which it is able to reproduce. A diagrammatic picture of the flow of parasites between the two principal populations is presented in Fig. 3.1.

3.3 MODEL FRAMEWORK

In the design of a mathematical framework to mimic the population biology of a human infection it is clearly important to match this framework, as closely as possible, to the structure of the available epidemiological data. In the case of nematode infections, for example, epidemiologists usually record the prevalence (proportion of the population infected) and the intensity (average worm burden) of infection in various age classes of the human population. Such records may be acquired by either sampling at one point in time (horizontal survey) or over a series of successive points in time (longitudinal survey). It is

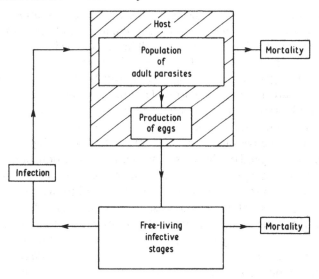

Figure 3.1 Diagrammatic flow chart of the principal populations and rate processes contained within the life cycles of directly transmitted nematode parasites.

important to measure the intensity of parasitic infection (often by indirect methods, such as the counting of helminth eggs in the faeces of the host) as well as the prevalence since, as mentioned earlier, for macroparasites the severity of clinical symptoms is usually associated with the number of worms harboured by an individual.

To facilitate the measurement of population parameters, and to enable a comparison to be made between theory and observation, our model framework must be designed to incorporate the epidemiological variables, parasite prevalence and parasite intensity. In order to meet this requirement, the model development described in this chapter centres on the mathematical description of the dynamics of the sexually mature worms in the human population and the free-living infective stages in the external habitat. The biology of development via the other stages in the parasite's life cycle will be reflected by the time delays and the mortalities associated with transmission between the two principal populations.

Our model is based on a framework developed by Anderson and May (1978) and consists of two coupled differential equations which mimic the dynamics of the total number, P_t, of sexually mature parasites in a human population of density, N, and the number, L_t, of free-living infective stages in the habitat of the human community. Human density is assumed to be constant on a time scale appropriate to changes in the parasite populations.

The equation for P_t consists of one gain and two loss terms. The gain term portrays the recruitment of parasites to the sexually mature population. We assume that the rate at which hosts acquire infection is directly proportional to the density of hosts times the density of infective stages, namely $\beta L_t N$, where β is a transmission coefficient which is proportional to the rate of contact between hosts and infective stages. After the larva enters the host, a given time interval, T_1, will elapse before the parasite completes development to the sexually mature state and during this interval a certain proportion of the invading organisms will die. We use the parameter D_1 to denote the proportion that survive through the time interval T_1. At time t, therefore, the net recruitment to the sexually mature worm population is $\beta L(t - T_1) N D_1$.

The two loss terms denote parasite mortalities due to natural causes and/or host-induced effects (immunological attack) and natural host mortality. If the host's per capita death rate is b, where $1/b$ denotes host life expectancy, and $p(i)$ is the probability that a host contains i parasites then the net loss of parasites due to host deaths is

$$bN \sum_{i=0}^{\infty} ip(i)$$

The natural death rate of helminth parasites within their host is invariably a function of parasite density. Such density-dependence may be due to competition for limited resources such as food or space, or, more commonly, to the mode of action of the hosts' immunological defences. If we denote the per capita density-dependent death rate as $\mu(i)$, then the net rate of loss due to such mortalities is

$$N \sum_{i=0}^{\infty} \mu(i)ip(i)$$

With these assumptions the equation for P_t takes the form:

$$dP/dt = \beta NL(t - T_1)D_1 - bN \sum_{i=0}^{\infty} ip(i) - N \sum_{i=0}^{\infty} \mu(i)ip(i) \qquad (3.1)$$

The equation for the number of infective stages, L_t, at time t also consists of one gain and two loss terms. As was the case for the death rate of adults, the production of eggs by mature female worms is usually a function of parasite density within the host. We denote the per capita rate of egg production as $\lambda(i)$ in a host with i parasites such that the net output of transmission stages by the total population of mature parasites is

$$s\Phi N \sum_{i=0}^{\infty} \lambda(i)ip(i)$$

where s represents the proportion of female worms in the population and Φ denotes the probability that a female worm has been mated and is able to produce fertile eggs. Of this output of eggs only a certain proportion, D_2, will survive to attain the infective state. If we denote the average time taken to reach this state from the birth of an egg as T_2, then the net recruitment to the population of infective stages at time t is

$$sD_2 \Phi N \sum_{i=0}^{\infty} \lambda(i)ip(i, t-T_2)$$

The two loss terms represent deaths due to natural mortalities, at a per capita rate μ_2, and losses due to infection at a net rate $\beta N t$. These assumptions lead to the following equation for L_t.

$$dL/dt = sD_2 \Phi N \sum_{i=0}^{\infty} \lambda(i)ip(i, t-T_2) - \mu_2 L - \beta NL \tag{3.2}$$

Three of the components contained in the model defined by Equations (3.1) and (3.2) require further explanation, namely, density-dependence, the mating probability Φ and the probability distribution of mature worms within the host population. These topics are examined in the following three sections of this chapter.

3.4 DENSITY-DEPENDENT POPULATION PARAMETERS

Quantitative information on the functional form and magnitude of density-dependent constraints on worm population growth within human hosts is at present very limited. In qualitative terms, however, such effects are known to operate on both worm survival and fecundity, since in their absence parasite populations would either grow or decay exponentially in an unconstrained fashion. A striking feature of the dynamics of nematode infections in human communities is the constancy of the parasite populations through time and their robustness to perturbations, whether induced by man's activity or climatic factors. This observed stability implies that the parasite populations within individual hosts are tightly regulated by density-dependent checks. These constraints are probably generated by the immune system of the host.

Indirect evidence of the existence of such responses in man is provided by experimental work on closely related parasitic species in laboratory animals. The work of Krupp (1962), for example, on the dog hookworm, *Ancylostoma caninum*, demonstrated that worm survival and fecundity both declined as the density of worms within the host increased (Fig. 3.2). In the case of worm survival, the per capita death rate appears to increase approximately linearly as parasite density rises (Anderson, 1980).

More direct evidence is provided by studies of the relation between the number of *Ascaris* harboured by children and young adults in a rural community in Iran and the density of nematode eggs in their faeces (Croll *et al.*, 1982). As illustrated in Fig. 3.3, worm fecundity declines as parasite density per host increases. Some examples of similar studies of the relationship between

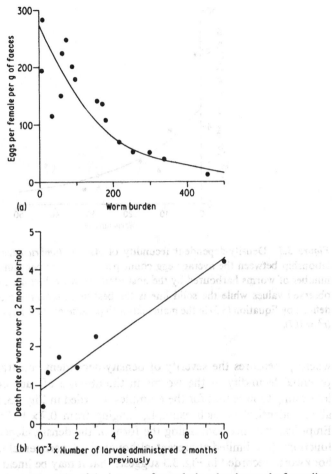

Figure 3.2 Experimental results of the impact of population density on the fecundity and survival of the dog hookworm *Ancylostoma caninum* (data from Krupp (1962)). (a) records the relationship between egg production per female worm (eggs per g of faeces) and the number of worms within the dog host. The dots are observed values while the solid line denotes the best-fit exponential model of the form defined by Equation (3.3) in the main text with parameter values $\lambda_0 = 278.8$ and $\gamma = 0.6 \times 10^{-2}$ ($r^2 = 0.9$). (b) records the instantaneous death rate of the parasites (per 2 month period) plotted against the number of larvae administered to the dog host. The dots are experimental results and the solid line is the best-fit linear model of the form defined by Equation (3.4) in the main text with parameter values $\mu_1 = 0.891$ and $\alpha = 0.34 \times 10^{-3}$ ($r^2 = 0.9$).

the fecundity of hookworms and worm burden are recorded in Fig. 3.4. In these examples fecundity decays exponentially as worm burden increases such that the function $\lambda(i)$ is of the form:

$$\lambda(i) = \lambda_0 \exp\left(-\gamma i\right) \tag{3.3}$$

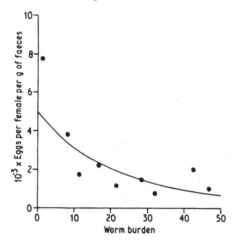

Figure 3.3 Density-dependent fecundity of *Ascaris lumbricoides* in man. The relationship between the average egg count per g of faeces per female worm and the number of worms harboured by the host (data from Croll *et al.*, 1982). The dots are observed values while the solid line is the best-fit exponential model (of the form defined by Equation (3.3) in the main text) with parameter values $\lambda_0 = 4.7$ and $\gamma = 0.04$ ($r^2 = 0.7$).

where γ measures the severity of density-dependent constraints and λ_0 the potential fecundity of the worms in the absence of such constraints. It is interesting to note that for the examples recorded in Fig. 3.3, the value of γ is almost identical in each example, ranging from 0.7×10^{-3} to 0.9×10^{-3}. Empirical evidence concerning the form of the density-dependent mortality function $\mu(i)$ is limited at present, although the experimental work on the dog hookworm recorded in Fig. 3.3 suggests that it may be linear in form where:

$$\mu(i) = \mu_1 + \alpha i \qquad (3.4)$$

Here, $1/\mu_1$ denotes adult worm life expectancy in the absence of regulatory constraints and the parameter α measures the severity of the density-dependence.

On the basis of the available empirical evidence it appears probable that density-dependent factors are of greater significance to worm fecundity than to worm survival. In the light of this, the models examined in this chapter are principally concerned with density-dependence in parasite reproduction.

3.5   THE DISTRIBUTION OF PARASITES WITHIN THE HOST POPULATION

It is clear from the structure of Equation (3.1) that the dynamical behaviour of the population model is critically dependent on the precise form of the

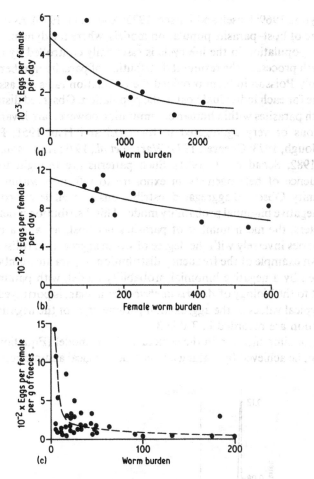

Figure 3.4 Some examples of density-dependent fecundity of hookworm parasites of man. (a) *Necator americanus* in man (data from Hill (1926)). The solid line is the best-fit exponential model (as defined in Equation (3.3) in the main text) with parameters λ_0 = 4.8 and $\gamma = 0.7 \times 10^{-3}$ ($r^2 = 0.7$). (b) *Necator* and *Ancylostoma* infections in man (data from Stoll (1923)). The solid line is as described for graph (a) but with parameter values $\lambda_0 = 10.3$ and $\gamma = 0.7 \times 10^{-3}$ ($r^2 = 0.5$). (c) *Necator americanus* in man (unpublished data from N. A. Croll). The dashed line is fitted by eye to illustrate the general trend in the data.

statistical distribution of parasite numbers per host (the $p(i)$ terms in Equation (3.1)). The model is of hybrid structure containing both deterministic and stochastic components (Anderson, 1979). It is sometimes possible to make assumptions that permit the distribution of parasite numbers per host to be deduced theoretically; the precise form of the distribution depending on the type and number of population processes incorporated in the model (Tallis and Leyton, 1969; Nasell and Hirsch, 1973; Anderson, 1976). As a result of the structure of host–parasite population models, where the dynamics of any one parasite population in the life cycle is essentially controlled by immigration and death processes, the resultant distribution of parasite numbers per host is invariably Poisson in form provided the population rates are assumed to be the same for each individual host in the population. Observed distributions of helminth parasites within human communities, however, are invariably highly contagious or very aggregated in form (Li and Hsu, 1951; Bradley and McCullough, 1973; Cheever, 1977; Warren et al., 1979; Anderson, 1980; Croll et al., 1982; Schad et al., 1981). Such patterns are thought to arise as a consequence of heterogeneity in exposure to infection within the human community. Observed aggregated distributions are well described empirically by the negative binomial probability model. This distribution is defined by two parameters, the mean number of parasites per host, M, and a parameter k which varies inversely with the degree of worm aggregation (Bliss and Fisher, 1953). An example of the frequency distribution of parasite numbers per host generated by a negative binomial probability model, with parameter values relevant to the biology of *Ascaris lumbricoides* in man, is portrayed in Fig. 3.5. Some typical values of the aggregation parameter, k, of the negative binomial distribution are recorded in Table 3.2.

A major simplification in the structure of our model (Equations (3.1) and (3.2)) can be achieved by making a phenomenological assumption concerning

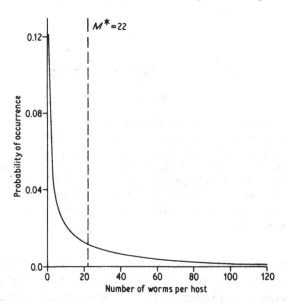

Figure 3.5 An illustration of the negative binomial probability distribution. The parameter values are set so as to mirror those observed for *Ascaris* in a rural community in Iran, namely $M^* = 22$ worms/host, $p^* = 0.88$ and $k = 0.57$ (Croll et al., 1982).

Table 3.2 Typical values of the negative binomial parameter k for hookworm and roundworm parasites of man.

Parasite	Location	k value	Reference
Ascaris lumbricoides	Iran	0.2–2.9	Croll et al. (1982)
Necator americanus	India	0.03–0.6	Anderson (1980)
N. americanus and Ancylostoma duodenale	Taiwan	0.05–0.4	Anderson (1980)

the form of the distribution of parasite numbers per host. On the basis of empirical evidence it is reasonable to assume that the probability terms in Equation (3.1)|(the $p(i)$'s) are distributed in negative binomial manner with mean M, where $M = P/N$, and aggregation parameter k (Anderson, 1980; Croll et al., 1982).

If we assume that density-dependence acts principally on worm fecundity as opposed to parasite mortality, where the functional form of $\lambda(i)$ is as defined in Equation (3.3), then Equations (3.1) and (3.2) may be expressed in a somewhat simpler form as follows:

$$dM/dt = \beta L(t - T_1)D_1 - (b + \mu_1)M \tag{3.5}$$

$$dL/dt = zsD_2\Phi NM(t - T_2)\left[1 + \frac{M(t - T_2)(1 - z)}{k}\right]^{-(k+1)} - (\mu_2 + \beta N)L \tag{3.6}$$

where $z = \exp(-\gamma)$ (see Equation (3.3)).

3.6   THE MATING PROBABILITY

Directly transmitted nematode parasites of man are dioecious (separate sexes) and hence the probability that an individual female worm successfully pairs with a mature male to produce fertile eggs (the mating probability, Φ) is dependent on the distribution of male and female parasites within the host population. At low parasite densities per host the average frequency of contact with potential partners may fall to such low levels as to adversely influence the net transmission success of the parasite within the host population. Aside from the distribution of parasites, other factors such as the sexual habits of the parasite and sex ratios within the population, influence the mating probability. With respect to sexual habits, whether a species is monogamous or polygamous is clearly important. Nematodes are thought in general to be polygamous such that if one male and three female worms are present in a host, all three females will be fertilized by the single male. Other aspects of mating behaviour are less well understood. For example, it is not known at present whether a mature female worm requires fertilization more than once to maintain egg production throughout her life span. In the absence of any information to the contrary we assume that a single act of copulation is adequate.

Sex ratios of species such as the human hookworms and the roundworm *A. lumbricoides* appear to lie close to unity (Stoll, 1923; Arfaa and Ghadirian, 1977; Hoagland and Schad, 1978; Croll *et al.*, 1982).

In recent years various studies have examined the significance of sexual habits, and the statistical distribution of parasite numbers per host, to the precise form of the mating function Φ (Macdonald, 1965; Leyton, 1968; Tallis and Leyton, 1969; Nasell and Hirsch, 1973; May, 1977). Table 3.3 lists the form of the function Φ given various assumptions concerning mating behaviour and the distribution of parasites. In all these cases it is assumed that the distributions of female and male worms are identical. The relationships between Φ and the mean worm burden, M, for the assumptions catalogued in Table 3.3 are portrayed graphically in Fig. 3.6. This figure illustrates a number of general points. First, irrespective of whether or not the parasites are monogamous or polygamous, aggregated or clumped distributions of parasites are advantageous to reproductive success when compared with random distribution patterns. This observation makes intuitive sense and also underlines the advantage of contagion to transmission success when average worm burdens are low (M small). Second, polygamy is beneficial to mating success when compared with monogamy. This effect is also most apparent at low worm densities. Third, and finally, it is important to note that reproductive

Table 3.3 The mating probability function Φ (see May, 1977).

Type of sexual behaviour	Mating function Φ
Hermaphroditic, self-fertilization possible	$\Phi = 1$
Dioecious, worms monogamous (a) Random distribution of parasites	$\Phi(M) = 1 - \dfrac{e^{-M}}{2} \displaystyle\int_0^2 (1 - \cos\theta)\, e^{-M\cos\theta}\, d\theta$
(b) Negative binomial distribution of parasites	$\Phi(M,k) = 1 - \dfrac{(1-\gamma)^{1+k}}{2} \displaystyle\int_0^2 \dfrac{(1-\cos\theta)}{(1+\gamma\cos\theta)^{1+k}}\, d\theta$ where $\gamma = \dfrac{M}{M+k}$
Dioecious, worms polygamous (a) Random distribution of parasites	$\Phi(M) = 1 - e^{-M/2}$
(b) Negative binomial distribution of parasites	$\Phi(M,k) = \left[1 - (1 + M/2k)^{-1-k}\right]$

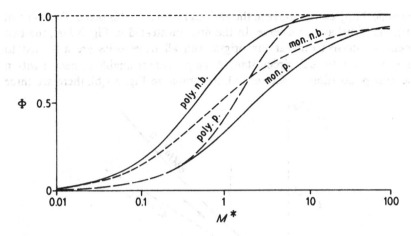

Figure 3.6   The dependence of the probability that a female worm is mated, Φ, on the average worm burden within the host population, M, for various assumptions concerning parasite distribution and sexual habits (the functional forms of Φ are listed in Table 3.3). Poly. n.b. denotes polygamous parasites distributed in a negative binomial manner; poly. p. denotes polygamous worms distributed in a random manner; mon. n.b. denotes monogamous worms distributed in a negative binomial manner and mon. p. denotes monogamous worms distributed in a random manner (see May, 1977).

success will be severely curtailed under conditions of low average worm burdens irrespective of mating behaviour or the distribution of parasites. The mating probability function, Φ, acts as a form of inverse density-dependence to create (as outlined in a later section of this chapter) a critical density of parasites per host below which mating success is too infrequent to ensure transmission of the parasite within the host population. Self-fertilizing hermaphroditic parasites, such as various species of tapeworms (see Chapter 4), are unaffected by these problems.

3.7   DYNAMICAL PROPERTIES OF THE MODEL

An analytical solution of Equations (3.5) and (3.6) for arbitrary Φ is unfortunately not feasible. The qualitative dynamical behaviour of the model, however, can be explored by the consideration of equilibrium properties. This approach is especially appropriate for the study of endemic helminth infections in regions where the prevalence and intensity of infection remain relatively stable from year to year. If desired, of course, numerical methods may be employed to generate time-dependent solutions of the model equations.

The equilibrium analysis described below follows standard methods (Maynard–Smith, 1978; May, 1977). By constructing isoclines in the L–M plane (setting dM/dt and $dL/dt = 0$) it can be seen in which directions the dynamical trajectories move in the various regions on this plane. Two general patterns of behaviour emerge. In the first, illustrated in Fig. 3.7 (a), the two isoclines intersect only at the origin, and all trajectories are attracted to $M = 0$, $L = 0$. In such circumstances the parasite is unable to persist within the host population. In the second, illustrated in Fig. 3.7(b), there are three

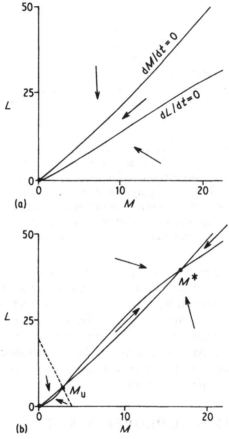

Figure 3.7   The arrows indicate how the dynamical trajectories of L and M behave in the various regions into which the L–M plane is dissected by the isoclines $dL/dt = 0$ and $dM/dt = 0$. The parasites are assumed to be polygamous and distributed in a negative binomial manner with parameter $k = 0.34$. (a) corresponds to the population parameters being below the transmission threshold $(R < 1)$, when the infection cannot maintain itself and all trajectories are attracted to the origin $(L = M = 0)$. (b) corresponds to the population parameters being above the transmission threshold $(R > 1)$ in which case there are two alternative stable states (one at M^*, one at $M = 0$), each with its own domain of attraction. The dotted line indicates the boundary between these two states which passes through the unstable state M_u. When $\mu_2 \gg \mu_1$ this boundary becomes a vertical line through M_u and we can speak of the 'breakpoint' at a worm load M_u (see text).

points of intersection of the isoclines, corresponding to two stable points at $M = 0$ and at $M = M^*$, separated by an unstable point at $M = M_u$. The directions of the trajectories in the various regions are as follows: points (i.e. initial values of M and L) originating to the left of the dashed line are attracted to the origin; points originating to the right of the dashed line are attracted to the point M^* at which the parasite maintains itself at a stable equilibrium (stable endemic disease) within the human population.

The case illustrated by Fig. 3.7(a) corresponds to the population parameters of the parasite being below a *transmission threshold*, where the infection cannot be maintained. The case illustrated by Fig. 3.7(b) corresponds to the population parameters being above the *transmission threshold* and in this event there are two alternative stable states (one at $L = 0, M = 0$ and one at $L = L^*, M = M^*$). The dashed line in Fig. 3.7(b) divides the L–M plane into the two points' respective domains of attraction. The value M_u is referred to as the *breakpoint* worm burden in the context of disease control (Macdonald, 1965).

The isoclines in Fig. 3.7 have been constructed on the assumption that the mating function Φ corresponds to a polygamous parasite which adopts a clumped, or aggregated, distribution within the host population (see Table 3.2). This situation corresponds to most directly transmitted nematode infections of man. One special case is worth noting, namely, that of hermaphroditic worms which are able to self-fertilize. In this case $\Phi = 1$ and provided the parameter values combine to place the system above the transmission threshold, the isoclines of Fig. 3.7(b) will intersect at two points ($M = 0$ and $M = M^*$) corresponding to one stable point at $M = M^*$. In other words the point M^* is globally stable for all positive values of L and M. This special case makes clear that the existence of multiple stable states in the more general model (Equations (3.5) and (3.6)) is a consequence of the mating function Φ (May and Anderson, 1979; May, 1977; Macdonald, 1965).

The transmission threshold concept outlined above is identical to that described in Chapter 1 for directly transmitted microparasites. The threshold corresponds to the situation in which the *basic reproductive rate* of the parasite, R, is equal to unity. For macroparasites, however, our definition of this reproductive rate changes as a consequence of the basic unit of study employed to examine the dynamics of disease behaviour. For microparasites, this unit was an infected host and hence R was defined in terms of the number of secondarily infected hosts produce by one primary infection. For macroparasites, however, our basic unit of study is the individual parasite; hence R is now defined as the number of female offspring which are produced on average by one female parasite throughout her reproductive life span and which themselves survive to achieve sexual maturity in a population of N uninfected hosts (in other words in the absence of density-dependent constraints on worm survival). At equilibrium, of course, the effective reproductive rate $\hat{R}$ will equal unity.

An expression for R, in terms of the various population parameters, can be derived directly from Equations (3.5) and (3.6) by considering the conditions under which positive equilibrium values of L and M arise. This approach yields the expression:

$$R = \frac{zs\lambda \Phi D_2 N D_1}{(b+\mu_1)(\mu_2 + \beta N)} \tag{3.7}$$

This expression is simply the net reproduction of the parasite in each segment of its life cycle (including transmission) multiplied by the product of the expected life spans of the mature adult worm and the infective stage.

As illustrated in Chapter 1, this expression for R can be rearranged to define a critical host density, N_T, below which the parasite will be unable to persist within the community, namely;

$$N_T = [(\mu_1 + b)\mu_2]/[zs\lambda \Phi \beta D_1 D_2 - (\mu_1 + b)\beta] \tag{3.8}$$

This condition is directly analogous to the classical threshold theorem derived from models of viral and bacterial disease by Kermack and McKendrick (1927). It is of less significance, however, with respect to helminth infections, since unlike the viral and bacterial diseases, most are able to persist endemically in low-density human communities owing to their high transmission efficiencies (see CIBA (1977) for examples of helminth persistence in low-density human communities).

The concept of a basic reproductive rate, and its estimation from epidemiological data, are of central significance for both microparasitic and macroparasitic infections. In the case of helminths, control measures should be designed to reduce the value of R (ideally below the transmission threshold, $R = 1$), since this will, as illustrated in the following section, act to lower the incidence and intensity of infection. In addition, however, we have a further option, namely, to lower the average worm burden, M, below the unstable breakpoint, M_u. This feasibility of this approach, however, will depend on the precise numerical value of M_u within a given population. We will examine this issue in more detail later in this chapter.

3.8 TIME SCALES

Some additional simplification in model structure can be achieved by reference to the relative time scales on which the dynamics of the various populations operate (i.e. P, L and N) and by noting the relative magnitudes of the time delays (T_1 and T_2 in Equations (3.5) and (3.6)) involved in nematode life cycles.

For the majority of nematode infections of man the expected life span of the mature parasites is many orders of magnitude greater than that of infective stage, whether larvae or eggs. The former has a life span of the order of a few years while the latter has a life span of the order of a few weeks to a few months. Mature adults of the human hookworm, *Necator americanus*, for example, are thought to have a life span of roughly 3 to 4 years while the L_3 infective larvae live, under optimum conditions, for a few weeks (Sturrock, 1967; Muller, 1975). The dynamics of both parasite populations operate on a much faster time scale than that of the human host population, N, human life expectancy in endemic regions being of the order of 50 years or more. It is therefore not unreasonable to regard N as a constant when considering the dynamics of L and P (or M).

The developmental time delays T_1 and T_2 are also often short in relation to the life span of the mature adult parasite. For example in the case of N. *americanus* T_1 is approximately 40–50 days while T_2 is roughly 5–10 days. These time delays are therefore of limited significance to the dynamics of the parasite populations over a time scale relevant to the human host. A summary of the various time scales involved in the dynamics of hookworm and roundworm infections of man is presented in Table 3.4.

Table 3.4   A summary of the time scales involved in the dynamics of hookworm and roundworm parasites of man.

Parasite	Life expectancies			Developmental time delays (days)	
	Man	Adult parasite	Infective stage	T_1	T_2
Ascaris lumbricoides	50 years	1–2 years	1–3 months	50–80	10–30
Necator americanus	50 years	3–4 years	3–10 days	40–50	3–6

It is clear from Equations (3.5) and (3.6) that the characteristic dynamical response times of M and L are roughly $1/(b + \mu_1)$ and $1/(\mu_2 + \beta N)$ respectively. In these two expressions the parameters μ_1 and μ_2 dominate, as discussed in the preceding paragraphs, and furthermore $\mu_2 \gg \mu_1$. It follows that L has a much faster response time than M, and the dynamical trajectories tend to become vertical lines in the L–M plane, parallel to the L-axis. The dashed 'breakpoint' line in Fig. 3.7(b) straightens to a vertical line through M_u. In such cases, which are appropriate for most human helminth infections, we may effectively assume that the density of infective stages are essentially instantaneously adjusted to the stationary value L^* for all values of M. Given also that the time delays T_1 and T_2 are short in relation to the expected life span of the mature parasite, the model can be reduced to a single dynamical equation for the variable M, where:

$$dM/dt = \frac{M}{l}\left\{R\left[1 + \frac{M}{k}(1 - z)\right]^{-(k+1)} - 1\right\} \qquad (3.9)$$

The parameter R is as defined in Equation (3.7) and l denotes the life expectancy of the adult parasite, namely $1/(b + \mu_1)$. The form of this equation is not quite as simple as it first appears since R is a function of the mating probability Φ which is itself a function of M and k (see Table 3.3). The special case where Φ = 1 is appropriate for hermaphroditic self-fertilizing worms and for polygamous species which are highly aggregated in their distribution within the host population (k small) in regions of endemic disease where the mean worm burden is greater than two to three parasites per host (see Fig. 3.6). In areas where hookworm and ascariasis are endemic this latter case is invariably true and hence the value of Φ can be taken to be effectively equal to unity. Under these circumstances two equilibrium states may arise (found by setting dM/dt = 0). Where $R < 1$ the infection cannot persist and M^*, the equilibrium mean worm burden (the average intensity of infection), is equal to zero. If $R > 1$ then

$$M^* = (R^{1/(k+1)} - 1)\frac{k}{(1-z)} \tag{3.10}$$

Given that the parasite distribution within the human community is negative binomial in form with clumping parameter k, the equilibrium prevalence of infection (the proportion of the community infected), p^*, is simply:

$$p^* = \left[1 - \left(1 + \frac{M^*}{k} \right)^{-k} \right] \tag{3.11}$$

When Φ is effectively equal to unity the intensity of infection, M^*, rises linearly as R increases, while the prevalence, p^*, approaches an asymptote whose value is determined by the degree of worm aggregation within the host population (Fig. 3.8). For random distributions the asymptote is unity where all hosts are infected. For contagious distribution the asymptotic level of p^* is inversely related to the degree of parasite aggregation within the host population and, irrespective of the degree of transmission success (the value of R), the proportion of the population infected will never approach unity (Fig. 3.9). This relationship has important practical implications for the interpretation of observed age–prevalence curves within human communities. The asymptotic prevalence of infection provides an inverse measure of the degree of worm aggregation within the community.

In the derivation of Equation (3.9) we assumed that the density-dependent constraints acted solely on worm fecundity. In the more general case where they act on fecundity (as defined in Equation (3.3)) and adult worm mortality (as defined in Equation (3.4)) the rate of change of M with respect to t becomes:

$$dM/dt = \frac{M}{l}\left\{ R\left[1 + \frac{M}{k}(1-z) \right]^{-(k+1)} - 1 - \frac{\alpha l(k+1)M}{k} \right\} \tag{3.12}$$

Or, alternatively, if density-dependence acts solely on worm mortality (as defined in Equation (3.4)), then the model is of the form:

$$dM/dt = \frac{M}{l}\left[(R-1) - \frac{\alpha l(k+1)M}{k} \right] \tag{3.13}$$

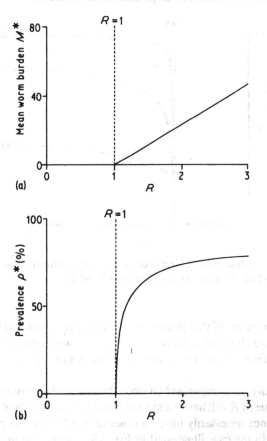

Figure 3.8 The relationship of the mean equilibrium intensity of infection M^* and the equilibrium prevalence of infection (expressed as a percentage), p^*, with the basic reproductive rate R. The vertical dashed line denotes the transmission threshold $R = 1$. In (a) and (b) the mating function Φ is assumed to be equal to unity while in (b) the negative binomial parameter k is set at $k = 0.34$.

In this case the equilibrium intensity of infection, M^*, is given by:

$$M^* = \frac{(R-1)k}{l\alpha(k+1)} \tag{3.14}$$

It is clear from Equations (3.10) and (3.14) that the magnitude of the equilibrium intensity of infection, M^*, is essentially determined by the value of R and the severity of density-dependent constraints on worm population growth within an individual host. The severity of these constraints is a function of either α or z, or both, and the degree of worm aggregation within the host population (measured inversely by k). Note that worm aggregation essentially acts to increase the severity of density-dependent constraints; the smaller the value of k the smaller will be the equilibrium intensity of infection. The

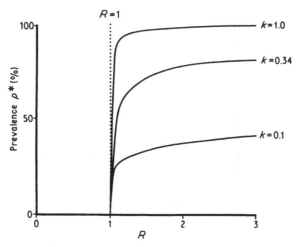

Figure 3.9   The influence of the degree of parasite aggregation (measured inversely by the parameter k) on the relationship between p^* and R.

intuitive explanation of this phenomenon is that as k gets smaller, more and more worms are clumped together in fewer and fewer hosts and thus density-dependent effects influence a greater proportion of the total parasite population.

More broadly, it is important to note that control measures which act to reduce the value of R will have an immediate effect on the intensity of infection M^*, but may not necessarily have an observable effect on the prevalence, p^*. For example, in the case illustrated in Fig. 3.8, a reduction in the value of R from 3 to 2 will have little impact on the equilibrium prevalence of infection. In practical terms, therefore, any assessment of the efficiency of control measures should be based on observable changes in M^* rather than on changes in the prevalence p^*.

For the general case where $\Phi \neq 1$ the relationship between R, M^* and p^* is more complex, as a consequence of the breakpoint concept discussed earlier. The general issues, however, concerning the influence of contagion on the relationship between R and p^* and the impact of control measures on M^* and p^* remain unchanged. The relationships between M^* and R, and p^* and R, are illustrated in Figs 3.10 and 3.11 respectively.

3.9   CONTROL

The control of directly transmitted nematode infections is based on two different approaches often used concomitantly in areas of endemic disease. The first involves the improvement of sanitation and hygiene standards within the community, in parallel with education to inform individuals about the life

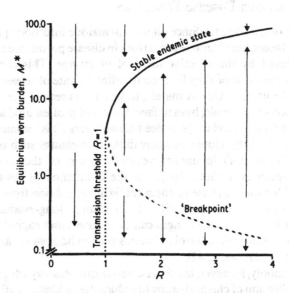

Figure 3.10 The relationship between the equilibrium mean worm burden, M^*, and the basic reproductive rate R for a polygamous species which is distributed in a negative binomial manner within the host population ($k = 0.34$). The dashed line denotes the unstable 'breakpoint' M_u and the arrows indicate how the dynamical trajectory of M will behave following a perturbation from one of the two equilibrium states M^* and $M = 0$. The vertical dotted line denotes the transmission threshold ($R = 1$) below which the infection cannot be maintained. As the value of the clumping parameter k decreases, the breakpoint moves towards the horizontal axis.

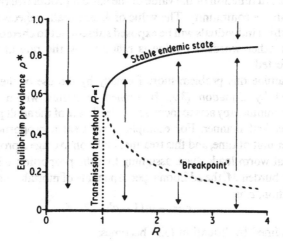

Figure 3.11 Similar to Fig. 3.10 but portraying the relationship between p^* and R.

cycles of the disease agents. Since all such nematode infections pass infective stages in the faeces, considerable reductions in disease prevalence and intensity can be achieved by the effective disposal of sewage. This acts to reduce substantially the value of R by limiting the effective rate of release of infective stages into the habitat. Unfortunately, however, in areas of the world where such infections are endemic, human faecal material is often used as a fertilizer for the production of food crops. Indeed in many areas it is the major source of crop fertilizer. It is therefore extremely difficult to change such practices (i.e. the use of 'night soil') in underdeveloped regions of the world without enormous capital expenditure (both for the installation of sewage disposal facilities and for the purchase of chemical fertilizers). Aside from the issue of capital expenditure, it is also difficult to change long-established social patterns and habits. If such changes can be induced, and capital is available, then sanitation alone will control infections such as hookworm and ascariasis (Smillie, 1924; Andrews, 1942).

More commonly, however, the short-term control strategy adopted involves the mass application of chemotherapy to reduce the incidence of disease within the population (the frequency of disease symptoms being directly proportional to the mean worm burden within the community). In the short term, chemotherapy is a comparatively cheap method of control and it can produce immediate improvements in health. Such short-term benefits, however, can be very misleading. In the long term, to suppress permanently the average worm load, continual treatment is necessary since once an individual's worm burden is removed he or she is then immediately susceptible to reinfection.

In population terms, the proportion of the population treated and the frequency of treatment required to induce a given reduction in the average worm burden, is a function of the value of the basic reproductive rate, R, of the parasite within the community. The value of R essentially reflects the force of infection to which individuals will be exposed subsequent to chemotherapeutic treatment. In other words, its value is reflected by the rate at which they become reinfected.

We can examine this problem more formally by the use of the population model defined by Equation (3.9). If applied randomly within the human population, chemotherapy acts to increase the death rate of the adult parasites in a density-independent manner. For example, if we treat a proportion g of the population per unit of time, and this treatment kills on average a proportion h of their individual worm loads, then, assuming that the proportion g harbour the average worm burden M, the additional per capita rate of mortality applied to the worm population, c, is:

$$c = -ln(1 - gh) \qquad (3.15)$$

The model defined by Equation (3.9) becomes:

$$dM/dt = \frac{M}{l}\left\{ R\left[1 + \frac{M}{k}(1-z) \right]^{-(k+1)} - 1 - cl \right\} \qquad (3.16)$$

The new effective reproductive rate, $\hat{R}$, under the impact of control is defined by:

$$\hat{R} = \frac{zs\lambda\Phi D_2\beta D_1 N}{(b+\mu_1+c)(\mu_2+N)} \qquad (3.17)$$

To eradicate the helminth infection from the community it is necessary to reduce the value of $\hat{R}$ to less than unity and this may be achieved by treating a proportion $\hat{g}$ of the community (where the individuals to be treated are selected at random) per unit of time where:

$$\hat{g} = \{1-\exp[(1-R)/l]\}/h \qquad (3.18)$$

This equation makes clear the significance of the value of R to the degree of control required to eradicate a helminth infection (Fig. 3.12). If chemotherapy ceases before the mean worm burden falls below the breakpoint level, M_u (see Fig. 3.10), the parasite population will return to its precontrol level. The rapidity of the parasite population's ability to recover is inversely proportional to the value of R. These issues are illustrated in Fig. 3.13 in which numerical simulations are presented mimicking changes through time of the mean worm burden, M, for various levels of chemotherapy and for low and high R values. A further point to note, concerning the action of chemotherapy on the population dynamics of the parasite, concerns its differential influence on the prevalence and intensity of infection. As displayed in Fig. 3.14, the equilibrium

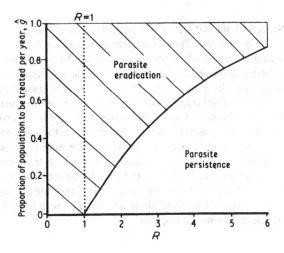

Figure 3.12 Control by chemotherapy. In the shaded region of the graph the proportion of the population treated each year, $\hat{g}$, is sufficient to eradicate the infection. In the unshaded region the parasite persists. The boundary between the two regions is defined by Equation (3.18) in the main text. The life expectancy of the mature parasite was assumed to be 3.5 years and the chemotherapeutic agent was taken to be 90% effective ($h = 0.9$).

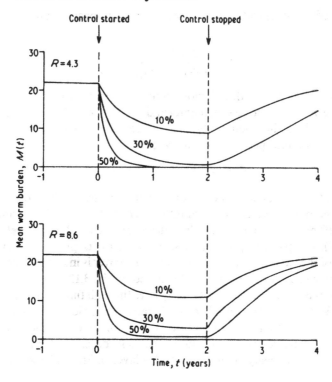

Figure 3.13 Numerical simulations of the impact of chemotherapy on the mean worm burden of the population. Time-dependent solutions are depicted for various levels of drug treatment recorded as the percentage of the population treated per month. The simulations are based on the numerical solution of Equation (3.16) in the main text. The mean intensity of infection, M^*, prior to control is set at 22 worms per host, and at time $t = 0$ chemotherapy is administered on a continual basis to varying proportions of the population for a period of 2 years. After 2 years control ceases and the graphs portray the rate of return of the mean worm burden to its precontrol level. In the terminology of Equation (3.11) in the main text in (a) the value of h is set at 0.9, R is set at 4.3 and a range of g values are used, namely, 0.1, 0.3 and 0.5. In (b) h is again set at 0.9, R is set at 8.6 and the g values are 0.1, 0.3 and 0.5. The life expectancy of the mature worms was assumed to be 1 year in all simulations (the value of the density-dependent parameter z was set at 0.96). The simulations are designed to mimic the impact of chemotherapy on the dynamics of ascariasis.

worm burden decays approximately exponentially as the intensity of chemotherapeutic application increases. The prevalence, however, remains relatively high until the rate of application (the g of Equation (3.15)) approaches the critical rate $\hat{g}$ (Equation (3.18)). In other words to assess the impact of control measures within a community it is important to monitor the intensity of

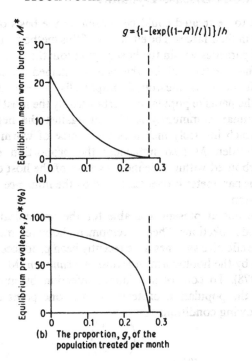

Figure 3.14 This figure illustrates the impact of chemotherapy, as expressed on the horizontal axis by, g, the proportion of the population treated per unit of time, on the equilibrium mean worm burden, M^* (a) and the equilibrium prevalence of infection, p^*, (b). The parasite is eradicated when $g = \{1 - \exp[(1 - R)/l]\}/h$. Parameter values: $R = 4.3$, $l = 12$ months, $k = 0.57$ and $h = 0.9$.

infection as opposed to just simply the prevalence. This latter parameter does not provide a good indication of the impact of control measures.

If the object of control is disease suppression, rather than parasite eradication, we can reformulate the problem in a slightly different manner. For example, if clinical symptoms of disease are known to be absent at a specified average worm burden within the community, say $\bar{M}$, then the aim of control may be viewed as the reduction of M^* (the mean intensity prior to control) below the critical level $\bar{M}$. If the burden, $\bar{M}$, is a proportion q of the mean worm load M^* prior to control, then the proportion $\hat{g}$ of the population that must be treated per unit of time to reduce M^* below $\bar{M}$ is given by:

$$\hat{g} > \{1 - \exp[(1 - R)(b + \mu_1)(1 - q)]\}/h \qquad (3.19)$$

So far we have assumed that the individuals who receive chemotherapy are chosen at random from the population. A better approach, however, is to treat selectively the most heavily infected members of the community (Smilie, 1924; Warren and Mahmoud, 1976; Anderson and May, 1982b). In practical terms, the individuals to be treated could be chosen on the basis of the density of nematode eggs in their faeces. The efficiency of this method will depend on the distribution of parasites within the host population; the more aggregated the distribution, the greater will be the benefits gained from adopting this approach. This point is illustrated graphically in Fig. 3.15 where the percentage of the parasite population harboured by the most heavily infected 10% of the human community is plotted against the negative binomial parameter k which inversely measures the degree of worm clumping. The mean worm burden M also influences the proportion of the parasite population harboured within a defined segment of the host community, but the effect of this parameter is overshadowed by the influence of the degree of worm aggregation.

Vaccines are not at present available for the immunization of humans against nematode infections. Their development, however, may be possible in the future since effective vaccines have recently been produced to protect dogs from infection by the hookworm, *Ancylostoma caninum* (Miller, 1978; Clegg and Smith, 1978). To control a helminth infection by immunization, the proportion of the population protected at any one point in time, f, must satisfy the following condition:

$$f > \left(1 - \frac{1}{R}\right) \tag{3.20}$$

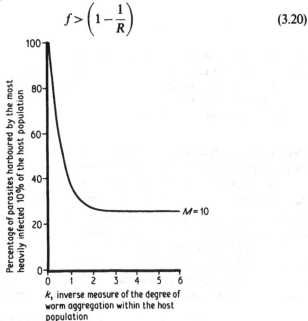

Figure 3.15 The relationship between the percentage of the total parasite population harboured by the most heavily infected 10% of the human community and the degree of worm contagion (measured inversely by the negative binomial parameter k). The worms are assumed to be distributed in a negative binomial manner with the mean worm burden set at 10.0.

Note that this condition is identical to that described in Chapter 1 for the control of microparasitic infections. There is, however, one complication in the case of helminth infections. In contrast to viral diseases such as measles, it appears unlikely that it will be possible to develop a vaccine which provides life-long protection to reinfection. More probably, as in the case of the dog hookworm vaccine, the duration of artificially induced acquired immunity will range from a few months to a maximum of a few years. In this case individuals would have to be revaccinated at successive intervals throughout their life. For example, if the vaccine provides protection for V years, then the proportion of the population that must be immunized each year, $\hat{f}$, must satisfy the following condition:

$$\hat{f} > \left(1 - \frac{1}{R}\right)/V \qquad (3.21)$$

This result is also applicable to the control of helminth infections by a slow release chemotherapeutic agent which provides protection against infection for a defined period of time (the parameter V in Equation (3.21)).

3.10   AGE–PREVALENCE AND AGE–INTENSITY CURVES

Epidemiological surveys of nematode infections within human communities are usually designed to measure the prevalence and intensity of infection within various age classes of the population. Prevalence is assessed by the examination of faecal samples for the presence or absence of eggs, while intensity may be measured indirectly by reference to the density of eggs in such samples or, more accurately, by the use of chemotherapeutic agents to expel the worms from a sample of the human population. This latter method enables direct estimates to be made of the distribution of worm numbers per individual and of the average worm burden (average intensity of infection) in a range of age classes. The data obtained in this manner are often plotted in the form of age–prevalence and age–intensity curves, some examples of which are shown in the next two sections of this chapter. The rapidity with which the prevalence and intensity rise with host age is a direct reflection of the force of parasite transmission within the community (the magnitude of R).

The population model defined in Equation (3.9) may be used to gain qualitative insights into the factors which determine the shape of these curves. Specifically if the infection is endemic within the population such that the total parasite population has remained relatively stable through time, then in a community with an approximately stable age distribution, the rate of change of the mean number of parasites per host, $M(a)$, with respect to host age, a, may be described by the following equation:

$$\frac{dM}{da} = \Lambda - \frac{M}{l} \qquad (3.22)$$

where Λ is defined as:

$$\Lambda = \frac{RM^*}{l}\left[1 + \frac{M^*}{k}(1-z)\right]^{-(k+1)} \tag{3.23}$$

and M^* is as given in Equation (3.10) (Anderson and May, 1982b). In the derivation of Equation (3.22) it is assumed that the various population parameters, such as the rate of infection, β, and the degree of worm clumping, k, are constant and independent of host age. The parameter Λ represents the constant 'force of infection' in the endemic community in which the disease is at its stable state M^*.

When $\Phi \neq 1$, numerical methods are required to solve Equation (3.22). However, in many areas of endemic hookworm and ascariasis the mean worm burden $M(a)$ rises rapidly with host age, a, such that $\Phi = 1$ for all but the very young age classes of the community. In such cases Equation (3.22) has the general solution:

$$M(a) = \Lambda l(1 - e^{-a/l}) \tag{3.24}$$

The average intensity, $M(a)$, therefore approaches an upper asymptote in the older age classes of the community where the asymptote is M^* as defined in Equation (3.10). An expression for the prevalence of infection, $p(a)$, at age a can be derived from the zero probability term of the negative binomial distribution where:

$$p(a) = 1 - \left[1 + \frac{M(a)}{k}\right]^{-k} \tag{3.25}$$

The shape of the age–intensity curve is determined by two parameters: the basic reproductive rate, R, and the life expectancy of the adult worms, l. The severity of density-dependent constraints largely determines the value of Λ (mediated by the degree of worm aggregation k) which itself sets the equilibrium average intensity of infection, M^*, in the older age classes of the community where:

$$M^* = \Lambda l \tag{3.26}$$

The magnitude of the value of R will in part dictate the rapidity with which this worm load is approached as individuals in the community age.

The shape of the age–prevalence curve (Equation (3.25)) is determined by the change with age of the mean worm burden and the degree of worm clumping within the community. The prevalence will approach an asymptote as individuals age where the level is set by the value of k. If k tends to infinity (random distribution of parasites), the asymptote will be unity. As k gets smaller, where the degree of aggregation increases, the level of the asymptote will decrease. In other words if the degree of worm clumping is high the asymptotic prevalence will never approach unity even if the mean worm load is extremely large.

In the derivation of Equation (3.24) we assumed that density-dependent constraints acted on worm fecundity. If they instead act on worm survival (as defined in Equation (3.4)), then the differential equation for the rate of change of $M(a)$ with respect to a is of the form:

$$\frac{dM}{da} = \Lambda - \frac{M}{l} - \frac{\alpha(k+1)M^2}{k} \tag{3.27}$$

where $\Lambda = RM^*/l$.

When $\Phi = 1$, the solution of this equation is:

$$M(a) = M^*(1 - e^{-Aa})(1 + Be^{-Aa})^{-1} \tag{3.28}$$

where $A = (zR - 1)/l$, $B = 1 - 1/R$ and M^* is as defined in Equation (3.14). As a becomes large $M(a) \to M^*$. It should be noted that Equations (3.27) and (3.28) differ from those presented in Anderson (1980) to mimic the dynamics of the acquisition of infection with respect to host age. Equations (3.27) and (3.28) are the more general results since those given in Anderson (1980) are only appropriate for the dynamics of the introduction of infection into an uninfected community.

3.11 PARAMETER ESTIMATION

A central problem in the application of mathematical models to the study of disease epidemiology concerns the estimation of the many parameters which determine the population behaviour of the disease agent. In Chapter 1 we saw how age–prevalence data could be used to estimate the basic reproductive rate of microparasitic infections.

The age–intensity and age–prevalence data can also provide a means for obtaining crude estimates of the population parameters of helminth infections. Specifically, the age–intensity model defined in Equation (3.24) can be fitted to observed data by means of non-linear least-squares techniques (Conway, Glass and Wilcox, 1970; Anderson, 1980). Only two parameters are involved in such methods, namely, Λ and l. If independent estimates are available for the parameters, k (worm aggregation), l (worm life expectancy) and z (inverse measure of the magnitude of density-dependent constraints on worm fecundity), then the estimation of Λ from age–intensity curves can produce crude estimates of the basic reproductive rate R. More formally R is given by the following equation:

$$R = \frac{\Lambda l}{M^*}\left[1 + \frac{M^*}{k}(1-z)\right]^{(k+1)} \tag{3.29}$$

where M^* is given by the value of the upper asymptote of the age–intensity curve.

The methods described in this and the preceding sections are employed in the following two sections in the study of the population biology of two specific nematode infections, namely, hookworm and ascariasis.

3.12 HOOKWORM INFECTIONS

The two most intensively studied directly transmitted human helminths are the two species of hookworm, *Ancylostoma duodenale* and *Necator americanus*. These species occur sympatrically over much of the Indian subcontinent and over much of the world, including parts of South America, the Far East and Africa. In the Ganges region of West Bengal, for example, 79 % of the human population is infected with at least one species and 95 % of this infected population harbours both species (Schad, 1971). In regions where hookworm is endemic, the prevalence of infection rises rapidly during early childhood and remains very high (often close to 100 %) through to old age. Some examples of such patterns are recorded in Fig. 3.16.

The basic life history patterns of both species are well understood as is the pathology associated with infection. Quantitative information concerning the population processes which determine observed epidemiological patterns, however, is very limited at present (Hoagland and Schad, 1978; Chandler, 1929).

Two of the most detailed epidemiological studies are those concerned with *N. americanus* in a rural community near Calcutta in India by Nawalinski, Schad and Chowdhury (1978a, b) and with the same parasite in a rural district of the Kaohsiung area of Taiwan by Hsieh (1970). The patterns of infection in the two communities are similar in overall form but differ in magnitude. Analyses of both studies are reported in Anderson (1980). In both instances the average intensity of infection rises to a plateau in the adult age groups, but the level of this plateau differs substantially, being approximately 51 worms in the Indian community but only 6–7 worms in the Kaohsiung area of Taiwan (Anderson, 1980). Crude estimates of the R values for each community were obtained by fitting the age–intensity and age–prevalence models defined in Equations (3.24) and (3.25) to the observed data. The values are approximately 2.7 in the Indian community and 1.5 in the Taiwanese community. The shapes of the age–intensity and age–prevalence functions generated by the model equations, however, only crudely approximate to the observed trends in each community. This is illustrated in Fig. 3.17 where the age–intensity and age–prevalence curves for hookworm infections (both *N. americanus* and *A. duodenale*) in the Taiwan community are recorded. The dotted lines in graphs (a) and (b) in Fig. 3.17 record the predictions of Equations (3.24) and (3.25) respectively. The discrepancies between observation and theory are a consequence of age-dependence in the force of infection, Λ. This parameter, as illustrated in graph (c) of Fig. 3.17, is in reality a function of host age where the rate of infection increases during early life to reach a plateau in the adult age groups. The age-dependence in Λ is probably a consequence of age-

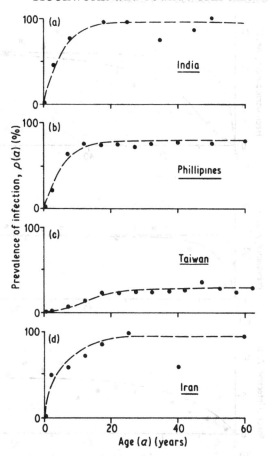

Figure 3.16 Some examples of age–prevalence curves for hookworm infections in various regions of the world. (a) *A. duodenale* and *N. americanus* in a rural community in India (data from Chowdhury and Schiller, 1968). (b) *A. duodenale* infections in a rural community in the Phillipines (data from Pesigan *et al.*, 1958). (c) *N. americanus* infections in a rural community in Taiwan (data from Hsieh, 1970). (d) *A. duodenale* and *N. americanus* infections in a rural community in Iran (Croll and Gyorkos, unpublished data).

dependence in the transmission coefficient, β, which is a component of the basic reproductive rate R. As illustrated in Fig. 3.17 a model incorporating Λ as a function of age provides much more accurate predictions of the observed trends.

In both populations the degree of aggregation of parasite numbers per host was also dependent on host age. Aggregation was most marked in the very young children but decreased with age, reaching a plateau in the early teens. The degree of aggregation was severe in both populations but of much greater

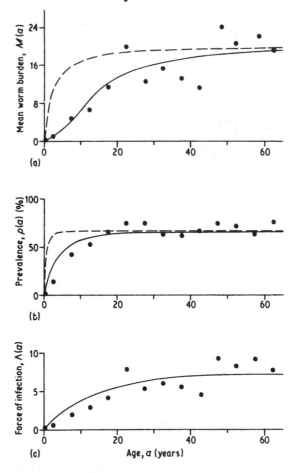

Figure 3.17 Age–intensity (a) and age–prevalence (b) curves for hookworm infections in a rural community in Taiwan (data from Hsieh, 1970). The solid points are
observed values and the dashed lines are the predictions of the model defined by
Equations (3.24) and (3.25) in the main text. (Parameter values, $R = 1.3$, $M^* = 17.5$,
$l = 2.5$ years, $z = 0.99$, $k = 0.08$). The solid lines in (a) and (b) represent the predictions
of a model which is a modification of that defined in Equations (3.24) and (3.25) and
includes an age-dependent force of infection $\Lambda(a)$. The estimates of this age-dependent
rate, for hookworm in the Taiwan community are presented in (c). The solid line in this
graph represents the function $\Lambda(a) = C(1 - e^{-Da})$ where $C = 7$ and $D = 0.08$.

severity in the Taiwan community (Fig. 3.18). The average values (over all age
classes) of the negative binomial parameter, k, were 0.34 and 0.08 respectively
in the Indian and Taiwanese communities. These average values were
employed to obtain the model projections recorded in Fig. 3.17.

The data available for the rural community near Calcutta, some of which is

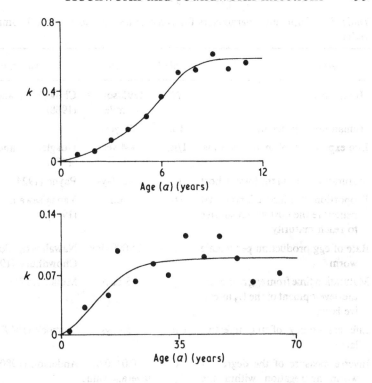

Figure 3.18 The degree of parasite aggregation, measured inversely by the negative binomial parameter k, within different age classes of the human population. In (a) the k values are for *N. americanus* infections in a rural community in India while in (b) the k values are for the same hookworm species in a rural community in Taiwan (Anderson, 1980). The solid points are the estimated k values while the solid lines are fitted by eye.

recorded in Table 3.5, is sufficiently detailed to provide a rough estimate of the location of the 'breakpoint' worm burden, M_u. For the parameter values listed in Table 3.5 the predicted relationship between the equilibrium mean worm burden, M^*, and the basic reproductive rate, R, is displayed in Fig. 3.10. Given an R value of 2.7 and a degree of parasite aggregation reflected by a k value of 0.34, the 'breakpoint' worm burden is approximately 0.3 parasites per host. In the Taiwan community, the breakpoint will be even lower since its level is primarily determined by the severity of parasite aggregation within the population. As the degree of contagion increases, the breakpoint, M_u, declines until it reaches zero worms per host as $k \rightarrow 0$ (Bradley and May, 1978; May, 1977).

These observations suggest that the stable endemic mean worm burden, M^*, is effectively globally stable to perturbation since the region of attraction to the stable state of parasite extinction ($M = 0$) is extremely small.

Table 3.5 Population parameters for *Necator americanus* in a rural community in India.

Parameter	Symbol	Value	Data source
Human density	N	1895/square mile	Chowdhury and Schiller (1968)
Human life expectancy	$1/b$	50 years	–
Life expectancy of mature worms	$1/\mu_1$	3–4 years	Hoagland and Schad (1978)
Maturation time in the human host	T_1	42 days	Payne (1924)
Proportion of infective larvae that penetrate the host which survive to reach maturity	D_1	0.1	Yanagisawa and Mizuno (1963)
Rate of egg production per female worm	λ	15 000/day	Nawalinski, Schad and Chowdhury (1978a,b)
Maturation time from egg release to the development of the L_3 infective larva	T_2	5 days	Muller (1975)
Life expectancy of the infective larva	$1/\mu_2$	5 days	Sturrock (1967)
Inverse measure of the degree of worm aggregation within the host population	k	0.01–0.6 (average value 0.34)	Anderson (1980)
Proportion of female worms in the population	s	0.5	Stoll (1923)
Sexual habits	–	Dioecious and polygamous	–
Basic reproductive rate	R	2–3	Anderson (1980)

In the Indian community, for example, the region of attraction to the state of stable endemic infection (M^*) is 0.3 → ∞ worms per host, while the region of attraction to the state of parasite extinction is 0 → 0.3 worms per host. This suggests, therefore, that the 'breakpoint' concept is of little significance to the design of control policies and attention should instead be focused on the reduction of the force of transmission below the transmission threshold ($R = 1$).

3.13 ASCARIASIS

Epidemiological studies of ascariasis have yielded a great deal of information concerning the abundance and prevalence of roundworms in various regions of the world (Sadun and Vajrasthira, 1953; WHO, 1967; Chowdhury, Schad and Schiller, 1968; Cross *et al.*, 1970; Chen, 1971; Obiamiwe, 1977; Arfaa and Ghadirian, 1977; Croll *et al.*, 1982). The life cycle of *Ascaris lumbricoides* is basically similar to that of the hookworm parasites. One major difference, however, is that transmission between hosts is achieved by the ingestion of an egg which contains an infective larvae, rather than by a free-living larval stage. One consequence of this difference is that the egg is to some extent resistant to extreme climatic conditions and hence the expected life span of the transmission stage in the external habitat is longer than that of the hookworm larvae.

In regions with endemic disease the prevalence and intensity of infection rise rapidly during early childhood and reach a plateau in the adult age groups (Fig. 3.19). In certain areas, the intensity of infection appears to decline in the

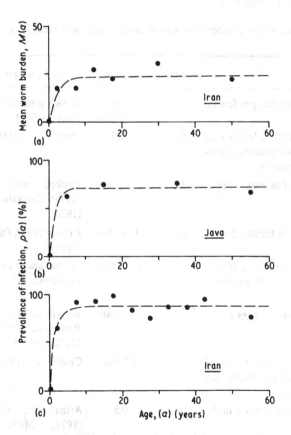

Figure 3.19 Some examples of age–intensity and age–prevalence curves for *Ascaris* infections in various human communities. (a) A rural community in Iran (data from Arfaa and Ghadirian, 1977). (b) A rural community in Java (data from Cross *et al.*, 1970). (c) A rural community in Iran (data from Croll *et al.*, 1982). The dots are observed values while the dashed lines are fitted by eye.

older age classes, although it is not clear at present whether this trend is the result of acquired immunity or a change in the pattern of contact with infective stages. The parasite is endemic in both tropical and temperate regions of the world where there is adequate moisture and low standards of hygiene and sanitation.

Current knowledge of the population biology of *A. lumbricoides* is less detailed than that concerning the hookworm parasites (as illustrated by the information recorded in Tables 3.5 and 3.6). One particular study, in a series of rural communities in Iran, however, has provided detailed information on the average intensity and distribution of worms within different age classes of the populations (Arfaa and Ghadirian, 1977; Croll *et al.*, 1982). This study also yielded data on the rate at which individuals reacquired infection after chemotherapeutic treatment.

Table 3.6 Population parameters for *Ascaris lumbricoides* in a rural village Jazin in Iran.

Parameter	Symbol	Value	Data source
Rate of egg production per female worm	λ	7300–22 700/day	Brown and Cort (1927); Cheng (1973)
Proportion of infective larvae that gain entry to the host that survive to reach maturity	D_1	0.02	Woodruff (1974)
Life expectance of mature worms	$1/\mu_1$	1–2 years	Binford and Connor (1976); Cruikshank *et al.* (1976)
Maturation time in human host	T_1	50–80 days	Koino (1922); Pawlowski (1978)
Maturation time from egg release to the development of an infective larva	T_2	10–30 days	Brown and Cort (1927); Pawlowski (1978)
Maximum life span of eggs in external habitat	–	1 + years	Brown and Cort (1927); Pawlowski (1978); Muller (1975)
Inverse measure of the degree of worm aggregation within the host population	k	0.5–0.8	Croll *et al.* (1982)
Proportion of female worms in the population	s	0.5	Arfaa and Ghadirian (1977); Mello (1974); Delgado *et al.* (1970)
Sexual habits	–	Dioecious and polygamous	
Basic reproductive rate	R	4–5	Croll *et al.* (1982)

The age–prevalence and age–intensity curves (from a horizontal study) for one village community (Jazin near Esfahan) are recorded in Fig. 3.20. The prevalence and intensity of infection rose rapidly during early childhood and reached their respective plateaus in children of between 10 and 15 years of age (Fig. 3.20).

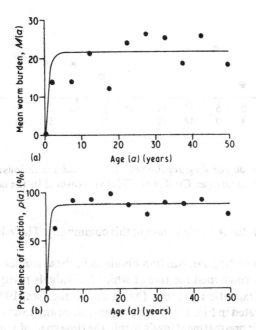

(a)

(b)

Figure 3.20 The intensity (a) and prevalence (b) of infection with *Ascaris lumbricoides* in various age classes within a rural community in Iran (data from Croll *et al.*, 1982). The solid points are observed values while the solid lines are the predictions of Equations (3.20) and (3.21) in the main text with R set at 4.3, $k = 0.57$, $l = 1.0$ and $z = 0.96$.

In contrast to the hookworm example described in the previous section, the simple model defined in Equations (3.24) and (3.25) provides a good description of the observed age-related trends in prevalence and intensity for ascariasis in the Iranian community (Croll *et al.*, 1982) (see Fig. 3.20). The assumption that the force of infection, Λ, is constant and independent of age is therefore a reasonable approximation of events in the community. In addition, the degree of aggregation of the parasites within the population also appears to remain approximately constant throughout the different age classes with an average k value of 0.57 (Croll *et al.*, 1982) (Fig. 3.21). Heterogeneity in parasite burdens within the population is probably a consequence of differences in personal hygiene and eating habitats.

Given this information, Croll *et al* (1982), were able to make a crude estimate

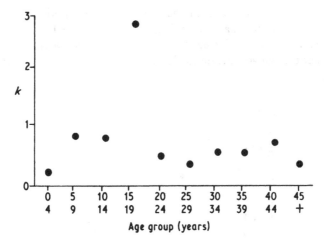

Figure 3.21   The degree of aggregation of *A. lumbricoides* in various age classes of the Iranian rural community (see Croll *et al.*, 1982) as measured by the negative binomial parameter *k*.

of the value of *R* for *A. lumbricoides* in this community. The value is between 4 and 5.

The most interesting information obtained in these studies of ascariasis in Iranian villages concerned the rate at which individuals reacquired infection after chemotherapeutic treatment (Arfaa and Ghadirian, 1977; Croll *et al.*, 1982). As illustrated in Fig. 3.22, both the prevalence and intensity of infection returned to their pretreatment levels within the time span of 1 year. The simple model defined by Equations (3.24) and (3.25) again provides a good description of the observed trends in prevalence and intensity with an *R* value of between 4 and 5 (Fig. 3.22). These results suggest that to control infection within these villages the frequency and intensity of chemotherapeutic treatment must be high, and remain so for a number of years in order to reduce the prevalence and average intensity to very low levels. If control measures cease before the parasite is eradicated, theory and observation indicate that the parasite population will rapidly 'bounce' back to its precontrol equilibrium level.

3.14   SEASONAL AND SPATIAL FACTORS

Many of the population parameters which influence the dynamics of directly transmitted nematode parasites in human communities will fluctuate in magnitude on a regular seasonal basis. Such fluctuations may be the result of the influence of climatic factors on the development, survival and infectivity of free-living transmission stages, or a consequence of seasonal patterns in human behaviour. In certain regions of the world, for example, the transmission of hookworm parasites may cease altogether at certain times of the year as

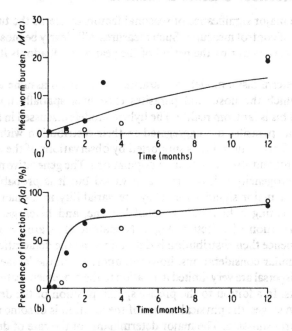

Figure 3.22 The change in the intensity (a) and prevalence (b) of infection through time after treatment with a chemotherapeutic agent. The data are for *Ascaris* infections in a rural community in Iran and represents two separate studies (the open and solid circles) (see Croll *et al.*, 1982; Arfaa and Ghadirian, 1977). The solid lines represent the predictions of Equations (3.24) and (3.25) in the main text with parameter values as follows: $R = 4.3$, $l = 1$ year, $M^* = 22$, $k = 0.57$ and $z = 0.96$.

a consequence of hot dry climatic conditions adversely influencing the survival of the L_3 infective larvae (Nawalinski *et al.*, 1978a, b; Augustine, 1923).

Seasonal fluctuations in the prevalence and intensity of infection have been recorded for both hookworm and roundworm parasites. These fluctuations, however, are of limited significance to the long-term stability of the parasite populations since the expected life spans of the longest lived stage in the parasite life cycles, namely the mature adult worms, are invariably greater than 1 year. This is certainly the case for hookworm and roundworm parasites. Seasonal changes in climate will induce seasonal trends in the value of the basic reproductive rate, which may even fall below unity at certain times of the year. However, provided the average value, on a year to year basis, is greater than unity, the parasite will persist endemically. The procedures outlined earlier for the estimation of R essentially average out such seasonal trends since they rely on age–prevalence and age–intensity data which encompass the accumulation of parasites within individuals over periods of many years. Seasonal effects would assume much greater significance if the expected life span of the mature worms was significantly less than 1 year. For hookworm and ascariasis, perhaps the major significance of seasonal factors concerns the timing of the application of control measures. Such measures will clearly be most effective if applied intensively during the period of the year when R adopts its minimum value.

Simple deterministic models of parasite transmission assume an idealized world in which the hosts and parasites exist in a spatially homogeneous landscape. This is far from reality. The hybrid models discussed in this chapter assumed that parasites are aggregated in their distribution within the host population. This assumption is supported by observations of the distribution of hookworms and *Ascaris* in human populations. The generative mechanisms of such heterogeneity will be many and varied but it is probable that two factors are of major significance. They are variability in human behaviour, particularly eating habits and personal hygiene, and heterogeneity in the spatial distribution of infective stages. Nematode eggs are obviously non-motile and hence their distribution is determined by the defaecation habits of the host. Similar considerations, however, apply to motile larvae since their powers of dispersal are very limited in relation to the movement patterns of their human hosts. In addition to the precise spatial position of the deposition of transmission stages, the physical nature of the location is of some importance to parasite transmission. The major determinants of the rate of development and survival of nematode transmission stages are humidity and temperature and hence factors such as soil type and the degree of shading from direct sunlight influence transmission success. Recent experimental work on helminth transmission, using animal models, indicates that spatial heterogeneity in infective stage distribution can itself generate highly contagious distributions of parasite numbers within host populations (Keymer and Anderson, 1979). The significance of such factors to the dispersion patterns of human helminths is poorly understood at present.

3.15 CONCLUSIONS

The basic framework of the model described in this chapter can be adapted to mimic the dynamics of a wide range of direct life cycle helminth infections (see Chapter 4). In general it appears likely that the dynamical properties of the model will be fairly robust to changes in biological detail induced by variations in life cycle structure. The concepts of *transmission thresholds* and *unstable breakpoints* will still emerge as central to an understanding of the parasite's population biology.

The observed stability, and robustness to perturbation, of many directly transmitted nematode infections of man is a consequence of three principal factors. First, in regions of endemic infection these parasites appear to have basic reproductive rates which are much greater than unity. This point is well illustrated by the example of ascariasis in the Iranian village community (Fig. 3.22). A rough guide to the magnitude of R may be gained by the rapidity with which the intensity of infection rises in the young age classes of the community. For hookworm and ascariasis this rise is typically fairly rapid. Second, tight density-dependent constraints appear to operate on the growth of parasite sub-populations within individual hosts. A good example is displayed in Fig. 3.3 in which the rate of egg production by female roundworms is shown to decline rapidly as population density rises. The net effect of density-dependent constraints within individual hosts, whether acting on parasite survival and/or fecundity, is to regulate the growth of the total parasite population within the human community and to enhance overall population stability. Third, and finally, the observed contagion of the worms in their distribution within the host population acts both to enhance the influence of density-dependent processes throughout the total parasite population and to reduce the value of the critical mean worm burden below which mating frequency is too low to maintain parasite transmission within the host population. A rough guide to the degree of aggregation in the distribution of the parasites may be obtained by inspection of the age–intensity and age–prevalence curves. For example, if the average intensity is high but prevalence moderate to low, the worms are highly clumped within the human population. Conversely, if intensity is low but prevalence high, the degree of contagion is low (Anderson, 1982b).

These conclusions have many implications for the design of methods and policies for the control of nematode infections. First, it is clear that the breakpoint concept, first described by Macdonald (1965), is of little relevance to the control of helminth infections as a consequence of their contagious distributions (May, 1977). Theory suggests that endemic equilibrium worm burdens will be effectively globally stable to perturbation. The observed histories of parasite populations after the cessation of chemotherapy support this conclusion (Fig. 3.22). A permanent reduction in disease prevalence will only be achieved by measures which induce a substantial and lasting suppression of the basic reproductive rate. Improved standards of hygiene and sanitation can clearly achieve this goal.

Although chemotherapy is unlikely to lead to the eradication of such parasites (unless applied very intensively over many years), the benefits gained from drug treatment can be substantially enhanced by selectively treating the most heavily infected proportion of the population. The greater the degree of parasite aggregation prior to control intervention, the greater will be the benefits gained from this procedure (Anderson and May, 1982b). Used in conjunction with improvements in sanitation and hygiene this approach appears to be the optimum method of control for gut-dwelling helminths. This point of view was first propounded many years ago by Smillie (1924) and has been restated recently by Warren (1981).

One of the major roles of theoretical work in the epidemiological study of infectious disease agents is to identify areas in which our biological knowledge is inadequate. There are many such areas relevant to our understanding of the dynamics of gut-dwelling nematodes. Hookworms and roundworms are the most intensively studied species and yet, as illustrated in Tables 3.5 and 3.6, our knowledge of many of their population parameters is extremely limited. Most epidemiological studies, for example, measure worm burdens indirectly by faecal egg counts. This approach is subject to error, however, since the rate of egg production is often dependent on worm density (see Figs. 3.3 and 3.4). There is a great need for more studies which record worm abundance and distribution by direct means (e.g. employing chemotherapeutic agents to expel individual worm burdens). If accurate egg–prevalence and age–intensity (obtained from both horizontal and longitudinal studies) data are available, quantitative estimates can be made of the basic reproductive rate within a given community. The measurement of this parameter is of central importance to the design of control policies since its magnitude reflects the degree of difficulty which will be experienced in the suppression of parasite abundance. This point is clearly illustrated in the section on parasite control in this chapter but is also stressed in many of the other chapters.

   Finally, concomitant with the need for improvements in the available data base there is also a requirement for more sophisticated statistical methods to aid in the estimation of parameters, such as R, from age–prevalence and age–intensity data.

4 Tapeworm infections

Anne Keymer

4.1 INTRODUCTION

Cestode parasites are the causal agents of significant public health and economic problems in many areas of the world, infecting both man and his domestic stock. The five most important species and their associated diseases are listed in Table 4.1.

Most species live as adult worms in the gut of a vertebrate host and release eggs into the external environment with the host faeces. The majority of cestode life cycles are indirect, larval stages being passed as a developmental necessity in one or more intermediate hosts. For example, both *Taenia solium* and *T. saginata* are specific adult parasites of man. Eggs are deposited with human faeces, and hatch to release oncosphere larvae on ingestion by a suitable intermediate host (cattle for *T. saginata* and swine for *T. solium*). The oncospheres develop to infective cysticercus larvae in the voluntary muscles, so initiating the disease 'cysticercosis'. Man becomes infected by consuming undercooked beef or pork, either by mistake or as a result of deliberate culinary procedures. An additional complication exists, since cysticerci of *T. solium* may develop in human intermediate hosts, probably by ingestion of eggs as a contaminant from the environment (Webbe, 1967). Cysticercus cellulosae is thus a disease of both man and pigs, whereas cysticercus bovis exists only in cattle. The rat tapeworm, *Hymenolepis diminuta*, has a life cycle similar in general pattern to that of *T. saginata*. Adult worms live in the small intestine of mammals, commonly rats, and cysticercoid larvae develop in a wide variety of insect intermediate hosts, commonly *Tribolium confusum* and *Tenebrio molitor*. *H. diminuta* has been widely used as a laboratory model and so forms the basis of much of the available experimental data relating to cestode population processes.

The other three species listed in Table 4.1 differ in some respect from the life cycle pattern just described. For example, although *Hymenolepis nana* may undergo larval development in an insect intermediate host, most transmission occurs as a result of a direct life cycle link, eggs being immediately infective to the final host (Witenberg, 1964), which may be man or one of a variety of other mammalian species. *Echinococcus granulosus* has a two-host life cycle, adults occurring in carnivorous mammals, commonly dogs, and larval hydatid cysts in other associated mammals such as cattle, goats, camels, buffalo and man (Smyth and Smyth, 1964). The interesting feature of the *E. granulosus* life cycle

Table 4.1 Tapeworms of public health significance in man and economic significance in animals.

Species	Order	Popular name	Final host	Intermediate host	Name given to disease	
					Adult	Larva
Diphyllobothrium latum	Pseudophyllidea	Broad fish tapeworm	Man	1st Copepod spp. 2nd Fish spp.	Diphyllobothriasis	
Taenia saginata	Cyclophyllidea	Beef tapeworm	Man	Cattle	Taeniasis saginata	Cysticercus bovis
Taenia solium	Cyclophyllidea	Pork tapeworm	Man	Pig or man	Taeniasis solium	Cysticercus cellulosae
Hymenolepis nana	Cyclophyllidea	Dwarf tapeworm	Man	None or beetle spp.	Hymenolepiasis	
Echinococcus granulosus	Cyclophyllidea	Bladder worm	Dog	Man, sheep, cow, goat camel, buffalo etc.		Hydatid disease

with respect to the parasite–host population dynamics is the asexual reproduction which occurs in the intermediate host. Each hydatid cyst, derived from a single egg, may contain up to a million infective protoscolices (Smyth, 1977). The cestode *Diphyllobothrium latum* has a three-host life cycle, eggs hatching in water to release a free-swimming coracidium larva. Two further stages of larval development are then necessary (in copepod and fish intermediate host species) before infection of the human definitive host can occur. Despite these differences, all cestode life cycles are similar in that transmission is always achieved by predator–prey links, either between two host species or between a host and a free-living infective stage.

An estimate of the world prevalence of cestode infections in man, as given by Peters (1978), is shown in Table 4.2, from which it may be calculated that approximately 3.4% of the total world population at this time was affected.

From Table 4.2, it can be seen that *T. saginata* is the most widespread and prevalent tapeworm infection in man. Moreover, it must be remembered that the estimates given are to a large extent based on the results of faecal sampling, a method notorious for consistent underestimation of true prevalence levels. Autopsy studies in Kenya, for example, have revealed a prevalence of more than 90% in areas where routine surveys indicated that only 10% of the population was infected (Joint FAO/UNEP/WHO Report, 1976). In addition, prevalence is extremely heterogeneous within large areas, the percentage infection in Kenya, for example, varying between 3 and 65% (Froyd, 1965).

By far the most serious tapeworm infection occurring in man, although by no means the most prevalent, is echinococcosis or hydatid disease. It has a worldwide distribution (Schantz and Schwabe, 1969), and although it has been eradicated in Iceland (Dungal, 1946) and successfully controlled in New Zealand (Burridge and Schwabe, 1977), Cyprus (Polydorou, 1977) and Tasmania (McConnell and Green, 1979), it still represents a major public health problem in many countries. For example, echinococcosis accounts for 0.85% of hospital admissions in Libya (Dar and Taguri, 1978) and 0.5% in Iran (Anon, 1976). The cost of surgical treatment for the removal of cysts is extremely high and is an unnecessary burden on the economy of countries in

Table 4.2 Estimates of the number of people infected with tapeworm parasites in different regions of the world in 1975 (figures in millions; data source: Peters, 1978).

	Africa	Asia (excl. USSR)	C. and S. America	Oceania	North America	Europe (excl. USSR)	USSR	World total
Taenia saginata	32	11	2	1	1	1	29	77
Hymenolepis nana	2	27	2		1	2	5	39
Diphyllobothrium latum		2				3	10	15
Others	1	2					1	4

which eradication is a feasible proposition by methods involving destruction of stray dogs and widespread use of chemotherapeutic agents such as mebandazole and bunamide.

Cases of tapeworm infection in man are relatively infrequent in areas with high standards of public hygiene. For example, 82 cases of *T. saginata* infection were reported in the United Kingdom in 1976, and 98 in 1977 (Crewe and Owen, 1978). Hydatid disease in Britain was formerly believed to be confined to sheep farming areas of Wales, where up to 37% of sheep may carry the infection (Walters, 1977) and where there were 98 human deaths from hydatidosis during the period 1957–1965 (Sullivan, 1977). Within recent years, however, a dramatic increase in the incidence of hydatid disease has become apparent, the adult worm being found in 29% of foxhounds, and the larval worm in 60% of associated horses throughout Britain in 1974 (Thompson and Smyth, 1974). Although human hydatid disease has not yet shown any increase in incidence, this obviously represents a potential health hazard in a country in which tapeworms are normally dismissed as a curiosity.

The cestode species of greatest economic significance are *T. saginata*, *T. solium* and *E. granulosus*. World prevalence data are not readily available, since the infections are extremely heterogeneous, but approximate figures are given in Table 4.3, based to a large extent on abattoir data from local regions of each country. It is likely that prevalence is, in reality, substantially higher than indicated here, since current methods of meat inspection vary between countries, and, in addition, there are no means by which disease incidence in animals slaughtered privately may be taken into account (Chambers, 1978, Dada, 1978). The economic loss sustained as a result of these infections is again difficult to assess realistically, but current figures from the United Kingdom indicate that annual losses due to cysticercosis and hydatidosis are £0.5 m and £0.1 m respectively (Crewe and Owen, 1978; Walters, 1977). In Nigeria, 500 tonnes of meat valued at US $1.8 m was condemned in 1978 (Alonge and Fasanmi, 1979), while losses in Botswana and Kenya were estimated to be £0.5

Table 4.3 Percentage prevalence of hydatidosis and cysticercosis in domestic stock in different regions of the world.

	Africa	Asia	C. and S. America	Oceania	N. America	Europe	USSR
Hydatidosis	6[a]	3.5[d]–48[c]	19–40[g]	12–30[g]	1–4[g]	1–37[h]	2–52[g]
Cysticercosis	10[b]–29[a]	0.3[e]–70[f]	1[h]–4[j]	0.21[h]	0.04[h]–1[j]	0.1[i]–1[j]	1–20[h]

[a] Basson *et al.* (1970)
[b] Griffiths (1979)
[c] Islam and Rashid (1977)
[d] Dajani (1978)
[e] Karim (1979)
[f] Rahman *et al.* (1975)

[g] Gemmell (1960)
[h] Walters (1977)
[i] Pawlowski and Schultz (1972)
[j] Crewe and Owen (1978)
[k] Grindle (1978)

and £1.0 m in 1977 (Grindle, 1978). In addition to the condemnation of heavily infected carcasses, further economic loss is sustained as a result of the treatment and subsequent depreciation of lightly infected meat, which is sold at approximately 60% of its true value (Grindle, 1978).

D. latum, the fish tapeworm, is of both economic and public health importance. As with many cestode species, the significance of infection as a human disease is compounded by the impact of the parasite on potential food-source populations. This species is somewhat unusual among tapeworms in that prevalence of the larval stage in second intermediate host fish species such as *Perca fluviatilis* and *Esox lucius* may reach 100% in the older age classes (see Fig. 4.1).

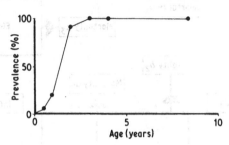

Figure 4.1 The prevalence of the tapeworm *Diphyllobothrium latum* in the fish *Esox lucius* (from Dogiel, 1962).

In spite of the high prevalence of tapeworm infections, and the considerable problems which they pose, surprisingly little is known about their population biology. This is in contrast to the substantial available literature relating to the dynamics of other parasitic diseases (e.g. Ross, 1911; Macdonald, 1965; Bradley and May, 1978; Yorke *et al.*, 1979; Anderson and May, 1979a, 1982a).

The present chapter describes some preliminary work concerning the population biology of cestode parasites, based on a model framework proposed by Anderson and May (1978) and May and Anderson (1978). The general properties of a model developed to describe the dynamics of a cestode infection are explored, and its relevance to cestode infections in the laboratory (*H. diminuta*) and in the field (*H. nana*) is discussed. Finally, the effects of seasonality and the implications of control measures are briefly considered, together with suggestions for future research.

4.2 GENERAL MODEL FRAMEWORK

A basic model is developed to describe the life cycle of tapeworms such as *T. saginata* or *H. diminuta*, in which three distinct developmental stages may be considered: the adult worm in the final host, the free-living parasite egg and the larval worm in the intermediate host. This life cycle may be represented by a flow chart as shown in Fig. 4.2. The model consists of coupled differential

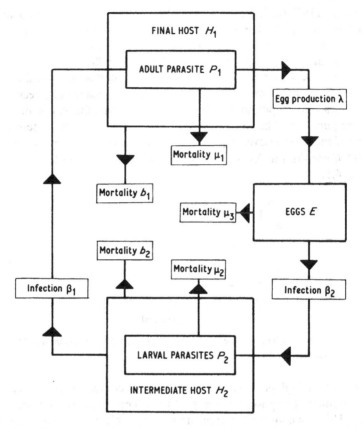

Figure 4.2 Diagrammatic flow chart of the populations and rate processes involved in the life cycle of a tapeworm such as *Taenia saginata* or *Hymenolepis diminuta*.

equations representing the dynamics of the parasite populations. It is assumed that both the final and intermediate host populations possess stable age distributions and are of constant sizes H_1 and H_2 respectively. The assumptions incorporated in the equations of the model are as follows.

4.2.1   Infection of the intermediate host

Infection of the intermediate host occurs as a result of ingestion of free-living infective stages, and so is governed by the dynamics of a predator–prey interaction. A functional response (i.e. a non-linear relationship between the rate of egg ingestion and egg density) has been demonstrated for the interaction between *T. confusum* and *H. diminuta* eggs under laboratory conditions (Keymer and Anderson, 1979; see Fig. 4.3(a)). In most natural situations, however, the density of tapeworm eggs relative to the density of the

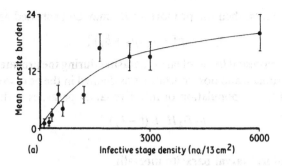

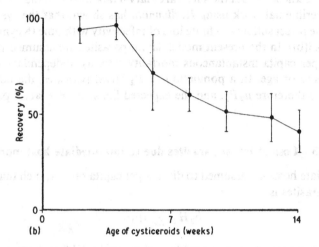

Figure 4.3 (a) The functional response between intermediate host infection and infective stage density, in the laboratory association between *Tribolium confusum* and *Hymenolepis diminuta* (from Keymer and Anderson, 1979). (b) Survival of *Hymenolepis diminuta* cysticercoids in *Tribolium confusum*, as measured by their infectivity to the final host (Keymer, 1981). The solid circles are observed means, and the vertical lines represent the 95% confidence limits of the means.

intermediate host population is unlikely to reach high enough levels to cause the generative mechanisms of a functional response (i.e. handling time and/or satiation; see Murdoch and Oaten, 1975) to become operative. In the present model, therefore, it is assumed that intermediate hosts acquire parasites at a rate proportional to the density of hosts, H_2, and the density of infective parasite eggs, E. The net rate of parasite acquisition is thus $\beta_2 H_2 E$, where β_2 is a coefficient representing the rate of transmission. Of those parasites acquired by an individual host, only a proportion, D_2, survive to reach infectivity. If the average prepatent period in the intermediate host (the time period from entry into the intermediate host to the development of the stage infective to the final host) is T_2 time units, then the proportion D_2 may be expressed as:

$$D_2 = \exp[-T_2(\mu_2 + b_2)] \tag{4.1}$$

where μ_2 and b_2 represent losses of larval parasites during the prepatent period due to natural parasite and host mortalities as defined in the next section. The net rate of gain to the population of infective larval parasites is thus:

$$\beta_2 D_2 H_2 E(t - T_2)$$

4.2.2   Natural larval parasite mortality

Very little is known about the survival of larval tapeworms in the intermediate host. Experimental work using *H. diminuta* has shown that the cysticercoid larva in the insect suffers a definite loss of infectivity with time (Keymer, 1981; see Fig. 4.3(b)). In the present model, larval parasites are assumed to have a constant per capita instantaneous mortality rate, μ_2, independent of either their density or age. In a population of P_2 larval parasites, the net loss of parasites is therefore $\mu_2 P_2$, and the expected life span of a larval parasite is $1/\mu_2$.

4.2.3   Loss of larval parasites due to intermediate host mortality

Intermediate hosts are assumed to die at a per capita rate b_2, such that the net loss of parasites is

$$b_2 H_2 \sum_{i=0}^{\infty} i p(i)$$

where $p(i)$ represents the probability that an individual host contains i parasites. It is assumed in the present model that there are no detrimental parasite-induced effects on host survival (either direct or indirect) or fecundity. Although the latter have been demonstrated in the laboratory for *H. diminuta* in the host *T. confusum* (Keymer, 1980a), it seems likely that few insect intermediate hosts would survive long enough in the natural environment for parasite-induced effects to be of significance. In addition, although several cestode species are clearly pathogenic to their mammalian intermediate hosts, there are as yet no reports of parasite-induced mammalian intermediate host mortality under natural conditions.

4.2.4   Loss of larval parasites due to final host infection

Final host infection is achieved by means of a second predator–prey association, this time between final and intermediate hosts. It is again assumed, however, that intermediate host density is unlikely to reach high enough levels to cause a reduction in ingestion rate to occur due to satiation or handling time effects, especially since the intermediate host species is often not the primary food source of the definitive host. Ingestion is thus assumed to be directly proportional to the density of final and intermediate hosts, H_1 and H_2 respectively, such that the net rate of loss to the larval parasite population is

$$\beta_1 H_1 H_2 \sum_{i=0}^{\infty} ip(i)$$

where β_1 is a coefficient representing the rate of transmission and $p(i)$ is the probability that an individual host harbours i parasites.

4.2.5   The acquisition of mature parasites: final host infection

As stated above, ingestion of intermediate hosts by prospective final hosts is assumed to be directly proportional to their densities, H_1 and H_2, such that the net rate of acquisition is

$$\beta_1 H_1 H_2 \sum_{i=0}^{\infty} ip(i).$$

Of those parasites acquired by an individual host, only a proportion, D_1, survive to reach sexual maturity, since some are lost due to parasite and host mortalities during the prepatent period (the time period from entry into the final host to reproductive maturity when worms begin egg production). If the average length of the prepatent period in the final host is T_1 time units, then the proportion D_1 may be expressed as:

$$D_1 = \exp[-T_1(\mu_1 + b_1)] \tag{4.2}$$

where μ_1 and b_1 are the instantaneous per capita rates of adult parasite and final host mortalities respectively. The net rate of gain of sexually mature adult parasites is thus:

$$\beta_1 H_1 D_1 H_2 \sum_{i=0}^{\infty} ip(i)(t - T_1)$$

4.2.6   Natural adult parasite mortality

The rate of natural adult parasite mortality is assumed in this paper to be dependent on the density of mature parasites within any given individual host. Little experimental evidence is available to support this assumption, although the observations of Ghazal and Avery (1974), and Hesselberg and Andreassen (1975) (Fig. 4.4) indicate that both survival and fecundity are density-dependent in *Hymenolepis* spp. In the present model, density-dependent constraints are limited for simplicity to parasite mortality. The per capita rate of natural parasite mortality is assumed to be linearly related to parasite burden, i, such that:

$$\mu(i) = \mu_1 + \delta i \tag{4.3}$$

where $1/\mu_1$ represents the expected life span of mature parasites in the absence of density-dependence, and δ is a coefficient measuring the severity of density-

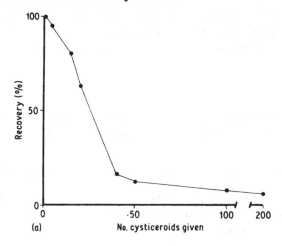

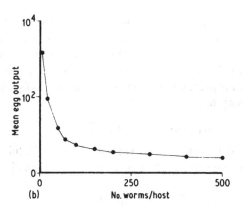

Figure 4.4 Density-dependent survival and fecundity in adult tapeworms. (a) The influence of the number of parasites given, on the percentage estalishment in *H. diminuta* in the rat (from Hesselberg and Andreassen, 1975). (b) The influence of worm burden on the mean egg output per worm in *H. nana* (from Ghazal and Avery, 1974).

dependent constraints on worm survival. The net rate of parasite losses due to such effects is therefore

$$H_1 \sum_{i=0}^{\infty} \mu(i) i p(i)$$

4.2.7 Adult parasite losses due to definitive host mortality

Hosts are assumed to have a constant, instantaneous, per capita mortality rate, b_1, such that the net loss of parasites is

$$b_1 H_1 \sum_{i=0}^{\infty} i p(i).$$

Adult tapeworms are often considered to be without serious pathogenic effects on the definitive host (Insler and Roberts, 1976; Rees, 1967), and in the present model it will be assumed that there is no parasite-induced host mortality.

4.2.8   The production of infective eggs

Most cestodes are hermaphrodite, and are thought in general to be able to carry out both self- and cross-insemination (Williams and McVicar, 1968; Nollen, 1975). It will be assumed in this chapter that all worms in the definitive host are equally capable of producing eggs, whether present singly or in multiple worm burdens. Assuming that the per capita instantaneous rate of egg production, λ, is constant and independent of worm age or density, the net rate of egg production is equal to λP_1. This is in direct contrast to dioecious helminths such as hookworms and schistosomes, where the production of viable eggs does not occur unless the worms are mated within the host. The 'mating function' in these parasites (i.e. the probability that any given female worm has been mated) has important consequences with respect to the overall dynamics of the host–parasite interaction (see Chapter 3). Since the eggs of cestode species belonging to the family Cyclophyllidea are immediately infective to the intermediate host, time delays in maturation (which are important for tapeworm species belonging to the family Pseudophyllidea such as *D. latum*), are not incorporated in the basic model.

4.2.9   Natural mortality of infective eggs

The population of infective eggs is subject to considerable mortality while in the external environment (Gemmell, 1977). Assuming that the instantaneous rate of mortality is μ_3 per egg per unit time, the net rate of loss is equal to $\mu_3 E$. Each egg thus has an expected life span of $1/\mu_3$.

4.2.10   Loss of infective stages due to host infection

Infective eggs are removed from the population as a consequence of ingestion by potential intermediate hosts. The rate of loss is equal to $\beta_2 H_2 E$, as described previously. Loss of eggs as a result of ingestion by animals unsuitable as intermediate hosts is assumed to be incorporated into the term denoting egg mortality.

4.2.11   The distribution of parasite numbers per host

The assumptions detailed above give rise to the following differential equations describing the changes through time of the adult parasite (P_1), larval parasite (P_2) and tapeworm egg (E) populations.

$$\frac{dP_1}{dt} = \beta_1 H_1 D_1 H_2 \sum_{i=0}^{\infty} ip(i)(t - T_1) - H_1 \sum_{i=0}^{\infty} \mu(i)ip(i) - b_1 H_1 \sum_{i=0}^{\infty} ip(i) \quad (4.4)$$

$$\frac{dP_2}{dt} = \beta_2 D_2 H_2 E(t - T_2) - \mu_2 P_2 - b_2 H_2 \sum_{i=0}^{\infty} ip(i) - \beta_1 H_1 H_2 \sum_{i=0}^{\infty} ip(i)$$
$$(4.5)$$

$$\frac{dE}{dt} = \lambda P_1 - \mu_3 E - \beta_2 H_2 E \quad (4.6)$$

It is clear from the structure of Equations (4.4), (4.5) and (4.6) that the dynamical behaviour of the model is dependent on the nature of the statistical distribution of parasites within the host population (as emphasized in Chapter 3). In the vast majority of parasite–host associations, the parasites have a clumped or contagious distribution within the host population, which may be empirically described by the negative binomial probability model, a distribution defined by the mean and a single parameter, k, which varies inversely with the degree of clumping (Crofton, 1971; Anderson and May, 1978; Anderson, 1979). This distribution has been found to provide a good empirical description of the distribution of *H. diminuta* in the intermediate host in both laboratory and field populations (Keymer and Anderson, 1979; Rau, 1979; see Fig. 4.5). In addition, the negative binomial can also be used to describe the distribution of adult tapeworms in the final host, for example *Caryophyllaeus laticeps* in the bream, *Abramis brama* (Anderson, 1974), and also larval tapeworms in the second intermediate host, for example, *Schistocephalus solidus* in the stickleback, *Gasterosteus aculeatus* (Pennycuick, 1971).

In the present model, it is assumed that the distribution of both the adult and larval tapeworms in the host populations may be described by the negative binomial probability distribution. By the use of its statistical moments, namely:

$$\sum_{i=0}^{\infty} ip(i) = \frac{P}{H} \quad (4.7)$$

and

$$\sum_{i=0}^{\infty} i^2 p(i) = \frac{P^2(k+1)}{H^2 k} + \frac{P}{H} \quad (4.8)$$

Equations, (4.4), (4.5) and (4.6) may be expressed as:

$$\frac{dP_1}{dt} = \beta_1 H_1 D_1 P_2(t - T_1) - P_1(b_1 + \mu_1 + \delta) - \frac{\delta P_1^2(k+1)}{H_1 k} \quad (4.9)$$

$$\frac{dP_2}{dt} = \beta_2 D_2 H_2 E(t - T_2) - P_2(\mu_2 + b_2) - \beta_1 H_1 P_2 \quad (4.10)$$

$$\frac{dE}{dt} = \lambda P_1 - \mu_3 E - \beta_2 H_2 E \quad (4.11)$$

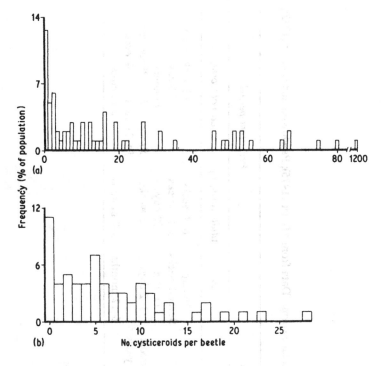

Figure 4.5. The frequency distribution of the cestode *Hymenolepis diminuta* in the intermediate host. The dotted lines represent the predictions of the negative binomial probability model. (a) *H. diminuta* in a field population of *Tribolium obscurus*; $k = 0.39$ (from Rau, 1979). (b) *H. diminuta* in a laboratory population of *Tribolium confusum*; $k = 1.04$ (from Keymer and Anderson, 1979).

where k is the parameter of the negative binomial distribution describing the adult worms in the final host.

4.2.12 Time scales

In common with many other parasitic organisms, the expected life spans of the majority of mature and larval tapeworms are many orders of magnitude greater than that of the infective egg (Anderson and May, 1979a; May and Anderson, 1979; see Table 4.4). The dynamics of the infective egg population thus operate on a much faster time scale than the dynamics of the other two parasite populations. In addition, the developmental time delays T_1 and T_2 are generally short in relation to the life span of the hosts and parasites. This suggests that the prepatent time delays are unlikely to be of significance to the dynamics of the parasite populations viewed over a number of generations. An exception to both these generalities is found in the life cycle of *E. granulosus*.

Table 4.4 The estimated life spans and prepatent periods of various tapeworms. Data from Muller (1975); Pawlowski and Schultz (1972); Dogiel (1962); von Bonsdorff (1977).

	Expected lifespan		Prepatent period		
	Adult worm	Larval worm	Egg	Adult worm, T_1	Larval worm, T_2
T. saginata	Many years	21–30 months	16 days	6–8 weeks	10–12 weeks
T. solium	10–15 years	Several years	Several weeks	5–12 weeks	60–75 days
H. nana	Few months	–	11 days	30 days	90 hours
D. latum	25 years	Procercoid several weeks Plerocercoid several years	1–2 days	3–5 weeks	Procercoid 14–21 days Plerocercoid 4 weeks
E. granulosus	6 months	Several years	6–12 months	6–7 months	5 months

4.3 DYNAMICAL PROPERTIES OF THE MODEL

The model may be considerably simplified by noting that the mean parasite burden per host, M, is given by P/H. By additional incorporation of the time-scale effects noted above, Equations (4.9), (4.10) and (4.11) may be reduced to give:

$$\frac{dM_1}{dt} = \beta_1 D_1 H_2 M_2 - M_1 (b_1 + \mu_1 + \delta) - \frac{\delta(k+1)M_1^2}{k} \tag{4.12}$$

$$\frac{dM_2}{dt} = \frac{\lambda H_1 \beta_2 D_2 M_1}{\mu_3 + \beta_2 H_2} - M_2(\mu_2 + b_2) - \beta_1 H_1 M_2 \tag{4.13}$$

The dynamical behaviour of the coupled Equations (4.12) and (4.13) may be examined by setting dM_1/dt and dM_2/dt equal to zero and constructing isoclines in the M_1–M_2 plane. Using this method, two general behaviour patterns emerge, as illustrated in Fig. 4.6. In the first (Fig. 4.6(a)), the two isoclines intersect only at the origin, indicating that the parasite is unable to persist within the host populations. In the second (Fig. 4.6(b)), the two isoclines intersect at the origin, and, in addition, at the point M^*, which represents a stable parasite equilibrium level to which all positive trajectories are attracted. In contrast to models of direct life cycle dioecious helminths (e.g. hookworm), where multiple stable states occur as a direct consequence of a worm mating function (see Chapter 3), the present model does not exhibit more than one positive equilibrium point for any combination of parameter values.

The two patterns of behaviour shown in Fig. 4.6 represent cases when the population parameters of the parasite are above (Fig. 4.6(b)) or below (Fig. 4.6(a)) a transmission threshold. The critical value of this threshold has been examined in detail by Anderson (1980), who has described an index of the number of offspring produced by a mature parasite during its egg-producing life span if introduced into a population of uninfected hosts (basic repro-ductive rate, R). The numerical value of R must be greater than unity in order for persistence of the parasite population to occur.

In the present model, the transmission threshold concept may be examined by first reducing the model to a single equation for the variable M_1, giving

$$\frac{dM_1}{dt} = M_1 \left[\frac{\lambda H_1 \beta_2 D_2 \beta_1 D_1 H_2}{(\mu_3 + \beta_2 H_2)(\mu_2 + b_2 + \beta_1 H_1)} - (b_1 + \mu_1 + \delta) - \frac{\delta(k+1)M_1}{k} \right] \tag{4.14}$$

The precise manner in which the various population parameters determine the probable persistence of the parasite are apparent from the structure of Equation (4.14). Essentially, for the transmission threshold to be exceeded, R must be greater than unity, where

$$R = \frac{\lambda H_1 H_2 \beta_1 \beta_2 D_1 D_2}{(\mu_3 + \beta_2 H_2)(\mu_2 + b_2 + \beta_1 H_1)(b_1 + \mu_1 + \delta)} \tag{4.15}$$

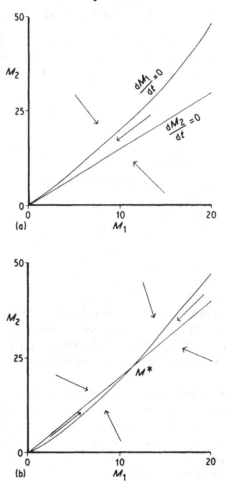

Figure 4.6 The arrows indicate how the dynamical trajectories of M_1 and M_2 behave in the various regions into which the M_1–M_2 plane is dissected by the isoclines dM_1/dt = 0 and dM_2/dt = 0. (a) Population parameters below the transmission threshold (parameter values, $\delta(k+1)/k = 0.01$, $\beta_1 D_1 H_2 = 0.5$, $b_1 + \mu_1 + \delta = 1$, $\lambda H_1 \beta_2 D_2$ = 1.5, $\mu_3 + \beta_2 H_2 = 1$, $\mu_2 + b_2 + \beta_1 H_1 = 1$) (b) Population parameters above the transmission threshold. Parameter values as for (a) except $\lambda H_1 \beta_2 D_2 = 2.0$.

The numerator of Equation (4.15) consists of the product of the model parameters involved in parasite transmission, and the denominator consists of the product of the accumulated rates of mortality in the adult parasite, larval parasite and parasite egg populations. Reproductive success is thus determined by the relative rates of transmission and loss. The concept of the basic reproductive rate is of considerable significance in the quantitative evaluation of the effects of various control options. The value of this and other similar techniques is, however, considerably hindered at the present time by the absence of suitable data on which to base an analysis.

Further insight into the dynamical behaviour of Equation (4.14) may be gained by evaluating the expression at equilibrium. The influence of the values of k and δ on the mean adult worm burden per host is shown in Fig. 4.7. Figure 4.7(a) shows the relationship between the degree of overdispersion in the frequency distribution of adult parasite numbers in the final host, and the mean worm burden of the final host population. When the level of overdispersion is high (i.e. when a few members of the host population harbour heavy worm burdens but the majority of the hosts are uninfected or carry only a few parasites), the mean worm burden will be relatively low. This relationship is due to the density-dependent constraints on parasite

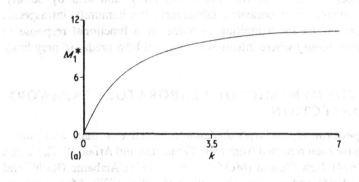

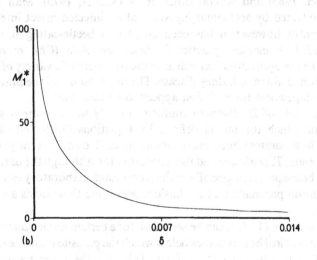

Figure 4.7 (a) The influence of k on the mean adult worm burden M_1. (parameter values, $b_1 + \mu_1 = 1$, $\delta = 0.02$, $\lambda H_1 \beta_2 D_2 = 2.5$, $H_2 \beta_1 D_1 = 0.5$, $\mu_3 + \beta_2 H_2 = 1$, $\mu_2 + b_2 + \beta_1 H_1 = 1$). (b) The influence of δ on the mean adult worm burden, M_1. Parameter values the same as (a) except $k = 0.3$.

population growth within individual hosts, which tend to cause heavy parasite mortality when the parasite population per host is high.

Figure 4.7(b) illustrates the effect of the degree of density-dependence on adult worm survival on the mean worm burden per host. It is apparent that density-dependence may exert stringent regulation on parasite population growth, and has the important consequence of stabilizing the dynamics of the host–parasite interaction (Anderson and May, 1978). When the severity of density-dependence is low, the equilibrium parasite population level is high, tending towards infinity as the severity of density-dependence becomes vanishingly small. Although, in the present model, density-dependence is restricted to parasite mortality, parasite population growth may also be regulated by factors such as density-dependent parasite fecundity, parasite-induced effects on host survival and/or fecundity, and also by density-dependent constraints on parasite establishment (i.e. immunity, intraspecific parasite competition for a limiting resource, or a functional response to infective-stage density where infection is achieved by a predator–prey link).

4.4   THE DYNAMICS OF A LABORATORY TAPEWORM INFECTION

The rat tapeworm, *Hymenolepis diminuta*, is infective to man, and human infections have been reported from Iran (Ghadirian and Arfaa, 1972), Ceylon (Kulasiri, 1954), New Guinea (McMillan *et al.*, 1971), Alabama (Ratliff and Donaldson, 1965) and several other areas (Muller, 1975). Man normally becomes infected by accidental ingestion of an infected insect intermediate host. Recently, however, it has been noted that beetle-eating is, in fact, a widespread folk medical practice in Southeast Asia (Chu *et al.*, 1977) prescribed as an aphrodisiac, as well as in the treatment of a variety of ailments ranging from asthma to kidney disease. The implications of the practice with respect to tapeworm transmission appear to be unknown.

The life cycle of *H. diminuta* conforms exactly to the pattern shown in Fig. 4.2 for which the model defined by Equations (4.12) and (4.13) was derived. The laboratory hosts most commonly used to support the parasite are the flour beetle, *T. confusum* and the laboratory rat, although the parasite is by no means host-specific, especially in the larval stage. Laboratory estimates for the population parameters of the basic model using these hosts are given in Table 4.5.

From Equation (4.15), it can be seen that, for a certain numerical value of R, there will be critical host densities below which the parasite is unable to persist. Since $\beta_1 H_1 \ll \mu_2 + b_2$ and $\beta_2 H_2 \ll \mu_3$ (see Table 4.5), the following approximation may be made:

$$H_1 H_2 > \frac{\mu_3(\mu_2 + b_2)(b_1 + \mu_1 + \delta)}{\lambda \beta_1 \beta_2 D_1 D_2} \tag{4.16}$$

Table 4.5 Approximate parameter estimates for *Hymenolepis diminuta* in the laboratory rat and *Tribolium sp.*

Parameter	Symbol	Value	Data source
Death rate of mature worms (single worm burdens)	μ_1	0.001/parasite/day	Keymer (1980b)
Constant relating to severity of density-dependence in adult worm mortality	δ	0.0004	Chappell and Pike (1976)
Adult worm prepatent period	T_1	17 days	Roberts (1961)
Rate of egg production per worm	λ	$70 \times 10^3/24$ h	Hesselberg and Andreassen (1975)
Rate of egg mortality	μ_3	0.09/egg/day	Keymer (1982)
Rate of infection of intermediate host	β_2	?	
Deathrate of larval worms	μ_2	0.01/parasite/day	Keymer (1981)
Larval worm prepatent period	T_2	9 days	Voge and Turner (1956)
Rate of infection of final host	β_1	?	
Final host mortality rate	b_1	?	
Intermediate host mortality rate	b_2	0.013/host/day	Keymer (1980b)
Negative binomial parameter relating to distribution of adult worms in the final host	k	1.27	Montgomery (personal communication)

Although experiments have not yet been designed to examine this relationship for *H. diminuta* (or for any other host–parasite interaction), Equation (4.15) may be used to estimate the threshold host densities required to maintain the parasite infection.

The population parameters which are not easily available from the literature are the final host mortality rate, b_1, and the two transmission parameters, β_1 and β_2. If it is assumed, on average, that laboratory rats live for about 2 years, then the final host mortality rate may be approximated by the value 0.001 per host per day. A rough estimate of the rate of infection of the final host, β_1, may be obtained from the results of experiments carried out by Coleman (1978) in which known numbers of beetles (with a known level of infection) were released into a 5 ft × 5 ft cage containing five uninfected rats. The remaining beetles were removed after 7 days, and the number of tapeworms which developed per rat was determined by dissection after a period of 3 weeks. Assuming that the rate of infection is proportional to the rat density, the cysticercoid density and distribution within the beetles introduced, and to the transmission parameter, β_1, then the change in the number of adult parasites in the rat population (P_1) through time may be represented by:

$$\frac{dP_1}{dt} = \beta_1 H_1 H_2 \sum_{i=0}^{\infty} i p(i) \qquad (4.17)$$

Similarly, the decrease in the cysticercoid population (P_2) through time, is given by:

$$\frac{dP_2}{dt} = -\frac{dP_1}{dt} \qquad (4.18)$$

Given that the initial number of larval parasites present in the beetle population is $P_2(0)$, the solution of these two simultaneous equations gives rise to the expression:

$$P_1 = P_2(0)\,(1 - e^{-\beta_1 H_1 t}) \qquad (4.19)$$

The average value of the parameter β_1 obtained from Coleman's data using Equation (4.19) is 4.3×10^{-6} per cysticercoid per day per host per hectare.

Similarly, an order of magnitude estimate of the transmission parameter β_2 may be obtained from the results of experiments in which adult *T. confusum* were exposed to known densities of *H. diminuta* eggs for varying periods of time, in an arena 13 cm^2 in basal area (Keymer, 1982). Again assuming no functional response between egg density and rate of predation, the changes through time in the number of cysticercoids (P_2) and eggs (E) present in the arena are given by the equations:

$$\frac{dP_2}{dt} = \beta_2 E H_2 \qquad (4.20)$$

$$\frac{dE}{dt} = -\mu_3 E - \beta_2 E H_2 \qquad (4.21)$$

where μ_3 is the instantaneous mortality rate of the eggs under experimental conditions (0.03 per egg per minute). Given that the number of eggs present in the arena at the start of an infection experiment is E_0, and that all the eggs are equally infective, Equations (4.20) and (4.21) have the solution:

$$P_2 = \frac{\beta_2 H_2 E_0}{(\mu_3 + \beta_2 H_2)} \left[1 - e^{-(\mu_3 + \beta_2 H_2)t} \right] \qquad (4.22)$$

From Equation (4.22), it is clear that as $t \to \infty$, $P_2 \to \beta_2 H_2 E_0/(\mu_3 + \beta_2 H_2)$, and so an estimate of β_2 may be obtained from the plateau of a graph of mean parasite burden plotted against exposure time. Using this estimation procedure in conjunction with results obtained experimentally, the value of β_2 obtained is 7.5×10^{-8} per egg per day per host per hectare.

Substituting these estimates, together with the values given in Table 4.5, into (4.16), the critical density of beetles for parasite persistence in an area where the rat density is 20 per hectare, may be estimated as 15 beetles per hectare. Bearing in mind that the parameter estimates used are only approximate values obtained under specific laboratory conditions, the main point of interest resulting from the above procedure is the extremely low critical host density required for parasite transmission. This may be typical of many indirect-life-cycle helminths which have the ability to persist endemically in low-density populations. Furthermore, Anderson (1982a) has argued that the ability of a low-threshold host density of one host species to be offset by a high density of the other host may have provided a major selective advantage for the acquisition of an indirect life cycle during parasite evolution.

4.5 THE DYNAMICS OF A HUMAN TAPEWORM INFECTION

Among the most intensively studied tapeworms of man is *H. nana*. Even for this species, however, quantitative estimates of the various population parameters are extremely scarce. *H. nana* has a life cycle very similar to that of *H. diminuta* except that man may act as both the final and intermediate host. This may be represented by the flow chart shown in Fig. 4.8, and it is assumed that, in human epidemiology, this type of transmission is likely to be more frequent than that involving a beetle intermediate host, although the latter may also occur. In the direct life cycle, the parasite undergoes larval

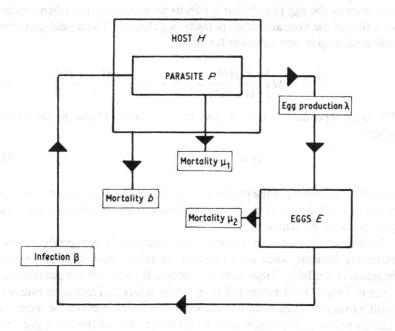

Figure 4.8 Diagrammatic flow chart of the populations and rate processes involved in the life cycle of *Hymenolepis nana*.

development in the intestinal wall of the host prior to emergence as an adult worm. This, however, may be effectively ignored with respect to the overall dynamics of the interaction, as long as the developmental time lag is increased to include both larval worm development and adult worm prepatency. Recapitulating the assumptions given for the basic model, the dynamics of *H. nana* may be represented by the following equations for E (parasite eggs) and M (mean parasite burden per host)

$$\frac{dM}{dt} = \beta DE - (b + \mu_1 + \delta)M - \frac{\delta M^2 (k+1)}{k} \tag{4.23}$$

$$\frac{dE}{dt} = \lambda MH - (\mu_2 + \beta H)E \tag{4.24}$$

where the population parameters are as shown in Fig. 4.8. The dynamical behaviour of Equations (4.23) and (4.24) is similar to that of the basic model, with two general patterns of behaviour. If the population parameters are below the transmission threshold, the parasite is unable to persist in the host population. If the parameters are above the transmission threshold, there is a stable equilibrium mean parasite burden, to which all positive trajectories are attracted.

Since the life span of the parasite egg is much shorter than the several-month survival period of the adult worm (see Table 4.4), it may be assumed that the dynamics of the egg population is effectively at equilibrium when compared with that of the host and adult parasite populations. The model may thus be collapsed to give one equation for M:

$$\frac{dM}{dt} = M \left[\frac{\beta \lambda HD}{(\mu_2 + \beta H)} - (b + \mu_1 + \delta) - \frac{\delta M (k+1)}{k} \right] \tag{4.25}$$

The basic reproductive rate, R, may be easily derived from Equation (4.25), where:

$$R = \frac{\beta \lambda HD}{(\mu_2 + \beta H)(b + \mu_1 + \delta)} \tag{4.26}$$

As before, R consists of the product of the transmission parameters divided by the compounded rates of mortality, and must exceed unity in order for parasite persistence to be achieved.

Evaluation of the parameters which constitute the basic reproductive rate is extremely difficult, since little quantitative information relating to human infection is available. Approximate estimates for some of the parameters are given in Table 4.6. The values of both the fecundity and mortality rates of the adult worm are taken from laboratory studies of *H. nana* in the mouse, and thus are unlikely to represent accurately the dynamics of the worm in a human host, although the estimate of mortality of 0.02 per day per worm does accord favourably with the expected life span of a 'few months' given for *H. nana* in

Table 4.6 Estimates of the population parameters involved in the life cycle of *Hymenolepis nana*.

Parameter	Symbol	Value	Data source
Death rate of mature worms (single worm burdens)	μ_1	0.02/day/worm	Ghazal and Avery (1974)
Constant relating to density-dependence in adult worm mortality	δ	?	–
Prepatent period (time from ingestion of egg to maturation of adult worm)	T	20 days	Muller (1975)
Rate of egg production per worm	λ	3400 eggs/worm/day	Ghazal and Avery (1974)
Rate of egg mortality	μ_2	0.09/day	Muller (1975)
Rate of infection	β	?	–
Host mortality rate (man)	b	0.000055/day	Based on an expected life span of 50 years

man by Muller (1975). In the absence of any quantitative information relating to the parameters δ (density-dependence in worm mortality) and β (transmission coefficient), no worthwhile evaluation of R can at present be attempted. This highlights the necessity for further epidemiological research in relation to cestode infections, especially since, by combination of Equations (4.25) and (4.26) to give:

$$\frac{dM}{dt} = M\left[(R-1)(b+\mu_1+\delta) - \frac{\delta M(k+1)}{k} \right]$$ (4.27)

it can be seen that the absolute numerical value of the basic reproductive rate in part determines the level of parasitism in the population. From Equation (4.27), the equilibrium average burden of parasites is simply:

$$M^* = \frac{k(R-1)(b+\mu_1+\delta)}{\delta(k+1)}$$ (4.28)

This corresponds to the special case of the direct-life-cycle helminth model proposed by Anderson in which the probability of a female worm being mated is unity. A discussion of the properties of this model is given by Anderson (1980). In a community in which the intensity of infection has been stable for a long period of time the mean worm burden, $M(a)$, at age a can be derived from the model defined in Equation (4.27) (see Chapter 3) where

$$M(a) = M^*[1-e^{-\gamma}][1+Ae^{-\gamma}]^{-1}.$$ (4.29)

Here $\beta = 1 - (1/R)$, $\gamma = (2R-1)(b+\mu_1+\delta)a$ and M^* is as defined in Equation (4.28). The age–prevalence curve (which is the form in which most epidemiological data are available) can be obtained from the zero probability term of the negative binomial distribution with mean $M(a)$ and parameter k, where the prevalence in age class a, $p(a)$ is:

$$p(a) = 1 - \left[1 + \frac{M(a)}{k} \right]^{-k} \qquad (4.30)$$

The general shapes of the predicted age–intensity and age–prevalence curves are shown in Fig. 4.9. Models of this form have been shown to provide reasonable qualitative predictions of observed trends in data relating to human roundworm infections (see Chapter 3), and therefore might be expected, also, to mirror the prevalence of tapeworm infections in man.

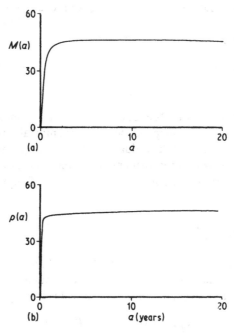

Figure 4.9 (a) The relationship between the average intensity of infection ($M(a)$) and the age of the host (a) predicted by the model defined in Equation (4.29). (b) The prevalence of infection $p(a)$ in different age classes of the population, as predicted by the model defined by Equation (4.30) (parameter values: $R = 2, k = 0.1, \delta = 0.002, (b + \mu_1 + \delta) = 1$).

Figure 4.10 shows age–prevalence data for *H. nana* infection in Iran (Sahba *et al.*, 1967). In contrast to the predicted results in which prevalence increases to a plateau in the older age classes, *H. nana* infection is highest in the 2–4-year age group, declining thereafter to extremely low prevalence levels in adults. These data are supported by qualitative assertions from many other areas of

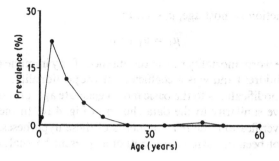

Figure 4.10 The prevalence of *Hymenolepis nana* in different age classes of a rural population in south-west Iran (from Sahba *et al.*, 1967).

the world in which *H. nana* is said to be primarily an infection of children (Witenberg, 1964). Clearly, the model described in Equation (4.30) is inadequate to describe the observed prevalence of *H. nana*, although it does crudely mirror the prevalence of certain other cestode infections, for example *D. latum* in the fish intermediate host (see Fig. 4.1). Although the generative mechanisms of the relationship shown in Fig. 4.10 are unknown, two potential explanations may be postulated.

4.5.1 Age-dependent variation in transmission

Given the life cycle of *H. nana*, it would seem reasonable to postulate that behavioural differences between children and adults may cause age-dependent variation in the rate of transmission of the disease to occur. Within the confines of the model, this may be described by making the transmission parameter β a decreasing function of age, a, such that:

$$\beta = \beta' e^{-\gamma a} \tag{4.31}$$

where β' is the rate of transmission in newborn children and γ is a coefficient of proportionality. Clearly, behavioural factors are likely to change in a manner much more complex than that described by this equation, which is used merely to gain qualitative insight into the influence of the transmission parameter on the dynamics of the infection.

4.5.2 Age-dependent development of immunity against infection

A high prevalence of infection in children could be the result of age-dependent immunity, whereby the ability of the immune system to react against helminth infections such as *H. nana* increases as the host becomes older. In the present model, this may be described by making the worm mortality rate. μ_1, an increasing function of host age, a, such that:

$$\mu_1 = \hat{\mu}_1 + wa \tag{4.32}$$

where $\hat{\mu}_1$ is the worm mortality rate in the absence of any immune reaction (i.e. in newborn children) and w is a coefficient of proportionality.

These two modifications to the basic model generate age–prevalence curves with qualitative similarity to the data shown in Fig. 4.10. In the absence of experimental verification, the relative merits of these hypotheses, and others which have not been discussed here, cannot at present be analysed.

4.6 SEASONAL FACTORS

In addition to the possibility that the value of certain population parameters may vary with age, it is also likely that seasonal patterns will occur. The survival of cestode eggs, for example, is critically dependent on temperature, humidity and microbial contamination (Gemmell, 1977). Larval development of tapeworms in poikilothermic intermediate hosts is also influenced by climate, both because the size of the host population may vary with the time of year, and also because developmental time may be inversely related to temperature (Heyneman, 1958). Many other factors such as seasonal changes in host behaviour, which may affect the value of the transmission parameter, β, and changes in host health (perhaps due to variation in diet or the presence of concurrent infections) which may alter the value of μ, the rate of parasite mortality, are also likely to be important.

Seasonal changes in the value of individual parameters may result in cyclical differences in the value of R, which may in turn be reflected in monthly variation in the prevalence of infection. An example is given in Fig. 4.11, which shows mean monthly worm burdens of the sheep tapeworm *Monezia expansa* in South Africa (Horak and Louw, 1977) and the United States (Stoll, 1938). In both cases, low prevalence during the cooler months is attributed to retarded development of the cysticercoids in the oribatid mites which serve as the intermediate host.

Seasonal parameter changes may be such that the value of the basic reproductive rate may fall below unity during certain periods of the year, indicating that parasite transmission may occur only at certain times. For parasite persistence in a defined region, however, the period during which R falls below unity must be less than the maximum life span of any one stage in the parasite life cycle. There are unfortunately insufficient data available to allow examination of these possibilities. In cestode infections, however, where the life span of the adult worms varies between 6 months in *E. granulosus* and many years in *T. saginata* and *D. latum* (see Table 4.4), seasonal changes in R are likely to be of little significance to the overall persistence of the parasite from year to year. The model development outlined in earlier sections may thus be used to explore the dynamics of the parasite on a yearly basis, as long as the parameter components are regarded as average yearly values.

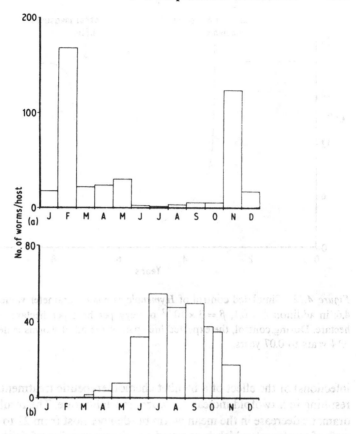

Figure 4.11. Seasonal prevalence in *Monezia expansa* in sheep. (a) Data from South Africa (Horak and Louw, 1977). (b) Data from USA (Stoll, 1938).

4.7 CONTROL

In recent years, several advances have been made in research for drugs of use in the treatment of both adult and larval tapeworm infections (FAO/UNEP/WHO, 1976; Heath and Lawrence, 1978; Kern, Dietrich and Volkmer, 1979). Within the confines of the model described in the present paper, chemotherapy acts to increase the parasite death rate in a density-independent manner, if applied randomly within the host population. As described earlier, this model generates a single stable equilibrium point for any combination of parameter values, and thus predicts that, while continued application of anthelminthics may be effective in reducing the mean worm burden per host, discontinuation of the treatment before total eradication has been achieved is likely to result in a return to the original intensity of infection. For example, Fig. 4.12 shows a simulation (using the parameter values given in Table 4.6, together with estimates of β and δ based on data from other cestode

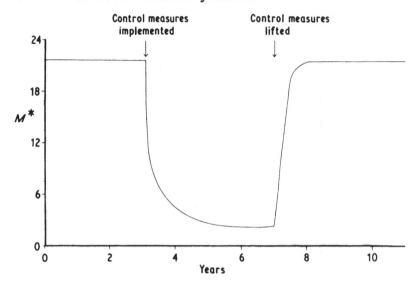

Figure 4.12 Simulated control of *Hymenolepis nana*. Parameter values: as in Table 4.6; in addition $\delta = 0.1$, $\beta = 3 \times 10^{-7}$ per egg per host per hectare, $H = 2000$ per hectare. During control, the expected life span of the adult worms is decreased from 0.14 years to 0.07 years.

infections) of the effect of a blanket chemotherapeutic treatment for *H. nana* resulting in a twofold increase in worm mortality rate. The results indicate a dramatic decrease in the mean worm burden per host from 22 to 4 in the first year of treatment, which is reversed on discontinuation of drug application; resumption of the initial level of parasitism occurs within a period of 6 months. In as far as the significance of this model formulation may be applied to parasite–host systems in the field, these results may indicate that chemotherapeutic treatment alone is not the best strategy for attempted long-term control of cestode infections.

The only tapeworm disease for which large-scale control has been attempted is echinococcosis. Control programmes have included the restriction of access of dogs to raw offal at abattoirs and farms, the reduction of the dog population in conjunction with mass dog treatment, and extensive anti-echinococcus education campaigns (Gemmell, 1979). The results of such programmes in Cyprus, Tasmania, Iceland and New Zealand are shown in Fig. 4.13. Interestingly, the successful echinococcosis campaign in Tasmania had no effect on the prevalence of *T. ovis* in dogs (Gregory, 1977), although the control measures included annual dog purging. Similarly, an 8-fold increase in the national prevalence of *T. ovis* was noticed during the implementation of an echinococcus programme in New Zealand (Burridge and Schwabe, 1977). These effects are thought to reflect the change in source of food for dogs from

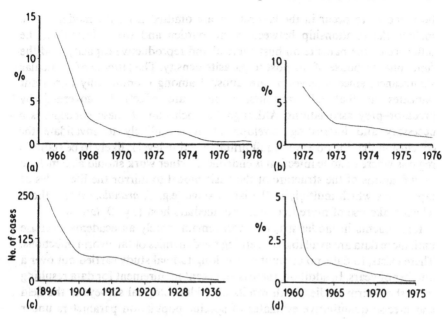

Figure 4.13 The results of control programmes for *E. granulosus*. (a) % prevalence in dogs in Tasmania (McConnell and Green, 1979). (b) % prevalence in dogs in Cyprus (Polydorou, 1977). (c) No. of reported human cases in Iceland (Dungal, 1946). (d) % prevalence in dogs in New Zealand (Burridge and Schwabe, 1977).

raw viscera to sheep carcasses, although the effects of cross-immunity (Gemmell, 1967) and the increased emphasis on diagnosis of infections may be involved. These observations, together with the fact that tapeworm infections are still present in many areas where the standards of education and public health are high, indicate that eradication may not always prove as easy as the foregoing results might suggest. It would be of interest to discover whether the success of *Echinococcus* control may be in any way explained by the behaviour of a model modified to include aspects of the *E. granulosus* life cycle such as asexual reproduction in the intermediate host, the relatively short life span of the adult worm and the long prepatent periods of both adult and larval parasites.

4.8   CONCLUSIONS

The basic model framework developed by Anderson and May (1978) and May and Anderson (1978) may be adapted to mimic the dynamics of a wide range of helminth parasites. In the present preliminary investigation, several aspects of host–tapeworm interaction have not been considered. For example, several density-dependent constraints on parasite population growth, which have been shown to occur in the laboratory, are omitted from the model. These include the relationship between worm burden and worm fecundity, the influence of the parasite on host survival and reproductive capacity, and the functional response of the host to parasite density. The latter is of particular significance, since tapeworms are unusual among economically important parasites in that all transmission links are effectively governed by predator–prey associations. Although the inclusion of these concepts is a necessary and interesting development, it is unlikely to invalidate the conclusion that the observed equilibrium infection level is likely to be stable in regions where cestode infection is endemic. Further work should also include modifications of the structure of the basic model to mirror the life cycles of tapeworms which multiply in the larval stage (e.g. *E. granulosus*) and those which make use of more than one intermediate host (e.g. *D. latum*).

Refinements in model structure will remain merely an academic exercise until more data are available concerning the dynamics of tapeworm infections. There exists, to date, no account of any longitudinal study carried out over a number of years. In addition, there is an urgent requirement for data resulting from short-term studies, both results of epidemiological surveys in the field and precise quantitative estimates of specific population parameters under controlled experimental conditions in the laboratory.

When used in conjunction with available data, theoretical techniques are of considerable value in the acquisition of conceptual insight into the processes affecting the dynamics of the host–parasite association. In addition, the manipulation of model frameworks is also of use in a predictive capacity, to forecast the effects of various control measures, and thus to evaluate the potential benefits of programmes proposed within specific economic boundaries.

5 The population dynamics of malaria

Joan L. Aron and *Robert M. May*

5.1 INTRODUCTION

This chapter deals with the transmission and maintenance of malaria, paying attention both to the overall dynamics and to the population biology of the infection in human hosts and mosquito vectors. We aim to combine some new work with review and synthesis (and, in some cases, reinterpretation) of existing work.

We begin with a brief sketch of the life cycle of the malaria parasite. The stripped-down, basic model for the transmission dynamics is then presented and analysed (using graphical, 'phase–plane' techniques that have not commonly been used in this context before). We emphasize the relation between the biology and the mathematics, focusing on the role played by the basic reproductive rate of the parasite, and on the dynamics of the prevalence of infection among humans and mosquitoes (including Macdonald's distinction between 'stable' and 'unstable' malaria).

Next, the model is elaborated to take more realistic account of the interplay between malaria and the mosquito population. Following Macdonald, we discuss the dynamical effects produced by the incubation period of the parasite in infected mosquitoes. We then examine the dynamical consequences of seasonal and other variation in the total mosquito population. Models which combine seasonal variation with year-to-year fluctuations in mosquito density can mimic observed patterns of steady seasonality or of episodic outbreaks in the monthly reporting of malaria cases; the different patterns depend on the basic reproductive rate of the parasite. Purely seasonal changes in the rates of mosquito emergence will produce annual cycles in mosquito density, in the number of infected mosquitoes, and in malaria prevalence in both mosquito and human populations; the relative phases of these cycles (the relative timing of their peaks), as deduced from this simple model, accord with observations.

The human side of the equation is then considered in more detail. The phenomenon of superinfection is discussed, and some of the models that have been proposed to describe it are reviewed; again, phase–plane techniques permit a transparent analysis of the similarities and differences among the models. Using Macdonald's original work as a point of departure, we consider ways in which data may be used to choose the correct model. We conclude that superinfection demonstrably exists, but that available data are too coarse to discriminate among the contending models.

Studies in hospitals and in natural settings show that humans acquire immunity as a result of infection. Moreover, both the maintenance of immunity and the degree of immunity depend on reinfections. We examine the dynamical consequences of these facts. In particular, we present a new model in which the rate of loss of immunity is explicitly related to the intensity of transmission; this model leads to age–prevalence curves that change with changing transmission rates in the same way as real age–prevalence curves do. An important conclusion is that reduction of transmission rates from initially high levels may actually result in increased prevalence of malaria among adults (prevalence among infants will always decrease, and prevalence will of course decrease for all age groups when transmission is brought to very low levels). This conclusion accords with the opinion of some malaria epidemiologists, and has significant implications for control programmes and public health. We also briefly review data indicating that the acquisition and loss of immunity is a gradual, rather than a discrete, process. There is a consequent need to develop models in which the effects of malaria on the human host depend on the intensity of infection, rather than simply on its presence or absence; in the terminology of Anderson and May (1978, 1979a), such continuum models would regard malaria as a 'macroparasite', as opposed to the discretized compartmental models which represent an adequate approximation for 'microparasites'. This part of the chapter ends with a short overview of current research directed towards elucidating the basic mechanisms producing immunity to malaria.

In conclusion, we emphasize that our account of the population biology of malaria has ignored population genetics and evolution. The co-evolutionary interactions among humans, mosquitoes and malarial parasites have repeatedly forced themselves to our attention, as control programmes have been confounded by the evolution of resistance to insecticides and drugs. We briefly discuss the many ways in which efforts to control or eradicate malaria are, in Joel Cohen's words, always efforts 'to hit a moving target'.

5.2 LIFE CYCLE OF THE MALARIA PARASITE

Malaria is caused by the multiplication of parasitic protozoa of the family Plasmodiidae within the blood cells or other tissues of the vertebrate host; the clinical symptoms in man arise from multiplication of the blood stages. Although there are several genera of malarial parasites associated with many kinds of hosts, this chapter focuses on the species of *Plasmodium* occurring in humans: *P. falciparum*, *P. vivax*, *P. malariae* and *P. ovale*. Of these, *P. falciparum* is the most common in tropical regions, and *P. vivax* in temperate zones.

Infection of a human host begins with the bite of a female anopheline mosquito and the injection of sporozoite stages into the bloodstream. These stages of the parasite are carried to the liver where they develop in the parenchymal cells. After an incubation period of several days (or months, as some authors have argued for *P. vivax*; Lysenko *et al.*, 1977), these exo-erythrocytic stages grow, divide and release merozoites back into the bloodstream. The merozoites penetrate red blood cells, where they grow and subdivide to produce more merozoites that rupture the host cells and invade other red cells. At some ill-understood point in this continuing process, a proportion of the merozoites develop into sexual stages, the gametocytes. Only gametocytes are infective to the mosquito. When a vector mosquito bites a human and ingests male and female gametocytes, these are freed from the blood cell, the female gamete is fertilized, and develops into an oocyst on the wall of the mosquito's gut. After 10 days or so (the actual development time is temperature-dependent), immature sporozoites migrate from the ruptured oocyst to the mosquito's salivary glands, mature to infectivity, and the cycle is ready to repeat itself. Figure 5.1 gives a schematic illustration of this cycle.

Notice that the overall cycle of the malaria parasite involves transmission both from mosquito to man, and from man to mosquito, by the bite of a female anopheline. The history of this discovery is entertainingly told by Harrison (1978), and good reviews of the current state of the malaria problem are given by Bruce–Chwatt (1979, 1980).

5.3 BASIC MODEL

The earliest attempt to provide a quantitative understanding of the dynamics of malarial transmission is the so-called Ross–Macdonald model, which still is the basis for much malarial epidemiology (Ross, 1911, 1916; Macdonald, 1952, 1957, 1973; Lotka, 1923; Fine, 1975a; Bailey, 1975).

This model, which captures the basic features of the interaction between the infected proportions of the human host population and the mosquito vector population, is defined as follows:

$$dx/dt = (abM/N)y(1-x) - rx \qquad (5.1)$$
$$dy/dt = ax(1-y) - \mu y \qquad (5.2)$$

where:

x is the proportion of the human population infected;
y is the proportion of the female mosquito population infected;
N is the size of the human population;
M is the size of the female mosquito population;
$m = M/N$ is the number of female mosquitoes per human host;
a is the rate of biting on man by a single mosquito (number of bites per unit time).
b is the proportion of infected bites on man that produce an infection;

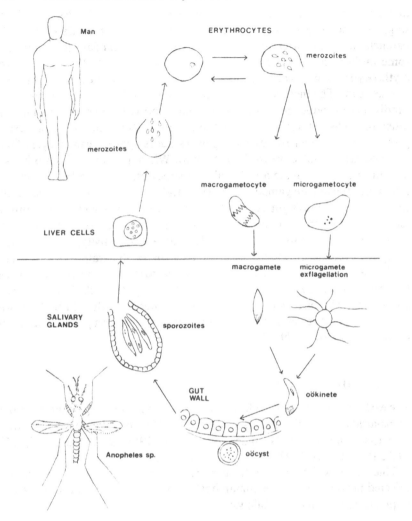

Figure 5.1 Schematic illustration of the life cycle of the malaria parasite (not drawn to scale).

r is the per capita rate of recovery for humans ($1/r$ is the average duration of infection in the human host);

μ is the per capita mortality rate for mosquitoes ($1/\mu$ is the average lifetime of a mosquito).

In this simple model, the total population of both humans and mosquitoes is assumed to be unchanging (N and M constant), so that the dynamical variables are the proportion infected in each population (x and y). The first equation describes changes in the proportion of humans infected; new infections are acquired at a rate that depends on the number of mosquito bites per person per unit time (aM/N), on the probabilities that the biting mosquito is infected (y) and that a bitten human is uninfected ($1 - x$), and on the chance that an uninfected person thus bitten will actually become infected (b); infections are lost by infected people returning to the uninfected class, at a characteristic recovery rate (rx). Similarly, the second equation describes changes in the proportion of mosquitoes infected; the gain term is proportional to the number of bites per mosquito per unit time (a), and to the probabilities that the biting mosquito is uninfected ($1 - y$) and that the bitten human is infected (x); the loss term arises from the death of infected mosquitoes (μy). More formally, the loss terms for infected humans and for infected mosquitoes both involve death and recovery. But for human hosts the recovery rate is typically faster than the death rate (by one to two orders of magnitude), whereas for mosquitoes the opposite is typically the case, so that the above formulation is a sensible approximation. (It is likely, however, that infected mosquitoes have a significantly higher mortality rate than uninfected ones (Schiefer et al., 1977), which means that appropriate μ values in Equation (5.2) may be larger than those estimated from healthy mosquitoes, or as population averages (for further discussion, see Anderson and May, 1979b.)) Less justifiable is the omission of a parameter, c say, in the gain term in Equation (5.2) (analogous to the parameter b in Equation (5.1)), to measure the probability that an uninfected mosquito will actually become infected after biting a malarious host. This probability c is certainly not unity (Ross, 1911).

This model is, of course, highly simplified. One of the most glaring omissions is the failure to distinguish between the various 'infected' categories of human and mosquito hosts to take account of the different developmental stages of the parasite. For instance, the model does not incorporate the incubation period of the parasite in the mosquito (during which period there are no sporozoites in the salivary glands of the 'infected' mosquitoes), even though this incubation period is comparable to the mean life span of the mosquito. This complication is pursued below. Likewise, there is no distinction between the pathological asexual merozoite blood stages and the infectious gametocyte sexual stages in the human. (The parameter c, mentioned above, could take some crude account of this aspect of the transmission dynamics.) Encounters between biting mosquitoes, and the humans they bite, are assumed to be random.

Notwithstanding these shortcomings, the simple model defined by Equations (5.1) and (5.2) is useful in laying bare the essentials of the transmission process, and in elucidating patterns in the diverse array of epidemiological data for different geographical regions.

In particular, the model makes plain the significance of the 'basic reproductive rate' of the parasite, R (Macdonald, 1950, 1952, 1957). The basic reproductive rate is essentially the number of secondary cases of infection generated by a single infective individual in a population of susceptibles: if this number is, on average, less than unity, the disease will be unable to maintain itself; if the number exceeds unity, the disease will be able to maintain itself. In general, the larger the basic reproductive rate, the greater the resistance of the infection to eradication. In this simple model, the basic reproductive rate (conventionally called Z_0, rather than R, in the literature on malaria) is:

$$R = ma^2b/\mu r \qquad (5.3)$$

This result, which is established below, is intuitively understandable. The mosquito biting rate, a, enters twice in the cycle (hence the a^2 factor). Transmission is helped by large numbers of mosquitoes per human host (large m) and by large b; transmission is hindered by high mosquito death rates or by fast recovery (large μ and r respectively).

The Equation (5.3) is usually derived algebraically, by analysis of the stability properties of the differential Equations (5.1) and (5.2) (Macdonald, 1957, 1973; Lotka, 1923; Fine, 1975a; Dietz, 1974; May and Anderson, 1979). A more transparent and more generalizable derivation can, however, be obtained by a geometrical 'phase–plane' analysis of the dynamical behaviour of the model. Here, as illustrated in Fig. 5.2, the x-axis corresponds to the dynamical variable x, the proportion of human hosts infected, and the y-axis to the dynamical variable y, the proportion of mosquitoes infected. In this figure, the variable y is unchanging along the isocline labelled $dy/dt = 0$; for given x, y is increasing below this isocline and decreasing above it. Similarly, the variable x is unchanging along the isocline labelled $dx/dt = 0$; for given y, x increases to the left of the isocline and decreases to the right of it. In the four domains of the $x-y$ plane thus defined by the isoclines in Fig. 5.2(a), the dynamical trajectories of this system will move in the general directions indicated by the arrows. The intersection of the two isoclines represents the equilibrium state, to which all trajectories will tend in Fig. 5.2(a). Clearly, the basic topological requirement

---

Figure 5.2 Depicted is the 'phase–plane' of the dynamical variables x (proportion of humans infected) and y (proportion of mosquitoes infected); each point in the plane corresponds to a particular pair of values x, y. As discussed more fully in the text, the variable x is not changing along the isocline $dx/dt = 0$, and y is unchanging along $dy/dt = 0$. The intersection of the two isoclines, if it exists, represents the equilibrium point of the system, and elsewhere trajectories move in the directions indicated by the arrows. In (a) the initial slope a/μ of the y-isocline significantly exceeds the initial slope r/abm of the x-isocline ($R \gg 1$), and the equilibrium point nestles in a relatively deep valley, corresponding to Macdonald's 'stable' malaria. In (b), the initial slope a/μ is relatively small, but still exceeds r/abm ($R > 1$); the equilibrium point exists, but now in a relatively shallow canyon, corresponding to Macdonald's 'unstable' malaria. In (c), the initial slope a/μ is less than r/abm ($R < 1$), so that the isoclines do not cross; all trajectories are attracted to the origin, and the disease cannot maintain itself.

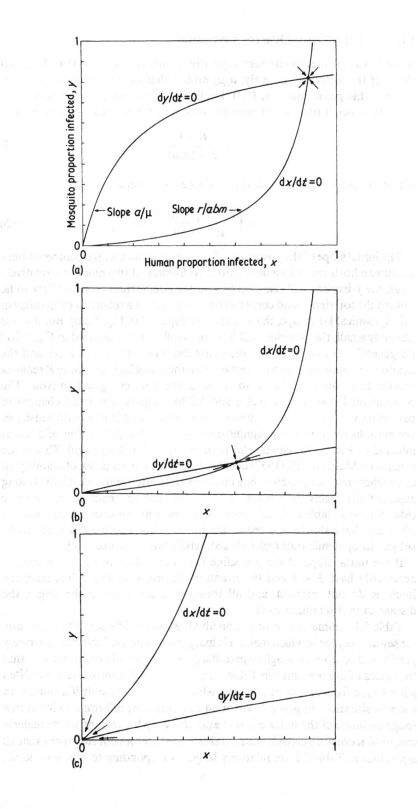

(a)

(b)

(c)

for the two isoclines to intersect at positive values of x and y is that the initial slope of the y-isocline (namely, a/μ) exceed that of the x-isocline (namely, r/abm). This gives Equation (5.3). Explicitly, the equilibrium proportion of humans infected (the equilibrium *prevalence* in the human population) is:

$$x^* = \frac{R-1}{R+(a/\mu)} \qquad (5.4)$$

The corresponding equilibrium prevalence for mosquitoes is:

$$y^* = \left(\frac{R-1}{R}\right)\left(\frac{a/\mu}{1+a/\mu}\right) \qquad (5.5)$$

The initial slope of the y-isocline, a/μ, represents the average number of bites on human hosts made by a mosquito in its lifetime. If this number is relatively large, the y-isocline will rise steeply, and the equilibrium point is likely to lie toward the top right-hand corner of the x–y plane, in a relatively deep valley in this dynamical landscape; this situation is depicted in Fig. 5.2(a). But if a/μ is relatively small, the y-isocline will have the shallow form depicted in Fig. 5.2(b) (in general, the maximum y value along the y-isocline is $a/(a+\mu)$), and the equilibrium point and the intersection with the x-isocline (assuming R remains greater than unity) is likely to lie in a shallow, elongated canyon. The comparison between Figs. 5.2(a) and 5.2(b) suggests that small changes in parameter values, such as changes in the biting rate a or in mosquito density m, are more likely to result in significant changes in the proportion of humans infected in Fig. 5.2(b) (small a/μ) than in Fig. 5.2(a) (large a/μ). This is the essence of Macdonald's (1957) conclusion that a/μ is an index of stability; in areas where mosquito vectors bite man relatively often and have relatively long expected life spans, this index is high and malaria tends to be endemic (Macdonald's 'stable malaria'); conversely, where mosquitoes bite on man less often and have shorter life spans, the index is low and malaria tends to be subject to epidemic outbreaks (Macdonald's 'unstable malaria').

If the initial slope of the y-isocline is less than that of the x-isocline, we necessarily have $R < 1$ and the situation illustrated in Fig. 5.2(c). Here the isoclines do not intersect, and all trajectories converge on the origin; the disease cannot maintain itself.

Table 5.1 summarizes information about Macdonald's 'stability index' a/μ, for several regions in which malaria is indigenous. The available data are rarely precise and complete enough to permit a good estimate of both μ and a, so that the values of a/μ presented in Table 5.1 are very rough approximations. Often μ is inferred from age–structure data, which is permissible only if dealing with a steady situation. In general, we found that sufficient information for even a rough estimate of the index a/μ was available only for regions where malaria was, in Macdonald's classification, 'stable'; it is therefore not surprising that all a/μ values in Table 5.1 are relatively large, corresponding to 'stable malaria'.

Table 5.1 Rough estimates of Macdonald's 'stability index', a/μ (the average number of bites made on humans in a mosquito's lifetime), from various geographical locations. The index is relatively high in all cases, agreeing with the observation that malaria is endemic in these places (the final result, for Sudan, is the exception; the figure of 0.47 is for a year of relatively high prevalence in this region, but malaria is more typically of Macdonald's 'unstable' kind). Where malaria is epidemic and 'unstable', consistent estimates of a and μ are hard to come by, which is part of the reason why the table contains no examples of low a/μ values (with the possible exception just noted).

Anopheles species	Place	Year	Daily survival probability, p	μ ($-\ln p$)	Gonotrophic cycle (days)	Human blood index	a (HBI/GC)	Stability index, a/μ	Reference
A. punctulatus	Maprik, New Guinea	1957–58	0.87	0.14	2	0.80	0.40	2.9	Peters and Standfast (1960)
A. balabacensis	Khmer	1964	0.95	0.05	3	0.75	0.25	4.9	Slooff and Verdrager (1972)
A. minimus	Bangladesh	1966–67	0.90	0.11	2	0.93	0.47	4.4	Khan and Talibi (1972)
A. gambiae	Kankiya, Nigeria	1967	0.94	0.06	3	0.75	0.25	3.4	Garrett–Jones and Shidrawi (1969)
A. gambiae	Garki, Nigeria	1972	0.89	0.11	2	0.87	0.44	3.9	Molineaux et al. (1979)
A. gambiae	Khashm El Girba, Sudan	1967	0.76	0.28	2	0.26	0.13	0.47	Zahar (1974)

(Details about the estimations and approximations involved in processing the data to arrive at the rough values of a/μ given in Table 5.1 are available on request.)

The table specifically excludes data from epidemic regions where new vectors have been introduced, or where there are mixtures of human populations owing to labor migration. In these circumstances, the simple assumptions of the model clearly do not apply. We also exclude data from regions where intervention with DDT has occurred, because there are now additional complicating factors in the interpretation of mosquito life-history parameters.

One such complication arises from inhomogeneities in the effects of insecticides, which are usually applied to interior surfaces and are more effective against mosquitoes that rest indoors after taking a blood meal. If insecticides do not affect all mosquitoes equally, measurements of the biting rate and of longevity may be severely distorted (Molineaux et al., 1979). For example, suppose after spraying there are two mosquito populations of roughly equal size: those that rest outdoors and are consequently relatively unaffected by the spraying and those that rest indoors and suffer greater mortality. For illustration let $a_1 = 0.25$ bites per day and $\mu_1 = 0.05$ per day for the exophilic mosquitoes, and $a_2 = 0.4$ and $\mu_2 = 0.2$ for the endophilic ones. The correct way to calculate the effective index, a/μ, is to take the appropriate arithmetical average of the separate indices: $\frac{1}{2}(a_1/\mu_1 + a_2/\mu_2) = 3.5$. But if the endophilic and exophilic categories are not properly distinguished, then a/μ is likely to be estimated using average values of a and of μ: $[\frac{1}{2}(a_1 + a_2)]/[\frac{1}{2}(\mu_1 + \mu_2)] = 2.6$. Molineaux et al. (1979) have analysed the consequences of this aggregation phenomenon in considerable detail. They emphasize that aggregating the groups will always underestimate the vectorial capacity of the mosquito population, and hence will always underestimate the basic reproductive rate R, and overestimate the impact of insecticides.

Further problems in the interpretation of these parameters arise, inter alia, from multiple biting per gonotrophic cycle (Boreham and Garrett–Jones, 1973), and in estimating the human blood index (Bruce–Chwatt et al., 1966). An excellent review of the methodology involved in the interpretation of epidemiologically relevant aspects of mosquito vector populations is by Garrett–Jones and Shidrawi (1969).

5.4 INCUBATION PERIOD IN THE MOSQUITO

Although the basic model above gives a good overview of the dynamics of malarial infection, some of its predictions are strikingly different from reality. In particular, it is clear from Fig. 5.2 that highly endemic areas (those where a high proportion of humans are infected, and where the stability index a/μ is relatively large) will show a high proportion of mosquitoes infected, on the basis of this model; this equivalently follows from Equation (5.5), where

Table 5.2 Prevalence of malaria ('sporozoite rates') in *Anopheles balabacensis* in various regions, at various times. These data were compiled by Slooff and Verdrager (1972).

Prevalences (%)	Country	Authority
2.4	Sabah	McArthur (1947)
2.9	Sabah	Colless (1952)
0.6–1.0	Khmer	Eyles *et al.* (1964)
2.4–7.6	Khmer	Eyles *et al.* (1964)
2.3	Vietnam	Hien (1968)
3.4	India	Clark and Choudhury (1941)
8.7	Thailand	Scanlon and Sandhinand (1965)
6.7	Thailand	Scanlon and Sandhinand (1965)
6.0	Thailand	Scanlon *et al.* (1967)
3.0	West Malaysia	Cheong (1968)

$y^* \simeq 1$ when R and a/μ are significantly greater than unity. But, as shown in Table 5.2, data on the sporozoite rates in mosquitoes – the percentage carrying infectious sporozoites – give values of at most a few per cent, even in very heavily endemic regions.

This particular fault can be remedied by taking explicit account of the incubation period, or latent period, of the parasite within the mosquito. The two categories of mosquito (uninfected and infected-and-infectious) are now replaced by three categories: a proportion, $1 - y - z$, that are uninfected; a proportion y that are infected and infectious; and a third, new proportion z that are latent (infected but not yet infectious). If the incubation interval in the mosquito has duration τ, Equation (5.2) in the basic model is replaced by the two dynamical equations:

$$dz/dt = ax(1 - y - z) - a\hat{x}(1 - \hat{y} - \hat{z})e^{-\mu\tau} - \mu z \qquad (5.6)$$
$$dy/dt = a\hat{x}(1 - \hat{y} - \hat{z})e^{-\mu\tau} - \mu y \qquad (5.7)$$

Here, the circumflex denotes evaluation at time τ in the past:

$$\hat{x} \equiv x(t - \tau); \text{ etc.} \qquad (5.8)$$

The proportion of latent mosquitoes increases, as before, at a rate proportional to encounters between infected humans and uninfected mosquitoes $(ax(1 - y - z))$, and decreases owing to deaths (μz) and transitions into the infective state by the surviving mosquitoes that were recruited into the latent class at time τ in the past $(a\hat{x}(1 - \hat{y} - \hat{z})e^{-\mu\tau})$. The proportion of infective mosquitoes increases by recruitment from the latent class, and decreases owing to deaths (μy).

The equation for the change in the proportion of humans infected remains unaltered, so that the dynamical system is now described by Equations (5.1), (5.6) and (5.7). The equilibrium solution is found by putting $dx/dt = 0$,

$dy/dt = 0$ and $dz/dt = 0$, and solving the ensuing set of algebraic equations. The basic reproductive rate of the malaria parasite is now:

$$\hat{R} = \frac{ma^2be^{-\mu\tau}}{r\mu} \qquad (5.9)$$

where b is now the proportion of bites by sporozoite-bearing mosquitoes that result in infection. That is, the effect of the latent period is to diminish the R of the earlier model (Equation (5.3)) by the factor $\exp(-\mu\tau)$. The expression for the equilibrium proportion of humans infected, x^*, is again given by Equation (5.4), except that $\hat{R}$ replaces R. The equilibrium proportion of mosquitoes infected, however, becomes:

$$y^* = \left(\frac{\hat{R}-1}{\hat{R}}\right)\left(\frac{a/\mu}{1+a/\mu}\right)e^{-\mu\tau} \qquad (5.10)$$

In effect, the earlier results are modified in two ways: the $\hat{R}$ of Equation (5.9) replaces the R of Equation (5.3) throughout, and the proportion of mosquitoes infected is rescaled by the factor $\exp(-\mu\tau)$. In other words, x^* can still approach unity, but y^* cannot exceed $\exp(-\mu\tau)$. As the average life span of infected mosquitoes is often significantly less than the latent period ($\mu\tau$ significantly greater than unity), y^* can be a few per cent even when $\hat{R}$ and a/μ are significantly greater than unity.

This relatively simple refinement, which goes a long way to making the model more realistic, has been discussed by Ross (1911) and Macdonald (1957). It is surprising that the similar latent periods exhibited by helminth parasites in their intermediate (arthropod or molluscan) hosts have only recently been incorporated into the corresponding basic models; in particular, theory and reality can thus be brought closer for the transmission dynamics of schistosomiasis (Anderson and May, 1979b; May, 1977b).

Macdonald (1957) drew from Equation (5.9) the important qualitative conclusion that imagicides are more effective than larvicides. The larval survivorship enters into $\hat{R}$ linearly, via the absolute mosquito population density M/N; in contrast, the adult mosquito survivorship enters in a highly non-linear way, via the factor $\exp(-\mu\tau)/\mu$ (or even, allowing for the concomitant effects on mosquito density, via the factor $\exp(-\mu\tau)/\mu^2$). Reduction of larval recruitment by a factor 2 would only halve the basic reproductive rate $\hat{R}$, but a doubling of the adult mortality rate (doubling of μ) would produce an exponentially severe decrease in $\hat{R}$. The change in emphasis in control measures directed against the mosquito vectors of malaria, largely as a consequence of Macdonald's insights, is described by Harrison (1978).

5.5   VARIABLE MOSQUITO DENSITY

Macdonald (1957) used the simple model to make broad geographical comparisons between the 'stable' malaria of Africa and the 'unstable' malaria of parts of India. On a more local scale, the model suggests that areas of greater transmission will be less sensitive to fluctuations in the transmission rate caused by large changes in the mosquito populations. An example illustrates this. In Ceylon (now Sri Lanka), before control by DDT, there was considerable local variation in the endemicity of malaria (as measured by the proportion of children with enlarged spleens, a conventional indicator of intensity of malarial transmission (see Boyd, 1949a, p. 595)). Figures 5.3(a) and 5.3(b) are hospital records of monthly malaria cases, over several years, from two different localities. Although Fig. 5.3(a), for the region of greater transmission, shows variability (and marked decline in the years following World War II), it nevertheless has a steady seasonal pattern from year to year. The region of lesser transmission, illustrated in Fig. 5.3(b), is prone to severe outbreaks which subside.

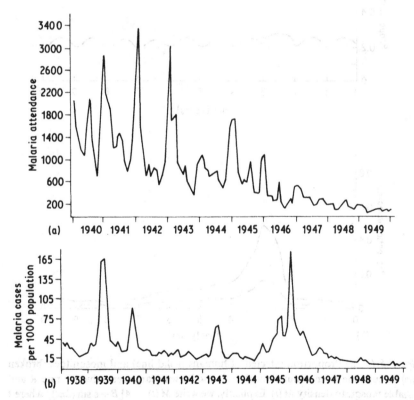

Figure 5.3 (a) Monthly malaria attendance at the Civil Hospital in Anuradhapura in the endemic zone of Ceylon (now Sri Lanka). Reproduced with permission from Rajendram and Jayewickreme (1951b), p. 93. (b) Monthly malaria attendance per 1000 population in the upper catchments of the Deduru Oya and Maha Oya basins in the epidemic zone of Ceylon (now Sri Lanka). Reproduced with permission from Rajendram and Jayewickreme (1951a), p. 29.

The basic model of Equations (5.1) and (5.2) demonstrates this pattern nicely if the total mosquito population, M, varies seasonally with an amplitude that fluctuates randomly from year to year. Figure 5.4(a) shows the dynamical behaviour of such a system when the transmission rate is very high (average value of $R \gg 1$), and Fig. 5.4(b) illustrates the behaviour when the transmission rate is just above the critical sustaining level (average value of R slightly above

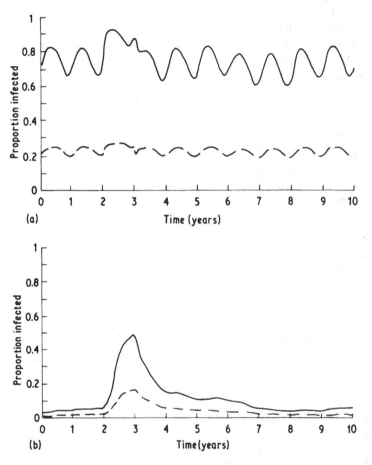

Figure 5.4 (a) Proportion infected of humans (solid line) and mosquitoes (broken line) versus time from simulation of basic model with large reproductive rate R and variable mosquito density $M(t)$. Explicitly, we write $M(t) = A[B + \varepsilon \sin (2\pi t)]$ where t is measured in years. Here, $B = 50$, $\varepsilon = 20$, and A is a random sequence which fluctuates around unity during the first half of the year (upper half of sine wave), but is otherwise equal to unity. The parameters used in the simulation are $a = 20 \, \text{year}^{-1}$, $\mu = 50 \, \text{year}^{-1}$, $r = 4 \, \text{year}^{-1}$, $N = 20$, $b = 1$. When $M = B$, $R = 5$. (b) Same as for (a) with small reproductive rate R. Here, $B = 10.5$ and $\varepsilon = 1$, and A, a, μ, r, N and b are the same as for (a). When $M = B$, $R = 1.05$.

unity). In both cases, the systems are subject to the same kind of (multiplicatively random) fluctuations, but the latter is much more affected than the former. Areas of low transmission are also more sensitive to sudden non-seasonal drops in the mosquito density, as happened when the plain of Philippi in Macedonia had a big drop in malaria following a dry year, while the neighbouring plain of Chrysoupolis (where malaria is more endemic) was scarcely affected (Boyd, 1949b, p. 642).

The regular changes in mosquito population density caused by seasonality also explain some interesting patterns in the overall dynamics of malaria. It is obvious that a rise in the mosquito population can lead to a malaria epidemic among the human hosts, but less obvious when the maximum prevalence of malaria among mosquitoes should occur. Peters and Standfast (1960, p. 251) note an inverse relationship, over the year, between mosquito population size and sporozoite rate. More detailed studies show the peak of mosquito density occurs either before (Boyd, 1949b, p. 636) or during (Christophers, 1949, p. 703) the peak of human malaria cases, but that the maximum prevalence (the peak sporozoite rate) among mosquitoes follows both the human peak (Boyd, 1949b, p. 637) and the peak of mosquito abundance (Boyd, 1949b, pp. 633, 634, 635). These observations are summarized in Table 5.3.

Boyd himself views the rise in the prevalence of malaria among the mosquito population as an epizootic, and sees a difficulty in having the mosquito prevalence peak after the human prevalence peaks; he suggests that the autumn epizootic may, in fact, be the delayed cause of the human epidemic in the following spring. We do not subscribe to this view. Although mosquitoes

Table 5.3 Results indicating the relative timing of peaks in annual cycles of total numbers of mosquitoes, proportion of mosquitoes infected (sporozoite rate), and prevalence of malaria in humans (from data summarized by Boyd, 1949b, pp. 634–637). Unfortunately, none of the studies gives information about all three quantities, but the pairwise comparisons suggest a consistent pattern, which is further discussed in the text.

Mosquito species	Geographical region and date	Peak in mosquito numbers	Peak in prevalence of malaria among humans	Peak in prevalence of malaria among mosquitoes
A. gambiae	Southern Nigeria, 1930	June–July*	–	Sept.
A. funestus	Philippines, 1931	Jan.–March*	–	May
A. quadrimaculatus	Alabama, 1924	Sept.	Oct.	–
	Alabama, 1925	July	Aug.	–
A. maculipennis	Holland, 1920–1922	–	June	Oct.–Nov.

* A crude estimate, assuming the number of mosquitoes examined roughly reflects their absolute abundance.

are often present during the season of relatively low transmission (in Boyd's case, winter in Holland), it is not necessary to invoke a mosquito reservoir to explain the gap between the rises in mosquito prevalence and human prevalence. Our view of the sequence of events is that, at first, mosquito density rises due to the seasonal increase in the number of emerging adults. As the total density rises, the density of infected mosquitoes also rises, followed by the peak in human cases. The rise in prevalence among mosquitoes occurs after the peak in human cases, not just from incubation delays, but because by then fewer mosquitoes are emerging into the population to swell the ranks of the uninfected mosquitoes, thus causing the proportion found infected to increase. This explanation has also been indicated by Peters and Standfast (1960) who, however, also implicate seasonal variations in longevity of mosquitoes as part of the explanation (whereas we do not believe this to be necessary).

This argument is set out schematically in Fig. 5.5. The mosquito population starts out with two classes of individuals: susceptible (s) and infected (i). The initial population comprises 400 s and 100 i, to give a prevalence of 20%; both classes undergo a mortality of 75% up to the next time interval. In Fig. 5.5(a), the immigration of new mosquitoes (i.e. emergence) into the uninfected class is high (500), and the infection rate from s to i is 10%. At the beginning of the next time interval, there will consequently be 590 s and 35 i, for a prevalence of 6% (the outcome of this calculation is independent of whether the infected individuals are transferred from s to i before or after applying the mortality factor). In Fig. 5.5(b), the infection rate is reduced to 5%, but the emergence is also drastically reduced to 20. Here, at the start of the next time interval, there will be 115 s and 30 i, for a prevalence of 21%. Although in Fig. 5.5(b) there is a lower rate of infection, there is actually an increase in prevalence, while in Fig. 5.5(a) there is a decrease in prevalence. The basic point is that prevalence in a population of mosquitoes, with short life spans, can vary very differently from that of the human population.

Exactly these patterns can be produced by the basic model of Equations (5.1) and (5.2) with a mosquito population that undergoes purely seasonal changes. For the dynamics of the mosquito population, M, we write:

$$dM/dt = E(t) - \mu M \qquad (5.11)$$

Here μ is as defined earlier, and $E(t)$ is the rate of emergence. We take $E(t)$ to vary sinusoidally over the year; the mosquito density will then also be sinusoidal, with a lag of about the mean life time of a mosquito. Note we have assumed the variation in mosquito density to arise from the periodicity in the rate of emergence; the mortality rate may also vary, but (as previously stated) the overall changes in emergence rate are likely to be more important. Equation (5.1), for the proportion of humans infected, is as before. Equation (5.2), for the proportion of mosquitoes infected, was derived under the assumption that the total number of mosquitoes was constant; this equation now becomes:

$$dy/dt = ax(1 - y) - [\mu + (dM/dt)/M]y \qquad (5.12)$$

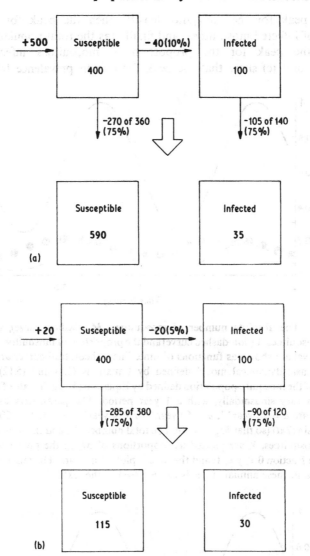

Figure 5.5 As discussed more fully in the text, this figure illustrates schematically how the number of susceptible and infected mosquitoes changes from one time interval to the next, under different assumptions about the rate of emergence of adult mosquitoes and about the infection rate. In (a), with a relatively high rate of emergence, the prevalence of infection is decreasing. In (b), with a low rate of emergence, the prevalence of infection is increasing, even though the infection rate in (b) is lower than in (a).

The steady annual cycles to which the solutions of this system of Equations (5.1), (5.11) and (5.12) tend are illustrated in Figs 5.6 and 5.7. Fig. 5.6 shows first the peak for the mosquito density, then the peak for the total number of infected mosquitoes, and finally (as the total population is declining) the peak for the proportion of mosquitoes infected. Figs 5.7(a), (b) and (c) show that the peak for human prevalence follows the

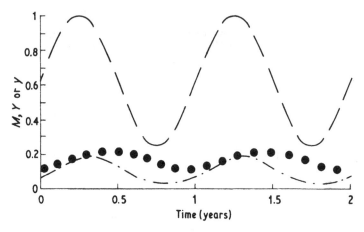

Figure 5.6 The absolute number of mosquitoes, M (dashed curve), number of infected mosquitoes, Y (dot–dashed curve) and the proportion of mosquitoes infected, y (dotted curve) are shown as functions of time. These theoretical curves are obtained from the basic dynamical model defined by Equations (5.1) and (5.12), with the dynamics of the mosquito population defined by Equation (5.11); the rate of emergence is taken to vary sinusoidally, with a 1 year period. The parameters used in this simulation are $a = 20$ year^{-1}, $\mu = 50$ year^{-1}, $r = 4$ year^{-1}, $b = 1$, $N = 20$ and $M(t) = 25 + 15 \sin(2\pi t)$ (so that $M_{max} = 40$). The total number, M, and the total number of infected mosquitoes, Y, are plotted as proportions of M_{max}; the prevalence y is by definition a fraction $0 \leqslant y \leqslant 1$; and the time is plotted in years. The relative timing of the maxima in these annual cycles is as discussed in the text.

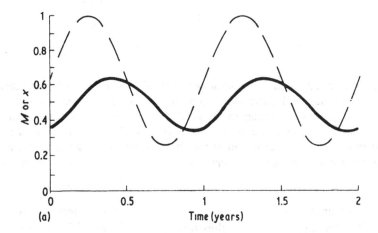

(a)

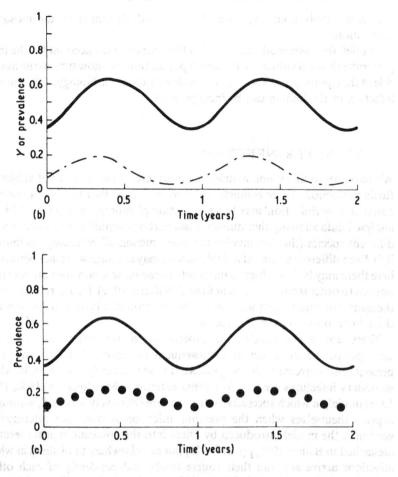

Figure 5.7 (a) The total mosquito population, M (dashed curve) and the proportion of humans infected, x (solid curve), are plotted as functions of time; the units are as in Fig. 5.6. (b) The absolute number of infected mosquitoes, Y (dot–dashed curve) and the prevalence of malaria among humans (solid curve) are shown together, as functions of time. (c) The prevalence of malaria among mosquitoes, y (dotted curve) and among humans x (solid curve) are shown together. In all three figures, the relative timing of the maxima in the annual cycles accords with observations, as discussed in the text and shown in Table 5.3.

maximum both for total density and for the number of infected mosquitoes, but precedes the maximum for the mosquito prevalence. This basic model does not incorporate incubation periods, the inclusion of which would accentuate the lags. Latency is important in determining the exact timing of the peaks and the nature of the reservoir for more realistic models of seasonal malaria transmission (Dietz *et al.*, 1974), but the relative timing during the transmission season is simply a consequence of the growth dynamics of the mosquito population.

In brief, the basic model can – with a few refinements – account for the main patterns exhibited within the mosquito population. We now turn to the human side of the equation and investigate how details about the biology of the parasite infection in the human can be incorporated.

5.6 SUPERINFECTION

We have, up to this point, assumed that an infected human is not subject to further infection. There is much evidence to suggest that this is not the case, and that 'superinfection' may be an important phenomenon. Cohen (1973) has analysed data showing that human hosts harbour simultaneous infections by different species (this can involve the phenomenon of 'heterologous immunity'). Even different strains of a single species may act somewhat independently; here there may be homologous immunity to the same strain after an infection, but not to other strains (at least at first; Taliaferro, 1949). Lastly, reinfection by the same strain may occur when homologous immunity is slow to develop, as is thought to occur with *P. falciparum*.

There are several models for superinfection, forming a continuum of descriptions for the effect of a subsequent infection when one already is present. One extreme is the original Ross model, already discussed, in which secondary infections are lost. The other extreme is Macdonald's (1950, 1957, 1973) model, in which successive infections are effectively 'stacked', waiting to express themselves when the previous infection is over. An intermediate version is the model introduced by Dietz into the epidemiological literature (described in Bailey, 1975, pp. 317–322; but not elsewhere published) in which infections arrive and run their course totally independently of each other. (Incidentally, Macdonald's version was intended to correspond to the situation described by Dietz, but there was a misunderstanding; see Fine, 1975b.) We have constructed yet other models, nested between those of Ross and of Dietz, in which superinfections are successively easier to shed, rather than being totally independent of each other; this may well be a more realistic class of models, but the above three are sufficient to illustrate the main points that arise. These various assumptions may be compactly written by replacing Equation (5.1) with the more general form:

$$dx/dt = h(1 - x) - \rho x \qquad (5.13)$$

Here h is the infection rate (Ross' 'happenings'), previously written in the more detailed form:

$$h = (abM/N)y$$

The quantity ρ is the rate of reversion to the uninfected state, and is defined variously as:

$$\text{Ross: } \rho = r \tag{5.14}$$

$$\text{Dietz: } \rho = h/[\exp{(h/r)} - 1] \tag{5.15}$$

$$\left. \begin{array}{ll} \text{Macdonald: } \rho = r - h & (r > h) \\ \rho = 0 & (r < h) \end{array} \right\} \tag{5.16}$$

As before r is the rate of recovery from a single infection.

Contrary to what is sometimes implied in Macdonald's writings, the different assumptions about the nature of superinfection make for quantitative, rather than qualitative, differences in the overall dynamical behaviour. This can be seen by returning to the phase–plane analysis of Fig. 5.2, and replacing the x-isocline (along which $dx/dt = 0$) of the original Ross model by the corresponding x-isocline generated by the Dietz and Macdonald formulae. This is done in Fig. 5.8. There is no difference among the models at low

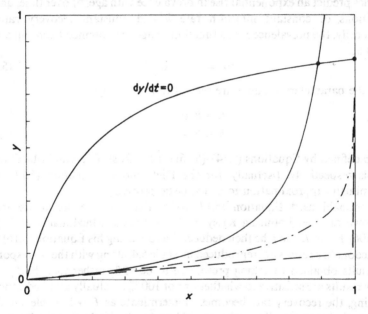

Figure 5.8 The phase–plane of the dynamical variables x and y is depicted, as in Fig. 5.2. Here the y-isocline, along which the proportion of mosquitoes infected is unchanging, is as before. The x-isocline, along which the proportion of humans infected is unchanging, is, however, calculated under various assumptions about the nature of superinfection: the solid curve, as before, assumes no superinfection (Ross model); the dashed curve makes the opposite extreme assumption of 'stacked' infections (Macdonald model); the intermediate dot–dashed curve corresponds to the Dietz model described in the text. Note that all three models are essentially the same at low prevalence levels, and that the qualitative dynamics are similar; the detailed locations of the equilibrium points are, however, different for the three models.

prevalence levels, so that the basic reproductive rate R is the same for all three, and all three have the same basic criterion for maintenance of the infection. This is intuitively obvious; superinfection is irrelevant at low prevalence levels. On the other hand, the equilibrium values of the proportions of humans and of mosquitoes infected, x^* and y^*, do depend on how superinfection is described. As one moves from the original Ross model, to that of Dietz, to that of Macdonald, both x^* and y^* increase somewhat. Thus the details, but not the overall stability properties, are affected by the specific assumptions made about superinfection (see also Dietz, 1980).

5.7 DISCRIMINATING AMONG MODELS FOR SUPERINFECTION

It is, however, difficult to test the differences among these theories. All three theories predict an exponential rise in prevalence with age, or over time, under conditions of constant infection rate h and constant recovery rate r. Specifically, the prevalence x as a function of age t is obtained from Equation (5.13) as:

$$x(t) = L(1 - e^{-kt}) \qquad (5.17)$$

Here the parameters L and k are related to h and r by:

$$L = h/(h + \rho) \qquad (5.18)$$

$$k = h + \rho \qquad (5.19)$$

with ρ defined by Equations (5.14)–(5.16) for the Ross, Dietz and Macdonald models respectively. (Actually, for the Dietz model, Equation (5.17) is a deterministic approximation to a stochastic process.)

Macdonald used Equation (5.17) to fit data on age–prevalence from Freetown and neighbouring Kissy in Sierra Leone (Macdonald, 1973, pp. 104–106). From L and k he then deduced h and r, using his Equation (5.16) for ρ. Macdonald's results are reproduced in Table 5.4, along with the corresponding results obtained by taking prevalence to be 99 % rather than 100 %. We see his results are sensitive to whether or not 100 % is actually attained; strictly speaking, the recovery rate becomes indeterminate as $L \rightarrow 1$. Table 5.4 also presents the corresponding estimates of h and r obtained using the Ross and the Dietz descriptions of superinfection. In principle, the different estimates of r given by the different models provide a means of distinguishing among them. We will return to this in a moment.

The difficulties inherent in extracting information from prevalence curves make it desirable to have some independent way of estimating rates. The infection rate can be so estimated if one knows the proportion of individuals ever infected, as a function of age. This quantity, $w(t)$, obeys the differential equation:

$$dw/dt = h(1 - w) \qquad (5.20)$$

Table 5.4 Values of infection rate h and intrinsic recovery rate r, deduced from various data (for L and k) under different assumptions about superinfection (as discussed in the text).

Data			Infection rate $h = kL$ (day^{-1}) for all models	Recovery rate r (day^{-1})		
Place and date	Value of L	Value of k (day^{-1})		Macdonald	Dietz	Ross
Freetown, 1925	0.41	0.005	0.0021	0.005	0.0039	0.0030
Freetown, 1933	0.88	0.005	0.0044	0.005	0.0021	0.0006
Freetown, 1947	0.065	0.005	0.0003	0.005	0.0048	0.0047
Kissy, 1933	1.0	0.013	0.013	(0.013)*	0	0
Kissy, taking L to be 99%	0.99	0.013	0.013	0.013	0.0028	0.0001

* Strictly, r is not determinable in the Macdonald model if $L = 1.0$.

whence

$$w(t) = 1 - e^{-ht} \qquad (5.21)$$

Thus longitudinal (cohort) studies of infants in heavily infected areas can be used to get a direct estimate of h (Pull and Grab, 1974). Combining Equations (5.18) and (5.19), we see that in all three models for superinfection h, L and k are simply related by:

$$h = Lk \qquad (5.22)$$

In brief, h, k and L obey a universal relation, independent of the model for superinfection. Thus independent measurement of the three quantities provides consistency checks, but no discrimination among the models. On the other hand, given any two of the above quantities, we can calculate a value for r, and this value does depend on the superinfection model chosen. Fig. 5.9 shows the general relation between r and the variables k and L. Note that for given k and L, the Ross model gives the lowest, and the Macdonald model the highest, value for r. Similar figures could be produced, and the same conclusion drawn, for r as a function of h and L or of h and k.

It follows that Fig. 5.9 could be used to determine the correct description of the superinfection process, provided that we had some independent way of estimating r. However, the measurement of natural recovery rates is fraught with difficulties, and there is a paucity of good data. Measurements in the field are beset with problems of detectability and reinfection. In hospitals, there are usually ethical barriers to the administration of controlled infections or the withholding of drugs (except, rarely, as a part of some other therapy, which will usually confound the results anyway).

Macdonald based his independent estimate of the recovery rate from *P. falciparum* on data from Puerto Rico by Earle *et al.* (1939), which gave

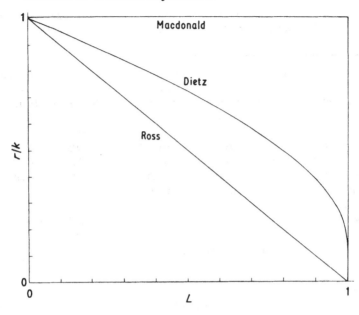

Figure 5.9 This figure shows the relation between the intrinsic recovery rate, *r*, and the quantities *k* and *L* that are obtained from data on age–prevalence curves, under various assumptions about the nature of the superinfection process. Under all assumptions, *r* is directly proportional to *k*, and we can therefore plot *r/k* as a function of *L*; the dependence of *r/k* on *L* differs among the Ross, Dietz and Macdonald models, as shown. Note that the inferred value of *r* will always be least for the Ross model, and greatest for the Macdonald model.

$r = 0.005$/day. On this basis, he concluded his model was superior to that without superinfection (the Ross model), because the recovery rates inferred from it (see Table 5.4) were closer to the actual rate of 0.005. This story is quite dependent on the choice of the independent value of *r*. Recently, Nájera (1974) and Fine (1975b) have commented that the actual number of people followed up in the Earle *et al.* (1939) study was fewer than Macdonald thought. Earle's own conclusion from the data was to set the recovery rate significantly lower than 0.005.

Given all the additional variation among parasite strains and among racial groups of people, it seems unlikely that *r* can be estimated to an accuracy sufficient to discriminate among models. However, the phenomenon of superinfection, *per se*, can be tested by comparative studies between two populations in which intrinsic recovery rates are essentially identical. All models of superinfection, except the original limiting case of no superinfection, have the property that observed recovery rates should decrease as infection rates increase, provided that the underlying recovery-rate-per-infected, *r*, is unchanged.

One kind of comparison is between closely adjacent villages with different transmission rates. Presumably, the racial groups are the same and the strains in the area are the same. The problem of mixing between the populations would tend to obliterate differences, making this a conservative test; if there are apparent differences, they are probably real. One such candidate is a longitudinal study of two villages in Thailand (Segal et al., 1974) in which infections in children in the area of greater transmission showed greater tendency to persist throughout the transmission season. The roughness of the resolution was such that it is impossible to say whether each individual infection was cleared before a new one started, but because infections in children tend to be long-lived, it is likely that the persisting positive samples represent continued infection. In other words, these data indicate that in the area of heavier transmission infections last longer, as any model of superinfection would predict. However, these data are at best suggestive, because of the complicating use of drugs and the greater transience of one of the populations.

Another, and usually easier, kind of comparison consists of obtaining information about the seasonal variation in recovery rates for a single group of people. If the apparent recovery rate depends on the inoculation rate, one would expect to see longer 'recovery times' during the transmission season, and shorter bouts during off season. There are two good sets of data for this kind of analysis: Krafsur and Armstrong (1978) from Ethiopia and Bekessy et al. (1976) from Nigeria. Both are longitudinal studies of recovery rates for different age groups. Interestingly, the pattern of superinfection is only partly proven. Only adults show the expected pattern, with the recovery rate being faster when transmission is reduced; there is little seasonality in the children's recovery rate. The apparent discrepancy arises because individual infections are longer-lived in children, and the infections acquired during the transmission season persist through the low-transmission season; the seasonal variation in transmission rate is being masked by the children's slow recovery rates. Because adults clear infections more quickly – itself an interesting phenomenon to which we turn below – seasonal variation in the apparent recovery rate has a chance to express itself.

In summary, the concept of superinfection is an important one that explains some general aspects of patterns of prevalence. The different models proposed to account for superinfection cannot, however, be crisply distinguished on the basis of existing data. Macdonald's model does not appear to be correct, because there is no evidence for an infection 'waiting' for another to leave, nor was this Macdonald's intention. Dietz's model, which does express Macdonald's original intention, is probably too simple by virtue of ignoring immunity and possible competition among parasites. Molineaux et al. (1980) have shown that parasite species do not seem to be independently assorted among individuals, but rather show a positive association. It is clear that immunity must be considered, if our understanding is to become more precise.

5.8 IMMUNITY: COMPARTMENTAL MODELS

One of the most important interactions between different infections is the acquisition of immunity as a consequence of infection. Models for the transmission dynamics of malaria have, however, only recently begun to take account of this phenomenon. The earlier models, discussed in the preceding sections, are oriented toward understanding how to eradicate the disease; the question is how to remove the last few infected members of a population, and therefore superinfection and immune processes are of little interest. Only since the WHO global eradication campaign based on application of DDT and drugs has failed has interest in the natural dynamics of the disease – including immunity – resurged.

This interest in immunity is further stimulated by the goal of inducing artificial immunity with vaccines. Experimental vaccination of non-human animals has already demonstrated the induction of immunity against various specific stages of malaria: sporozoites (Nussenzweig, 1977); merozoites (S. Cohen, 1979; Wellde et al., 1979); and gametocytes (Carter and Chen, 1976; Mendis and Targett, 1979). Vaccination with irradiated sporozoites has also been demonstrated to induce immunity in man (Rieckmann et al., 1974), although, as with all vaccinations of animals, the results are highly variable. These developments have motivated more detailed studies of the natural dynamics of immunity to malaria, as a prerequisite to any possible assessment of the efficacy of vaccines.

In natural situations, the result of acquired immunity in regions of intense transmission is a restriction of the clinical pathology of malaria to young age groups. One consequence is that, for example, eradication of malaria in Guyana reduced the number of malaria-related deaths among children, but had little effect on adult mortality rates (Giglioli, 1972). Genetic studies have shown that the sickle-cell trait, which protects heterozygous carriers from death or debility caused by severe bouts of malaria, confers its advantages mainly during the first few years of life (in natural circumstances, before control programmes; Fleming et al., 1979).

The standard characterization of the epidemiology of malaria is an age–prevalence curve, showing the proportion of each age group whose blood slides have parasites present. In hyperendemic areas, the prevalence peaks at an early age and then declines slowly; at the same time, the number of parasites found in those slides positive for parasites decreases relatively quickly with age (see Fig. 5.10). Such an age–prevalence curve is fairly easy to obtain, because it involves only one survey of a population; it is a single slice through time, a cross-sectional study.

Unfortunately, age–prevalence studies by themselves do not enable us to sort out the various components of acquired immunity, because the observed curves can be fitted by many different models, including some quite absurd ones. For example, consider the hypothetical circumstance in which everyone

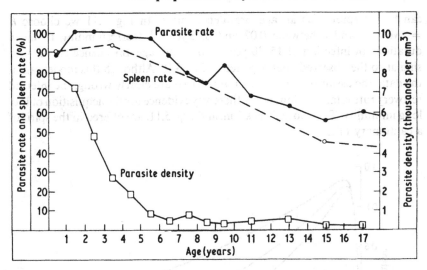

Figure 5.10 Malaria survey in hyperendemic area of Tanganyika (now Tanzania). The parasite rate is the percentage of the age group with blood samples positive for malaria. The spleen rate is the percentage of the age group with enlarged spleens. The parasite density is the number of parasites per cubic millimeter (in thousands) in those blood samples which were positive for the parasites. Reproduced with permission from Christophers (1949), p. 700.

is born susceptible, becomes infected (at some constant rate h) and then recovers (at some constant rate r) to become permanently immune to further infection. Letting x, y and z stand for susceptibles, infecteds and immunes respectively, we can describe the dynamics by the following 'catalytic model' (Muench, 1959):

$$dx/dt = -hx \qquad (5.23)$$
$$dy/dt = hx - ry \qquad (5.24)$$
$$dz/dt = ry \qquad (5.25)$$

The initial condition is $x(0) = 1$, and it follows that

$$x(t) + y(t) + z(t) = 1$$

for all times t. This set of equations can easily be integrated, to obtain an explicit description of the experience of a cohort moving through time. Moreover, if the rates remain constant for a few generations, the age–prevalence from a single cross-sectional survey should be equivalent to the life history of the oldest cohort. In other words, the expression for prevalence as a function of time,

$$y(t) = [e^{-rt} - e^{-ht}][h/(h-r)] \qquad (5.26)$$

can be interpreted as an age–prevalence curve. In Fig. 5.11 we choose h = 2 year^{-1} and r between 0.07 and 0.03 year^{-1} (corresponding to mean durations of infection of 15–30 years), to obtain age–prevalence curves very similar to the observed ones depicted in Fig. 5.10. Although this model can fit the data, the assumptions on which it is based are clearly wrong; the inferred recovery rate is far too slow, nor is there any evidence for the acquisition of life-long immunity. The above discussion, and Fig. 5.11, are offered in the spirit of a cautionary tale.

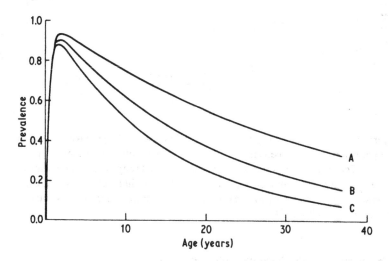

Figure 5.11   Prevalence of infection versus age in years according to Equation (5.26), derived from the simple model with life-long immunity. A single infection rate h is used with three different recovery rates r: h = 2.0 year^{-1}; and (A) r = 0.03 year^{-1}, (B) r = 0.05 year^{-1}, (C) r = 0.07 year^{-1}.

Bekessy *et al.* (1976) have analysed the epidemiology of malaria (mostly *P. falciparum*) in Nigeria, using a study in which individuals were followed over several years (a longitudinal survey). They argue that the decline in prevalence with age is due primarily to a decline in the intensity of the parasite burden, coupled with a greater ability of older hosts to suppress parasites once they are acquired. A marked seasonal pattern in parasitaemia continues even for the adults, indicating that they are still susceptible.

Dietz *et al.* (1974) have incorporated these ideas into a model of malarial epidemiology which is, to date, the most practical and realistic one. In it, there are two classes of individuals: one class has a slow recovery rate from malaria, and all infections can be detected; the other class has a fast recovery rate, and infections only have a 70% chance of being detected (owing to the low densities of parasites). Both classes repeatedly are exposed, become infected and recover, remaining within their own class except for a fixed rate of transition from the relatively susceptible class to the relatively immune class (with this transition rate being determined by fitting the model to the data). This model is illustrated schematically in Fig. 5.12. The model gives a good fit to the observed variation in malaria prevalence by age and by season in the Nigerian baseline study. Furthermore, the model applies fairly well to the epidemiology of another hyperendemic area, in Kenya (Molineaux *et al.*, 1978).

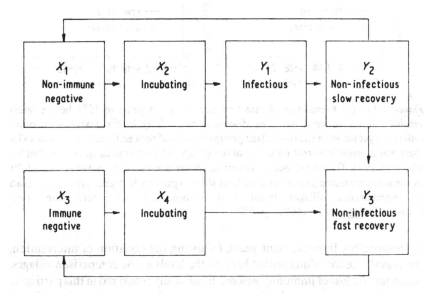

Figure 5.12 Schematic illustration of the malaria model of Dietz *et al.* (1974). As discussed more fully in the text, the diagram shows the various categories of individuals considered in the model, and possible transitions between categories.

There remains the question, however, of how well the model will apply as the epidemiological circumstances depart more and more from the natural and highly endemic areas in Africa. Such departures arise either in the consideration of quite different geographical regions, or from modification of the local epidemiology by massive intervention. One deficiency in the model of Dietz *et al.* is its failure to account for the loss of immunity that occurs when transmission is significantly reduced. For villages in the same Nigerian study used by Dietz *et al.* (1974), Cornille–Brögger *et al.* (1978) showed that two transmission seasons with massive intervention in the form of drug administration and anti-mosquito spraying were followed, in the next transmission season (lacking such intervention), by a higher-than-usual prevalence of malaria (measured as a proportion with positive blood slides). Figure 5.13 illustrates the results of these studies, showing the relative rise in prevalence in 1974 for those over 10 years old (younger individuals were still given drugs

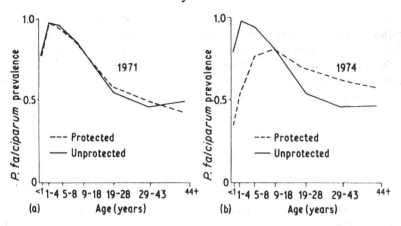

Figure 5.13 (a) Prevalence of infection versus age in years in 1971 before inter-vention, in an endemic area, as discussed more fully in the text. There is no difference yet between the two village groups (solid and broken line). In 1972 and 1973, there was massive intervention in one of the groups, which was subsequently halted for adults in 1974. (b) Prevalence of infection versus age in years in 1974. The adults in the once-protected group (broken line) show significantly higher prevalences than the comparative villages (solid line). Reproduced with permission from Cornille–Brögger *et al.* (1978), p. 582.

systematically). In subsequent years, following the cessation of intervention, the prevalence for adults settled back to the levels in the comparison villages. Although the loss of immunity was small and easily recovered in this particular study the phenomenon is clearly important for general models of epidemiological processes. Pringle and Avery–Jones (1966) have demonstrated similar effects in African children; after the children had been put on anti-malarial drugs for a few weeks, and then taken off drugs, they had larger parasitaemias than at the start of the study. In short, it seems that continued exposure helps maintain immunity.

A simple way to incorporate this mechanism is as follows. Suppose there are three classes of individuals: susceptibles, infecteds and immunes. Assume that immunity lasts for some fixed interval of time, τ, in the absence of re-exposure, but that if a person is further exposed before τ time units have elapsed, immunity is sustained and another interval of duration τ without exposure is required before immunity is lost (this model is also known as the process of particle counting with a type II counter: Karlin and Taylor, 1975; p. 179). If infective exposures arrive at a constant mean rate h, in an independently random way (a Poisson process), the average time spent in the immune state can be calculated. First, some definitions:

$$p = \text{probability of infection after time } \tau = \exp(-h\tau) \qquad (5.27)$$

$$q = \text{probability of infection before time } \tau = 1 - p, \qquad (5.28)$$

W = average interval between exposures given that the interval is
    less than $\tau = (1/h) - (\tau p/q)$ $\hspace{3cm}$ (5.29)

N = average number of infections until susceptible $= q/p$, $\hspace{0.5cm}$ (5.30)

T = average time interval in immune state $= WN + \tau$ $\hspace{1cm}$ (5.31)

The average rate of movement out of the immune state, γ, is then the inverse of the average time interval spent in the immune state; $\gamma = 1/T$. It follows that:

$$\gamma = hp/q \hspace{3cm} (5.32)$$

That is, substituting from Equations (5.27) and (5.28),

$$\gamma = h/[\exp(h\tau) - 1] \hspace{2.5cm} (5.33)$$

This result is illustrated in Fig. 5.14; the rate at which immunity is lost decreases as the infection rate increases.

This general description of the immune process can now be incorporated into a simple SIRS (susceptible-infected-recovered/immune-susceptible) catalytic model of the kind discussed earlier. Susceptible individuals are repeatedly infected, recover, enjoy temporary immunity, and again become susceptible (the model differs from the earlier SIR model of Equations (5.23)–(5.25) in that immunity is not permanent):

$$dx/dt = \gamma z - hx \hspace{3cm} (5.34)$$
$$dy/dt = hx - ry \hspace{3cm} (5.35)$$
$$dz/dt = ry - \gamma z \hspace{3cm} (5.36)$$

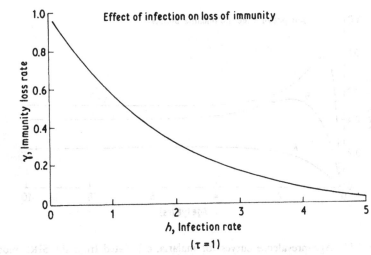

Figure 5.14 This figure shows the rate of loss of immunity, γ, as a function of the infection rate, h, for the model discussed in the text (Equation (5.33)). In this model, repeated infection helps maintain immunity. The 'immune interval', τ, is here taken to be 1.

As before, this linear set of differential equations can be integrated to construct age–prevalence curves, starting with 100% susceptibles [$x(0) = 1$]. The effect of varying the infection rate h can then be studied, under various assumptions about the immune processes.

Fig. 5.15 shows how variation in the infection rate h affects age–prevalence of malaria, when both the recovery rate r and the rate of loss of immunity γ are predetermined constants. As h increases, the prevalence increases in all age categories. In contrast, Fig. 5.16 shows how variation in h affects age–prevalence, when the immunity loss rate γ is coupled to h in the manner described by Equation (5.33) and Fig. 5.14. As the infection rate h increases, it remains true that the prevalence for children always increases, but the prevalence for adults at first increases and then decreases with increasing h; the age–prevalence curves for different values of h can now actually cross each other. The theoretical results displayed in Fig. 5.16 are similar to the patterns discussed and classified by Boyd, and illustrated in Fig. 5.17. In order to bring the curves in Fig. 5.16 into quantitative agreement with the data in Fig. 5.17, we have chosen the parameter values $r = 0.25\,\text{year}^{-1}$ and $\tau = 1.3\,\text{years}$. These parameter values are not unreasonable; the recovery time of roughly 4 years is a little too long, but the requirement for an immunity refresher within 1.3 years is consistent with the loss of immunity after a year and a half of intervention, as shown by Cornille–Brögger et al. (1978).

One important conclusion, with significant implications for control programmes, is illustrated in Fig. 5.18. This figure shows that, at relatively high

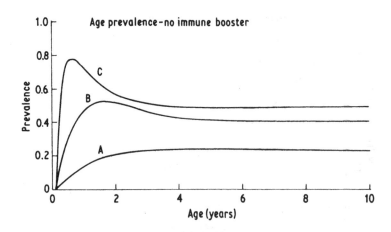

Figure 5.15 Age–prevalence curves for malaria, calculated from the SIRS model defined by Equations (5.34)–(5.36), assuming both the intrinsic recovery rate, r, and the rate of loss of immunity, γ, are constants, independent of the transmission rate, h (specifically, $r = 0.5\,\text{year}^{-1}$, $\gamma = 0.5\,\text{year}^{-1}$). The three curves, the general features of which are discussed in the text, are for: A, $h = 0.2\,\text{year}^{-1}$; B, $h = 1$; C, $h = 5$.

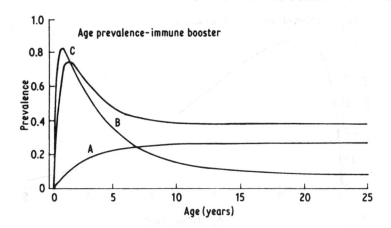

Figure 5.16 As for Fig. 5.15, except here the rate of loss of immunity, γ, depends on the transmission rate, h, in the manner described by Equation (5.33) and Fig. 5.14. Specifically, the figure is for $r = 0.25$ year^{-1} and $\tau = 1.3$ year; the three curves are for the different transmission rates; A, $h = 0.1$ year^{-1}; B, $h = 2$; C, $h = 4$. The features of these curves, and in particular the 'crossing over' phenomenon, are discussed more fully in the text.

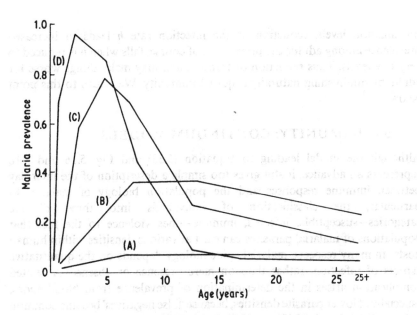

Figure 5.17 Prevalence of acture malaria infections versus age in years in stable indigenous populations for differing levels of endemicity: (A) low endemicity; (B) moderate endemicity; (C) high endemicity; (D) hyperendemicity. Reproduced with permission from Boyd (1949a), p. 571.

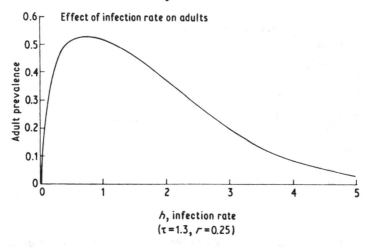

Figure 5.18 The prevalence of malaria among adults (people over the age of 20 years) is shown as a function of infection rate, h (plotted in units of year^{-1}), under the assumptions about the rate of loss of immunity that are defined by Equation (5.33) and Figs. 5.14 and 5.16. The parameters r and τ are chosen to be $r = 0.25$ year^{-1} and $\tau = 1.3$ years. The implications of this curve for public health and control programmes are discussed in the text.

transmission levels, reduction of the infection rate h leads to increased prevalence among adults; the prevalence, of course, falls when h is reduced to very low levels. Thus reduction of transmission may make things worse for adults by diminishing naturally acquired immunity. We return to this point below.

5.9 IMMUNITY: CONTINUUM MODELS

Although the model leading to Equation (5.33) and Fig. 5.16 and 5.18 represents an advance, it still gives too simple a description of the interplay between immune responses and the population biology of malaria. In particular, the classification of individuals into three discrete categories – susceptible, infected, immune – does violence to the fact that populations of malarial parasites can exist at various densities within human hosts. In many respects, malarial epidemiology depends on the quantitative aspects of infection, rather than on mere presence or absence. A related complication arises in the determination of prevalence from blood slides, especially at lower parasite densities, because 'false negatives' become common (Miller, 1958; Boyd, 1949a, p. 596). Aron (1982) has shown how such false negatives, which result in underestimation of the prevalence among older age groups, can also affect the statistics of infection and apparent recovery.

All detailed descriptions of the acquisition and loss of immunity, whether in the hospital or the natural environment, indicate that the phenomenon is gradual. In the studies of Cuica *et al.* (1934; cited in Brumpt, 1949, p. 102), in which *P. vivax* infections were administered for therapeutic reasons, there was a steady decline in the manifestation of clinical symptoms from the first inoculation to the fifth and last (which induced no clinical response). In natural settings in Nigeria, the age–prevalence curve rises over the first few years of life, but then shows a gradual decline until about the age of 20 years, after which the prevalence settles roughly to a chronic level (Dietz *et al.*, 1974). The gradual acquisition of immunity has also been demonstrated in rats by Zuckerman (1974), who showed that serum from immune rats (used to protect non-immune animals) became more and more effective as the number of infections given the immune donor rats increased. Conversely, Sergent and Poncet (1956) have shown loss of immunity in rats to be gradual; the longer the interval to a subsequent infection, the greater the proportion of rats producing para-sitaemias and the greater the intensity of the parasitaemias.

These facts suggest that an accurate model will need to abandon the approach of dividing people into discrete classes of infected and uninfected, and move toward a more detailed description in which the clinical symptoms and the immune response depend upon the magnitude of the parasite burden in the individual host. In the terminology of Anderson and May (1978, 1979a; see also May and Anderson, 1978, 1979), a rigorous discussion of the transmission dynamics of malaria will need to employ the continuum description appropriate to a 'macroparasite', rather than the simpler compart-mental models that typically serve as an adequate approximation for 'microparasites'. (A half-way house on this road could be to combine the above model relating immunity to infection rate with the model of Dietz *et al.* (1974), which has two different categories of infected individuals as well as loss of detectability in one of the immune classes.)

One such attempt to model the parasite population and the acquisition of immunity by continuum methods is by Elderkin *et al.* (1977), following a suggestion by Dietz. The dynamical variables in this model are: u, the population of asexual blood stages of malaria in the host; g, the population of gametocyte sexual stages in the host; and ω, the level of resistance (immunity) of the host. The system of partial differential equations permits all variables to be functions of both time, t, and the age, a, of the host. Under steady state conditions (when all time derivatives are zero) the model is then defined by the equations:

$$du/da = V \int_0^\infty \mu e^{-\mu a'} g(a') da' - \omega a \qquad (5.37)$$

$$dg/da = \gamma u e^{-\omega T} - \delta g \qquad (5.38)$$

$$d\omega/da = \alpha u - \beta(\omega - \omega_0) \qquad (5.39)$$

We make no attempt to discuss this model in detail, noting only that asexual stages are recruited from the gametocyte population indirectly via bites from infected mosquitoes (V is the 'vectorial capacity', proportional to the mosquito population density), and are destroyed by the immune process, whereas the sexual stages are recruited from the surviving asexual ones and decline by natural mortality. The essential feature is that resistance is boosted by stimulation from the asexual stages, but has an intrinsic decay rate in the absence of stimulation. These assumptions accord with the phenomenon of transmission-sustained immunity described above, and with the evidence that immunity is directed mainly against the asexual blood stages. The principal conclusion of this model is summarized in Fig. 5.19; this conclusion is qualitatively similar to that of our earlier model which gave Equation (5.33) and Fig. 5.16 and 5.18. Fig. 5.19 (based on a continuum model) and Fig. 5.18 (based on a compartmental model) agree in showing that the gametocyte reservoir increases with increasing transmission at low vectorial levels (low V), but that the reservoir eventually decreases with increasing transmission, as immune responses are evoked more and more strongly.

The conclusion that moderate reduction of transmission, from initially high levels, may actually increase the prevalence of malaria among adults is thus a robust one. This conclusion accords with the intuition of some malaria epidemiologists, and it has important implications for public health and control programmes.

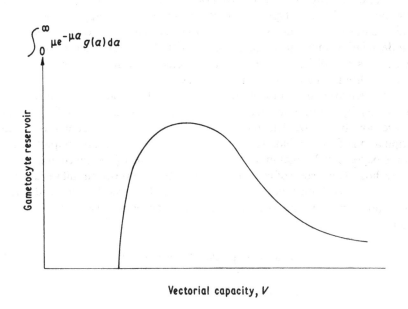

$$\int_0^\infty \mu e^{-\mu a} g(a)\, da$$

Gametocyte reservoir

Vectorial capacity, V

Figure 5.19 Gametocyte reservoir as a function of the mosquito vector's biting capacity. Reproduced with permission from Elderkin *et al.* (1977), p. 511.

5.10   BASIC MECHANISMS OF IMMUNITY

One underlying difficulty in incorporating immune processes in dynamical models of malaria is that the detailed mechanisms of the immune response are not well understood. Some of the major ideas are summarized here, with the caution that there is no consensus on how immunity to malaria is acquired.

One good candidate for characterizing immunity to malaria is the production of antibodies, which are large proteins with fairly specific ability to interact with antigens. Earlier studies of malarial immunity focused on the spleen (Boyd, 1949a; p. 589, 596), but the precision of spleen measurements is inherently limited. More recently, techniques have been developed for looking at antibodies in blood serum (Ambroise–Thomas, 1974; Meuwissen, 1974), thus permitting a more quantitative approach to immunity. Epidemiological studies have shown that antibodies are indeed produced in response to infection; in malarious areas, antibodies both to sporozoites (see Fig. 5.20; from Nardin et al., 1979) and to merozoites (see Fig. 5.21; from Cornille–Brögger et al., 1978) increase with age. Additional evidence is provided by the observed decrease in antibodies when the prevalence of malaria is substantially reduced, as illustrated in Fig. 5.22 (Ambroise–Thomas et al., 1974). Notice, incidentally, that gametocytes do not induce antibodies

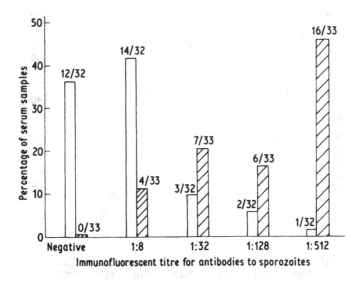

Figure 5.20   Percentage of blood serum samples from Keneba in the Gambia at each level of immunofluorescent titre for *Plasmodium falciparum* sporozoites. Increasing dilutions (maximum 1 : 512) indicate a greater density of sporozoite antibodies in the blood serum. The children aged 10–15 years (unshaded bars) have, on average, lower measurements for sporozoite antibodies than adults over 50 (shaded bars). Reproduced with permission from Nardin et al. (1979), p. 598.

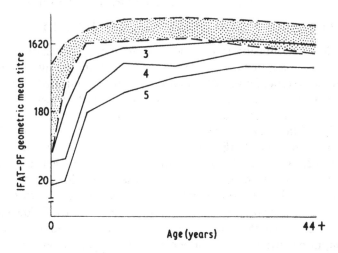

Figure 5.21 Geometric mean of the immunofluorescent antibody titres (IFAT) for *Plasmodium falciparum* merozoites for each age group in Garki, Nigeria. The shaded area represents the range of the unprotected population; 3, 4, 5, indicate different times (20, 50, 70 weeks respectively) after protection began. Reproduced with permission from Cornille–Brögger *et al.* (1978), p. 584.

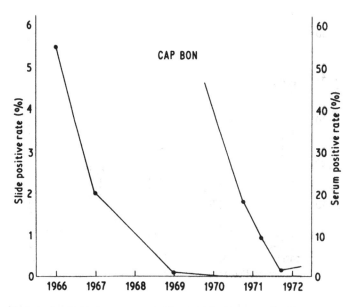

Figure 5.22 On the left, percentage of the population in Cap Bon, Tunisia with blood tests positive for malaria parasites. On the right, percentage positive for malaria (merozoite) antibodies as determined by the indirect immunofluorescent test with positive defined as greater than 1/20 titre. Reproduced with permission from Ambroise–Thomas *et al.* (1974), p. 53.

under natural conditions (Smalley and Sinden, 1977); gametocyte vaccines work when the gametes are exposed in the stomach of the mosquito. At the very least, these indicators can be used in epidemiological surveys, to get a better account of the history of the exposure of a population to malaria (McGregor, 1974). But it is also clear that some of the serum antibodies confer protection, because transfer of immune serum has been demonstrated to reduce parasitaemias in man and other animals (Brown, 1969).

Malaria parasites are complex cells, and there are several antigens producing different 'malaria-specific' antibodies. Recent studies with animals have begun to dissect the responses induced by the different stages in the life cycle of the parasite. Langreth and Reese (1979) have shown that *P. falciparum* in human and in monkey red blood cells produces antigens on the surface of the blood cell, so that the body may react to modified blood cell surfaces as well as to liberated merozoites. Deans *et al.* (1978) have shown that immune serum from monkeys, electrophoresed to demonstrate the presence of distinct antigens, responds both to the merozoites and to infected red blood cells; this issue is, however, clouded by Howard and Mitchell's (1979) demonstration that uninfected red cells from an immune mouse are cleared faster than ordinary red blood cells. More recently, techniques for producing monoclonal antibodies have enabled responses to individual antigens to be distinguished (Cox, 1980), demonstrating explicitly that certain antibodies can be effective against sporozoites (Yoshida *et al.*, 1980) and others against merozoites (Freeman *et al.*, 1980).

Antibodies are, however, not the whole story. Antibodies are produced by the so-called B-cells in the immune system, but evidence suggests that T-cells (other white blood cells which can act either directly on a foreign antigen, or by helping B-cells) can also be critical to the immune response. Chen *et al.* (1977) found that T-cells, and not B-cells, were necessary to induce the protective response against sporozoites in mice. Weinbaum *et al.* (1976) showed both T- and B-cells were needed to produce a complete immune response to the blood stages of the parasite. Other complicating aspects of the immune response include factors not specific to a particular disease, such as the general immune suppression caused by malaria (Taylor and Siddiqui, 1978; Weinbaum *et al.*, 1978), and the general immune stimulation caused by agents like BCG (Cox, 1978a). Sufficiently little is understood about the immune response to malaria that it remains a long-term research goal to build models as detailed as those constructed for the immune responses to simple, non-replicating antigens (as described, for example, by Bell *et al.*, 1978).

Further difficulties arise in moving from laboratory situations to natural populations. In addition to the shift from laboratory animals to people, there is the shift from the controlled conditions of the laboratory to a multitude of environmental complications. *Inter alia*, there is genetic variability among the malaria strains found in real populations of humans (Wilson, 1980) and of mice (Beale *et al.*, 1978), and there are interactions among different species of malaria (Molineaux et al., 1980) and among different kinds of blood parasites (Cox, 1975, 1978b).

Given all these difficulties, particularly in the comparison between laboratory and natural populations, it is our view that studies of the epidemiology of malaria in natural populations (of the kind reviewed in this chapter) – in which the characterization of immunity is admittedly phenomenological and imperfect – are at least as important as detailed studies of the mechanism of the immune response (at present mainly based on laboratory animals). Even in such studies of human populations, however, the heterogeneity of the host population must be kept in mind. Extrapolating from one country to another involves significant shifts in genetic and environmental backgrounds (possibly one reason why the European vaccine for tuberculosis has not yet been successful in India; Anon., 1980). Even locally, variation may be important, as in Armstrong's (1978) demonstration that two tribes living adjacently in Ethiopia had significantly different susceptibilities to *P. vivax*. Nold (1980) has shown formally how a single subpopulation can act as a core of infection, to sustain a disease in a population, thus re-emphasizing Yekutiel's (1960) warning that aggregating measurements over an entire population can obscure important epidemiological patterns.

5.11 EVOLUTION

Our discussion has dealt exclusively with the dynamics of the transmission and maintenance of malaria, ignoring evolutionary aspects of the association between the parasite and its hosts.

But for malaria, as for most other viral, bacterial and protozoan infections, evolutionary responses can profoundly complicate attempts to control or eradicate the disease. Thus the parasite has evolved drug resistance in response to anti-malaria drugs (Peters, 1974), the mosquito vectors have evolved resistance to insecticides (Harrison, 1978), and surface proteins may shift in response to the host's own immune response (Brown, 1977). More generally, relatively little is known about the importance of competition among malarial parasites, as opposed to host immune responses, in regulating their populations; such competitive effects arguably limit the populations of schistosomes and other parasites within human hosts (Bloom, 1979; Bradley, 1972). That the population genetics of host and parasite are linked is evidenced both by detailed studies showing that parasites multiply far more rapidly in an unnatural monkey host than in the natural one (see the review by S. Cohen, 1979), and by the broad geographical patterns of correlation between the sickle-cell trait and other human blood group polymorphisms and the prevalence of malaria (Birdsell, 1972, Chapter 12).

The co-evolution of parasites and hosts has received much attention recently (Clarke, 1976; Price, 1980; May and Anderson, 1979; Bradley, 1972, 1977), and a consideration of the selective pressures and co-evolutionary forces linking man, mosquitoes and malaria is only just beginning (J. Cohen, 1979; Pickering, 1980). The problems created by evolutionary responses must ultimately be confronted in any realistic, long-range planning to control malaria.

ACKNOWLEDGMENTS

We thank R. M. Anderson, J. C. Armstrong, R. Asofsky, J. E. Cohen, C. DeLisi, K. Dietz, L. Molineaux and D. W. Taylor for helpful conversations. This work was supported in part by NSF grant DEB77-01565, and by an NSF Postgraduate Fellowship (JLA).

6 Schistosomiasis

A. D. Barbour

6.1 INTRODUCTION

Schistosomiasis is a parasitic disease which is widespread in the tropics. The parasites, schistosomes, are digenetic trematodes, which normally inhabit the veins around the bladder or bowel. There are three principal varieties of human schistosome, each with its own peculiarities, broadly corresponding to the different continents in which the disease is found: *Schistosoma haematobium*, which is found throughout North and Central Africa, *Schistosoma mansoni*, found mainly in South America and Central Africa, and *Schistosoma japonicum*, which is found in China, Japan and the Philippines. Their life cycles are, however, sufficiently similar for them to be treated in the same way when building qualitative models of the transmission of the disease, even though the parameters in the models may differ substantially from one species to another; the following brief account of their natural history applies in general to all three. A detailed description of most aspects of the disease is given in the excellent book by Jordan and Webbe (1969).

The full life cycle of a schistosome involves two hosts, one human and the other an aquatic snail. A diagrammatic representation of the cycle is depicted in Fig. 6.1. Adult schistosomes live in pairs within their human hosts for a span of several years, during which time they steadily produce eggs. Many of the eggs, perhaps as many as 90 % or more (Nelson and Saoud, 1966), fail to complete their intended migration to the bladder or bowel, and become lodged in tissues elsewhere in the body, inducing more or less serious damage. Of the remainder, a proportion of those that reach water after excretion hatch into microscopic free-swimming miracidia. Each miracidium has a life span of around 1 day, which it spends searching for a snail host of the right variety; it is capable of recognizing an attractant secreted by the snail, and of locating it by swimming in a direction of increasing concentration of attractant. The miracidium penetrates the soft tissues of the snail, and initiates a process of asexual multiplication, which eventually results in hundreds of free-swimming cercariae, all of the same sex, being released into the water. The length of time that elapses between miracidial infection and the first release of cercariae is of the order of several weeks (roughly 5 weeks), and cercariae then continue to be released until the death of the snail (Anderson and May, 1979b). Cercariae, which, like miracidia, only live for a day or so, are also capable of locating their potential hosts, apparently by recognizing disturbance of the water surface,

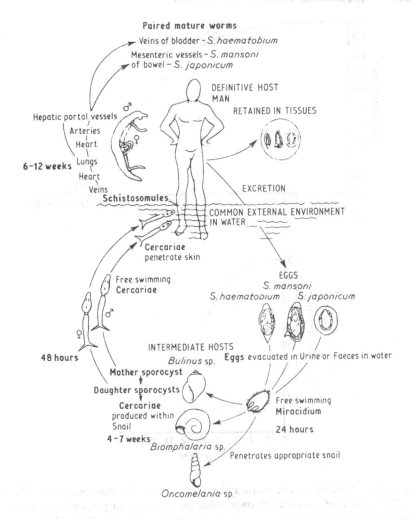

Figure 6.1 A diagrammatic representation of the life cycle of human schistosomes showing the two host species involved (man and snail) and the various developmental stages of the parasite (from Jordan and Webbe, 1969).

and enter the body through any skin exposed under water (Fig. 6.2). They then migrate via the lungs to the liver, where they develop into adult schistosomes, mate, and depart to their final home, in the mesenteric veins or the terminal venules of the vesical plexus, to lay their eggs, the whole phase of development within the human host lasting for 6 or more weeks.

One of the most awkward problems in gathering biological information about the disease is that it is virtually impossible to obtain any detail about schistosomes within the human host. For instance, the only effective way of

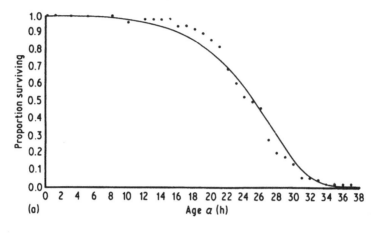

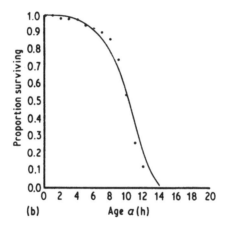

Figure 6.2 Survival of the cercaria and miracidium of *Schistosoma mansoni* at 25 °C.
(a) The survival of the cercarial stage. Solid points, observed proportion of cohort
surviving at age *t*; solid line, best-fit age-dependent survival model. (Unpublished data,
Anderson and Smith, Imperial College, London.) (b) The survival of the miracidial
stage. Solid points and solid line as for (a). (Unpublished data, Anderson and Smith,
Imperial College, London.)

determining the number of schistosomes living in a particular host, and their
distribution around the body, is by dissection. Thus much of what is thought
to take place within the human host relies on analogy with findings about
schistosomes in other animal hosts, such as mice, on autopsy studies, which, in
particular, are not suitable for measuring changes over time within a particular
host, or on indirect measurements, such as of immunological reaction or of the
rate of excretion of eggs. Questions about the life span of schistosomes and

about their mating habits, which could have a substantial influence on transmission, and hence on control, do not seem as yet to have reliable answers. Nor is it even possible, because of the character of the disease, to say in more than very general terms how serious are its effects, in comparison with those of other diseases, on the lives of the people exposed to it.

Perhaps the most surprising gap is the lack of information about immunity acquired by the human host. In any population system of this sort, there must be some mechanism that reduces the net reproductive rate as the population grows, because it readily develops in newly susceptible communities (i.e. has an initial net reproductive rate (R) greatly exceeding unity), but nonetheless subsequently attains an equilibrium within the community. Possible mechanisms within a parasitic system include *density-dependent* (crowding) effects induced by immune responses or competition for limited resources, within either host, increased host mortality and acquired host immunity. The classical explanation for schistosomiasis, advanced by Macdonald (1965), lies in the observation that a snail which has been infected by more than one miracidium releases cercariae no faster, and indeed sometimes slower, than a snail infected by precisely one miracidium. This rather extreme crowding effect implies that the total amount of infection that a community could sustain could be no greater than that fixed level which would result if its entire snail population were releasing cercariae at maximum rate. In practice, a lower level would be attained, because of the long (in terms of a snail's life) latent period of infection within the snail, and because the net reproductive rate in the system, which must be proportional to the chance that a successful miracidium has penetrated an as yet uninfected snail, must fall to its equilibrium value of unity before this chance reaches zero, which would be the case once all snails were infected. Increased snail mortality could possibly reinforce Macdonald's mechanism at high levels of transmission, if multiple miracidial infections tended to kill snails more quickly than single infections, but it seems unlikely that this is of any practical importance. Acquired immunity in snails is also unlikely to be significant, because of their short life span relative to the timescale of the transmission process, and it is, in any case, not observed. In the human host, increased mortality is difficult to assess, though it may, indirectly, play some part; but the long life span of the human host makes it unlikely to be very effective in controlling transmission. Crowding effects are, as indicated earlier, all but impossible either to substantiate or to disprove, and so must remain a possibility, though the apparent capability of some human hosts to sustain unusually large egg outputs perhaps tenuously suggests that such effects, if present, are not important in limiting transmission. There remains the possibility of acquired immunity in man. The importance of such a phenomenon for the control of schistosomiasis and the evidence for its existence are discussed in some detail later; it suffices for now to remark that no experiment has yet satisfactorily demonstrated the existence of such a mechanism in man.

6.2 A SIMPLE MATHEMATICAL MODEL

The earliest attempt to apply mathematical methods to explaining the transmission cycle of schistosomiasis was probably that of Hairston (1961), though its scope was rather limited. The first genuinely dynamic model of the system was proposed by Macdonald (1965), who used it to reach the celebrated conclusion that safe water supplies are more important than latrines. It is actually not easy to see how he could have reached this conclusion using only his model and the available data, and it is therefore very doubtful whether it should be accepted as an instance of the useful application of mathematics in epidemiology – it is rather more likely that it was a conclusion derived from a lifetime of experience in tropical medicine, and should properly be respected as such (see also Scott and Barlow, 1938). Macdonald's model is nonetheless the foundation for almost all subsequent models of transmission, and its essential importance lies in its clear statement of the mechanism of the effect of crowding within the snail host, which limits the reproductive capacity of the parasite population. Accepting this almost universal precedent, we shall start by considering a variant of Macdonald's model, in this case a rather simpler version, and then try to assess its success when considered in the light of the available data.

The basic model is derived by considering the flow of infection between man and snails in an isolated community. Starting with the flow from man to snail, it seems reasonable to suppose initially that the density of miracidia in the water around the locality should be proportional to a variety of different factors: the density of the human population, the number of egg-laying schistosomes per human host, the number of fertile eggs laid per schistosome per day, the chance of a given egg being excreted and reaching water, which itself is likely to be more or less related to the amount of water contact per person per day, and so on. Distinguishing each of these factors in the model would lead to very cumbersome expressions, and would very likely obscure its essential elements. Fortunately, many of them are, under Macdonald's assumptions, constant characteristics of the particular populations in question which are not materially influenced by the progress of transmission. For instance the human population density is not likely to vary greatly in response to different levels of infection, since schistosomiasis does not have too dramatic an effect on mortality, and the local inhabitants are not often willing or able to abandon infected areas. This is not intended to rule out the possibility of any dependence of the human population density upon the level of infection, but merely to propose that in an attempt at reasonable simplification of the model, it should be ignored as being less significant a feature of the transmission cycle than many others. Should there, however, be cause to suppose otherwise, or should this aspect be of particular interest for other reasons, as, for example, in May and Anderson (1979), it could then be explicitly incorporated into the model.

Making similar assumptions about some of the other factors mentioned above, we shall suppose that the density of miracidia is proportional to the ratio of the total number of egg-laying schistosomes in the population and the available water area. The constant of proportionality in the ratio depends only on the social habits of the human hosts, on biological parameters relating to the particular strain of the parasite, and on the local geography, but not on the level of infection or on the area of available water. Note that we are thereby implicitly assuming that the distribution of schistosomes within the human host population does not affect total egg output. Note also that constants of proportionality, such as the one discussed above, are normally the parts of the model that are affected by control measures. For example, providing safe water supplies for bathing and washing clothes might halve the amount of contact with hazardous water, and thereby reduce the constant of proportionality by half. If the model is to be useful, it should accommodate the effects of control measures within its existing structure. Just as biological reality may force one to abandon a simple model in favour of a more complex one, so may sometimes the need to describe the effects of particular control measures.

The next stage is to make some statement about how the density of miracidia is related to the rate at which snails are infected. Here, Macdonald's assumption about the effect of crowding within the snail host is introduced. It indicates that, for the purposes of transmission, it is the number of infected snails that is important, and not how often they have been infected, and hence that only miracidial penetrations of hitherto uninfected snails need to be taken into account. The simplest assumption, therefore, is to suppose that the rate at which new snail infections occur, per unit area of water, is proportional to the product of the density of miracidia, the chance that a given miracidium succeeds in penetrating a snail, and the chance that the snail penetrated was previously uninfected. This last is plausibly estimated as the current proportion of uninfected snails in the snail population, on the assumption that the miracidium does not distinguish between infected and uninfected snails. This is probably not strictly true, as the laboratory experiments of Disko and Weber (1979) would indicate, but should nonetheless constitute a reasonable first approximation. There remains the chance of successful penetration, which depends upon many environmental quantities, but principally, at least from a control point of view, upon the snail density. The particular form which the dependence takes in the field is not known, but, in view of the searching activity of the miracidium, it is reasonable to suppose that only at low snail densities does finding a snail present a problem, and that the chance of success is usually fairly close to its maximum value. Combining these assumptions, we arrive at an overall rate of new snail infections in the community of $\beta X q$, where X is the current total number of egg-laying schistosomes, q is the current proportion of uninfected snails, and β is a constant depending on biological, social and environmental factors, and which is susceptible to alteration by control measures.

The rate of flow of infection between snails and man is modelled in a similar way. In view of Macdonald's assumption, the rate of acquisition of egg-laying schistosomes by the human host population should be proportional to the size of the human population, the amount of water contact per person per day, and the density of infected snails. This leads to a rate of increase in the total number of egg-laying schistosomes of $\alpha\sigma Y$, where σ is the human population density per unit accessible water area, Y is the current number of infected snails, and α, like β, is a constant depending on biological, social and environmental factors. Both α and β are proportional to the amount of water contact per day, though, in view of the different mechanisms involved, the appropriate measures of water contact for the two parameters may well be different. In particular, β is the typical target for measures of improved sanitation, whereas safe water supplies are directed at reducing α. However, the fact that providing safe water can also lead to a corresponding reduction in the contamination constant β by reducing the amount of time spent by the populace in the neighbourhood of snail colonies, may account for the observation of Scott and Barlow (1938) on the relative merits of the sanitation and safe water strategies.

The rates of flow of infection so far computed have to be set against the rates of loss of infection from the various possible causes. The number of egg-laying schistosomes may be reduced both by the mortality of the schistosomes and by that of their human hosts. However, current estimates of the lifetime of a schistosome suggest that the former should be much the more important factor, and it therefore seems reasonable to describe the total rate of loss of egg-laying schistosomes as γX, where X is, as before, the current number of egg-laying schistosomes, and γ is the per capita death rate of schistosomes, so that $1/\gamma$ is a measure of the typical life span of a schistosome. Note that there are a number of assumptions implicit in this description, of which perhaps the most tenuous is that the schistosomes have independent life spans, so that there are no crowding effects within a particular human host. At any level of parasitization which leads rapidly to the death of the human host, this is clearly not the case, but, as mentioned before, it still probably represents a good first approximation. In the snail host, the situation is quite the opposite, with cercarial release usually continuing until the death of the snail. This leads naturally to an expression δY for the overall death rate of infected snails, where δ is the per capita death rate of infected snails.

Finally, it is necessary to make some assumptions about the behaviour of the host populations. The human population can usually be reasonably supposed to be constant, since the time scale over which it changes is much longer than any of the time scales in the infection process. In contrast, snails have a relatively short life span, and the size of a colony rapidly reaches an equilibrium in which their vigorous breeding capability is balanced by the limitations of the available ecological resources. Thus, though for quite different reasons, it is also plausible to assume that the snail population has a constant size, N say, and therefore implicitly that the death of a snail is on average balanced by the birth of another. The proportion q of infected snails is then given by $(N - Y)/N$. The sort of situation in which this assumption usually breaks down is one in which there is a substantial seasonal variation in the amount of water suitable for breeding, leading to dramatic changes in the snail population. Such variations may also change other parameters, in particular σ, the human population density per unit of accessible water area, but, as a first approximation, they are all taken to be constant.

The structure of the basic model, expressed in terms of the rates of increase and decrease of the numbers of infective units (here egg-laying schistosomes and infected snails) is now complete. The next stages in the argument would ideally be to estimate the various parameters in the model from field observations drawn from a number of communities (the parameters no doubt having different values in different areas, even when the strains of schistosome and snail are the same); to use these estimates to make predictions from the model of the effects on transmission of changing some of the parameters; and then to compare the predictions with the response actually obtained in the field. If satisfactory agreement, at least in qualitative terms, were obtained, the model could reasonably be used as a means of evaluating the likely effects of different control measures, as an aid to developing a strategy for control.

Unfortunately, few of the parameters in the model can be directly measured. The transmission parameters α and β, for instance, are particularly awkward to assess, and it is very difficult to imagine how to assign values to them from direct observation. Although efforts have been made to analyse some of their constituents, notably the water-contact rates estimated by Dalton and Pole (1978), the only satisfactory means of estimating them are indirect, and are based on the assumption that the model is, at least in part, a good one. It then becomes doubly important to check the validity of the model by testing its predictions against observation, since, with a minimum of four unknown parameters to play with, one can expect to find a reasonable fit to almost any set of data. It is possible that the forthcoming publications from the WHO project on Lake Volta may contain a sufficiently comprehensive body of data for such a quantitative exercise to be carried out. In the meantime, we shall attempt to examine the qualitative features of the model in the light of the less conclusive data at present available.

The first step in the analysis is to observe that when, as is usually the case where the disease is endemic, transmission is in equilibrium, the rates of increase and decrease in the numbers of each type of infective unit must balance. This gives two equations, the first from considering the egg-laying schistosomes and the second from considering infected snails:

$$\alpha\sigma\bar{Y} = \gamma\bar{X} \quad \text{and} \quad \beta\bar{q}\bar{X} = \delta\bar{Y} \tag{6.1}$$

where $\bar{X}$ and $\bar{Y}$ are the total numbers of egg-laying schistosomes and infected snails respectively in the community at equilibrium, and $\bar{q}$ denotes the equilibrium proportion of infected snails. The equations have two solutions: $\bar{X}$

and $\bar{Y}$ are either both zero, with the natural interpretation that there is no disease present, or both positive, corresponding to endemic transmission, in which case

$$(\alpha\beta\sigma/\gamma\delta)\bar{q} = 1$$

Note that, since $\bar{q}$ represents a proportion, and hence necessarily lies between zero and one, the latter possibility can only occur if

$$\alpha\beta\sigma/\gamma\delta > 1$$

The quantity $\alpha\beta\sigma/\gamma\delta$, which we shall denote by R, and which is usually referred to as the threshold parameter, is just the net (basic) reproductive rate of the parasite population under the ideal conditions when no snails are as yet infected; this last result merely states that the disease can be supported endemically if the parasite population, under uncrowded conditions, would tend to multiply, and not otherwise.

This simple statement, derived from quite elementary considerations, gives a clear indication of what is required if the disease is to be eradicated: R must be reduced to a value smaller than 1. Since R is just a product of the five parameters of the model, it is easy to deduce the qualitative effects upon it of various control measures. In particular, a given percentage reduction in any one of the parameters α, β and σ, or a corresponding increase in γ or δ, would have exactly the same effect on R. If also, as has been suggested, $\bar{q}$ is given in terms of $\bar{Y}$ as $1 - (\bar{Y}/N)$, the endemic values $\bar{X}$ and $\bar{Y}$ can be expressed explicitly as:

$$\bar{X} = N\left(\frac{\alpha\sigma}{\gamma} - \frac{\delta}{\beta}\right) \quad \text{and} \quad \bar{Y} = N\left(1 - \frac{1}{R}\right) \tag{6.2}$$

it is interesting here to note that α, β, γ, δ and σ are no longer symmetrically represented in the total worm burden $\bar{X}$, so that a given percentage reduction in α, σ or $1/\gamma$, if not enough to reduce R below unity, is more effective in alleviating worm burden than a similar reduction in β or $1/\delta$.

The model also illustrates that it is possible to have no disease present, even when $R > 1$. In order to assess the relative likelihood of the two equilibria, it is necessary to consider the dynamics of infective units when the system is not in equilibrium. The net rates of change in their numbers are then no longer zero, but are given by the two differential equations:

$$dX/dt = \alpha\sigma Y - \gamma X$$
$$dY/dt = \beta X(1 - Y/N) - \delta Y \tag{6.3}$$

of which Equation (6.1) are the special case when

$$dX/dt = dY/dt = 0$$

It is easy to analyse these equations, and to show that, if $R > 1$, the presence of any initial amount of infection ultimately leads to the endemic equilibrium. In practical terms, if $R > 1$, there is a considerable danger that casually imported disease will sooner or later become established, even if the community is currently uninfected.

Of the various methods of control currently employed, sanitation is aimed at reducing β and safe water supplies at reducing α, though, as mentioned earlier, safe water supplies may also have an appreciable benefit through β as well. In either case, R is thereby reduced. A single round of chemotherapy would reduce the current level of X without changing R, hence the endemic equilibrium would in due course be re-attained. In order to impinge upon R, chemotherapy has to be repeated regularly, in which case it can be considered to act by increasing γ, thus reducing R.

The effect of applying molluscicide is more complicated. A reduced number N of snails clearly leads to a corresponding decline in the equilibrium worm burden, as given by Equations (6.2). On the other hand, R is not obviously affected, so that killing snails is apparently of little use as a means of eradicating the disease. Clearly, this cannot strictly be the case, since, if there are no suitable snail hosts, there can be no transmission. The resolution of the difficulty lies in the discussion preceding the emergence of β, where it was noted that β does depend implicitly on snail density. Since this is the only way in which R is influenced by the killing of snails, it would be of great interest to know more precisely what form the dependence takes. Broadly speaking, any density of snails sufficient to make it almost certain that a given miracidium has at least one snail within its radius of operation would give rise to essentially the same value of β, and hence of R. Consequently, reducing the number of snails in each colony by, say, a factor of 10 would have little or no effect on β if the average snail density were not brought down below one or two snails per miracidial search area. Thus mollusciciding has to be directed at maintaining very low average snail densities, and, in view of the extremely resilient nature of snail populations, such an effort may often be rather difficult to achieve. In such cases, the killing of snails should probably be considered mainly as a means of alleviating worm burden, rather than as a potential aid in eradication.

There is a further problem associated with molluscicide, in that it kills many other organisms, as well as the snail hosts. A number of these organisms actively impede the miracidial stage of transmission, for instance by acting as decoys (Upatham and Sturrock, 1973). Since some of these species recover less quickly from the effects of molluscicide than do snail populations, there is a danger that miracidial efficiency could in some circumstances actually be improved as a result of mollusciciding campaigns, with a consequent increase in R.

6.3 COMPARISON OF THE MODEL WITH DATA

The discussion at the end of the previous section shows how useful a simple mathematical model can be in making qualitative judgements about control strategies. However, the value of such judgements depends on the model being a faithful representation of the transmission cycle, at least insofar as its broad outline is concerned. Unfortunately, there is one respect in which the current model is clearly deficient.

It has already been mentioned that most of the parameters of the model are difficult to estimate directly. However, if the model is valid, it immediately yields a means of estimating the value of R, the critical threshold parameter. This is because, at an endemic equilibrium, the proportion of uninfected snails $\bar{q}$ is equal to $1/R$, as follows from Equations (6.1). Now $\bar{q}$ is easily observed, and estimates, usually of $1 - \bar{q}$, the proportion of infected snails, have been derived from field observations in many parts of the world: summaries of the findings are presented in Jordan and Webbe (1969), pp. 145–150, and in Anderson and May (1979b). Characteristically, the proportions of infected snails observed range from levels of the order of less than 1 % in Egypt (S. haematobium) to around 7 % in the Philippines (S. japonicum) and, in peak months, to 10 % in Tanzania (S. haematobium), though much higher proportions were sometimes observed in individual colonies. The corresponding values for R are 1.01, 1.08 and 1.11, and it would require a proportion of infected snails of the order of 50 % to reflect a value of R around 2.

This sort of figure may be compatible with an ideal mathematical system, but the transmission of schistosomiasis is hardly that. Many of the factors involved in transmission can be expected to vary widely from one community to another, and, over a period of time, within a particular community. It would be very surprising if they always changed collectively in such a way as to preserve R at a value within the narrow range 1.0 to 1.1, especially when 1.0 represents the lower limit of endemic transmission; the partial rather than total success of control measures strongly reinforces the feeling that R is not at all susceptible to being reduced below unity by a small push in the right direction. What, then, is the explanation for the apparent discrepancy between theory and observation?

The most obvious source of error lies in the detection of infection in the snails sampled in the field. There are two methods of detection principally in use: a snail is either kept under observation in the laboratory, to see if it is releasing cercariae, or crushed and examined under a microscope for evidence of infection, in the form of sporocysts. In either case, a snail infected less than about 3 weeks before sampling would appear to be uninfected, if, as would usually be the case, the snail was examined immediately upon being brought to the laboratory. However, as far as Macdonald's model is concerned, a snail should be counted as infected as soon as it is penetrated by a miracidium, since all subsequent miracidial penetrations are wasted. The distinction is important numerically, because the time taken for a snail infection to develop to the point where it is detectable is of a similar order of magnitude to the natural lifetime of the snail. An analysis of a model similar to the basic model, but allowing for the latent period of infection in the snail, shows that the basic model remains valid, provided that an appropriate correction is made to allow for snails falsely recorded as uninfected. The precise correction for a sample drawn at random from the snail population, if only snails releasing cercariae are recorded as infected, is to multiply the proportion of snails observed to be infected by a factor of $1 + [\delta(e^{l\delta'} - 1)/\delta']$, where δ' is the death rate of uninfected snails and of snails with a latent infection, δ is the death rate of infected snails, and l is the length of the latent period (Barbour, 1978a; Anderson and May, 1979b).

The data given in Pesigan et al. (1958b), for S. japonicum in the Philippines, suggest the values $l = 9$ weeks, $1/\delta' = 16$ weeks, $1/\delta = 6$ weeks, which would lead to a correction factor of around 3.0. However, their method of sampling snails was known to be age-specific, and allowance for this reduces the correction factor to around 2.0. Furthermore, they used a crushing technique to examine for infection, which probably meant that a significant proportion of the latently infected snails were in fact detected and included in their estimates, with the result that the correction factor should probably have been further reduced. Even without this, applying a correction factor of 2.0 to their data on the proportions of infected snails gives an effective proportion of around 14%, which is still much too small to give a reasonable value for R.

Anderson and May (1979b) also discussed the effect of the latent period, in the light of a wide selection of data gathered from the literature. The example they chose to examine in numerical detail was that of S. mansoni in St. Lucia. Starting from the findings of Sturrock and Webbe (1971), who estimated $l = 5$ weeks, $1/\delta' = 6.6$ weeks and $1/\delta = 1.6$ weeks, and who observed proportions of infected snails close to 5%, they computed a correction factor of 5.5. Since Sturrock and Webbe tested for infection in snails by looking for cercarial release, and returned uninfected snails within 30 h of capture, they included no latent infections in their figures. However, their method of sampling snails was significantly age-specific, and a detailed analysis shows that, even allowing for latent infections, their data indicate that only 13% of snails were infected. It might conversely be argued that miracidia can reasonably be expected to be age-specific in their choice of host, but the age–prevalence curves of Sturrock and Webbe show no evidence of this. Other data relating to S. mansoni in St. Lucia give values $1/\delta' = 3.6$ weeks and $1/\delta = 2.7$ weeks (Sturrock, 1973), and proportions of infected snails of between 1% and 1.5% (Sturrock, 1973; Jordan, 1977), all of which would suggest even smaller corrections. Once again, the corresponding values of R are much too small. The above remarks also illustrate the need for a very careful determination of snail infection rates; the above considerations would be unnecessary if the snail samples were observed over a period long enough for latent infections to mature, and if those dying in the interim were crushed and examined.

The next most obvious candidate for explaining the unacceptably low values of R derived from the observed proportions of infected snails is heterogeneity: geographical, temporal, behavioural, or even among snails. Substantial geographical and temporal heterogeneity is clearly in evidence in almost every study of snail infection rates, with Webbe (1962), for example, recording overall proportions of infected snails of below 3 % for 14 months, of between 5 % and 8 % for 4 months, and of 12 % for 2 months, but with individual colonies frequently yielding samples of 200 or more snails of which more than 50 % were infected. It is also clear that a straight average of all the data recorded (number of infected snails/total number of snails) does not give an appropriate overall estimate. To take an absurd example to illustrate the point, it is obviously not right to include in the estimate any snails sampled from an area totally inaccessible to the native population. However, the fact that any such area must necessarily, in the absence of other host species, be free of infection points to the fact that it may be possible to compute an estimate of the overall effective proportion of infected snails, and hence of the parameter R, by using a suitably weighted average of the data, with weights deduced from observable quantities such as the local proportion of infected snails.

This is essentially the approach taken in Barbour (1978a). A model incorporating geographical and social heterogeneity is developed from the basic model, by making allowance for the varying intensities with which different hosts visit different water-contact sites. Its qualitative behaviour is broadly that of the basic model, though the exact representation of the threshold parameter R is now more complicated. Whilst it is no longer possible in general to estimate R exactly without first knowing the water-contact intensities, upper and lower bounds for R can be derived in terms of the observed values at the different water-contact sites of three measurable quantities: the snail density ρ, the proportion p of infected snails, and the accessible water area A. For instance, if L different sites are sampled, yielding the values ρ_j, p_j and A_j, $1 \leqslant j \leqslant L$, then a lower bound for R is given by:

$$\left[\sum_{j=1}^{L} p_j^2 \rho_j^2 A_j / (1 - p_j)^2 \right] / \left[\sum_{j=1}^{L} p_j^2 \rho_j^2 A_j / (1 - p_j) \right]$$

and an upper bound by:

$$\max_{1 \leqslant j \leqslant L} 1/(1 - p_j)$$

Similar formulae hold when ρ, p and A vary spatially in a continuous rather than a discrete manner.

The most important qualitative conclusion to be derived from the estimates is that assuming a homogeneous environment always leads to an under-estimate of R. A similar phenomenon was also noted in connection with the spread of influenza by McNamee (1978). It occurs here essentially because of the way in which increased water contact leads to an increase in both channels of infection, and hence has a non-linear effect on transmission. When actual data are considered, the effect can be dramatic. For instance, in Barbour (1978a), data from Pesigan et al. (1958b) were used to estimate R for the community around Malirong, the correction factor of 2.0 mentioned above being applied to the snail infection rates, to allow for under-recording of infected snails. If a direct average over time and space were used to assess the (corrected) proportion of infected snails, the value of R obtained would be about 1.1. However, the bounds above, used in conjunction with an analogous formula to allow for the substantial seasonal variation encountered, give a value for R of around 4.0.

A very noticeable feature of the results is that the upper and lower bounds for R, in both dry and rainy seasons, are very close together, indicating that transmission in Malirong was extremely focal in character, and that the relatively short season of high transmission was very much the most important part of the cycle. Indeed, if the data for May–June 1954 in Table XLVII of Pesigan et al. (1958b) were representative of dry-season transmission, and that for February–March 1956 of the wet season, the cycle would be broken if no transmission were allowed to take place at Malirong River Pocket No. 2 during the wet season. The proportion of infected snails observed there (39 % actual, 78 % corrected) overwhelmingly dominates the computation of the threshold parameter. The estimate of the threshold parameter is therefore very sensitive to this one particular measurement; if the actual proportion of infected snails observed there were read as 30 % instead of 39 %, an error apparently made during the calculations in Barbour (1978a), the estimate of the threshold parameter would be reduced to 2.0.

Since the figure of 39 % is exceptional in Table XLVII of Pesigan et al. (1958b), it is natural to try instead the figures for March–April 1955 as representative of the rainy season. If this is done, the (corrected) value of the threshold parameter is found to lie between 1.82 and 2.02, transmission now being almost entirely dependent on two sites, Malirong River Pocket No. 2 and Villaco Creek, during the wet season. This once again suggests that an energetic campaign for a limited period each year at just one or two sites would be enough to eliminate transmission. However, a value of R of around 2 still seems rather too small to account for the observed stability of transmission, and the high dependence on one or two sites and times seems much too good to be true. The focal dependence is in part related to an assumption in the model that an increase in water contact has a proportionate effect on both α and β, which is perhaps more appropriate to S. haematobium than to S. japonicum. But any more uniform average reduces the estimate of R, further detracting from the plausibility of the model. In summary, the qualitative findings, that it is important to concentrate attention on sites and times at which $p_j \rho_j$ is large, are useful, at least to the extent that Macdonald's model is valid; but, from the data in Pesigan et al. (1958b), stability of transmission, expressed by a reasonably large value of R, can only exceptionally be attained, and then only at the expense of accepting that transmission is highly vulnerable to a very limited eradication campaign. The clear implication is that the model does not give an adequate representation of reality.

There remains the possibility of heterogeneity within snail populations.

Anderson (1978) shows how a number of laboratory studies in the literature, concerned with the penetration of snails by miracidia, give indirect evidence that some snails are more prone to penetration than others. Further indirect evidence of this comes from the shape of the age–prevalence curves for the infection of snails, as for instance in Sturrock and Webbe (1971), in that prevalence begins to decline in the older age groups (Fig. 6.3). Should this indeed be the case in the field, it would have implications for estimating the proportion of infected snails relevant to Macdonald's model. For instance, if a certain part of the snail population were completely resistant to miracidia, it should not be treated as if part of the population of potential snail hosts. This in turn would imply that the estimates of R should be increased. However, a number of authors argue against heterogeneity being significant in the field, and the decline in prevalence observed by Sturrock and Webbe is very slight. In view of this, it is very unlikely that the effect would be large enough to resolve the difficulties described above.

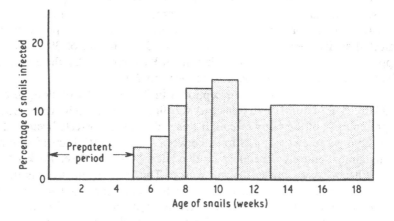

Figure 6.3 An example of an age–prevalence curve of schistosome infection in a snail population. The prevalence of *Schistosoma mansoni* infections in a population of *Biomphalaria glabrata* from a site in St. Lucia in 1970 (data from Sturrock and Webbe, 1971.)

Since it has proved awkward to reconcile the data of Pesigan *et al.* (1958a, b) with the models discussed so far, it is appropriate to mention that an important feature of *S. japonicum*, not explicitly accounted for in the model, is that it is also harboured in a number of animal hosts. Hairston (1961) was interested in assessing the parts played by the various hosts, and reached the conclusion that, whereas human beings made the most important contribution to transmission in Malirong, rats might not be far behind, and suggested rat control might be better than snail control. Curiously enough, Pesigan *et al.*

(1958a), arguing from the same data, deemed rats to be of little importance, and were much more concerned about dogs and cows. More recent models taking animal reservoirs into account include that of Lewis (1975b). In actual fact, the model of Barbour (1978a) discussed above, by making allowance for varying behaviour among definitive hosts, implicitly includes any animal hosts, so that no further changes are required. There is a slight objection to this, since the death rate of small animal hosts such as rats can be much greater than that of the schistosome, and this fact leads to a slightly different model. Nonetheless the presence of animal hosts cannot resolve the fundamental problem, which is that Macdonald's model requires much higher snail infection rates than are observed in practice.

6.4 IMMUNITY IN THE HUMAN HOST

With the stability of a model based on Macdonald's assumptions somewhat in doubt, it is natural to consider what other possibilities there are. In view of the discussion in Section 6.1, the only real alternative is one based on control exercised through the human, rather than the snail, host. The most likely form that this would take would be through some form of acquired immunity.

Evidence for acquired immunity comes mainly from two sources, experiments with animals and age–prevalence curves (see, for example, the discussions in Smithers and Terry, 1969 and in Warren, 1973). Immunity has been demonstrated in the laboratory in experiments on monkeys, baboons, rats and mice. It is thought to be stimulated by the presence of adult worms in the host, and is most effective in protecting against further infection rather than in destroying the worms which initiated the response (concomitant immunity). However, the detailed mechanism by which this is accomplished is obscure (Cohen and Sadun, 1976), and is probably different in different hosts, as, too, is the degree of concomitant immunity induced. There have been few experiments involving human beings, and no good evidence of the existence of immunity in man can be drawn from them.

The situation is apparently clearer as regards age–prevalence curves. It is almost always found that the prevalence of infection within the different age groups in a community follows a characteristic pattern, increasing to a peak around the early teens, and then declining to a lower level, which remains more or less constant beyond the age of 30 (Fig. 6.4). A similar pattern is obtained if egg output is plotted against age. Such curves are readily interpreted in terms of partial or total immunity to further infection conferred for a time by a certain degree of exposure. Bradley and McCullough (1973), in particular, were able to demonstrate that a model incorporating acquired immunity gave a good explanation of some data on *S. haematobium* drawn from a community in Tanzania. Unfortunately, studies also show that water contact varies with age in a broadly similar way. Since this could also give rise to the observed age–prevalence curves, it cannot necessarily be concluded that their

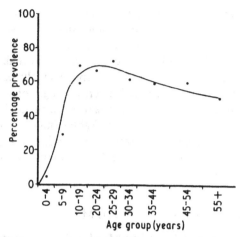

Figure 6.4 An example of an age–prevalence curve of schistosome infection in a human community; the prevalence of *Schistosoma japonicum* in various age groups of a human community at Palo in the Philippines (data from Pesigan *et al.*, 1958). Solid points, observed values; solid line, curve fitted by eye.

characteristic shape is evidence of acquired immunity. Indeed, in the recent paper by Dalton and Pole (1978), with data on *S. haematobium* in Ghana, the authors concluded that 'age was less important than degree of exposure as a contributory factor to variations in infection rates'. On the other hand, the evidence of Kloetzel and da Silva (1967) (*S. mansoni* in Brazil) shows that the characteristic curves are obtained in populations of adults, following their arrival as immigrants in an endemic area, if 'age' is measured starting from their arrival in the area. This observation represents the most direct evidence to date that a controlling mechanism is at work in the human host.

Just as with the earlier models based on snail moderation, there are many possible ways in which to go about specifying a model incorporating human immunity. As before, we shall begin by erring on the side of simplicity, and then see what sort of modification may be necessary to account for the available data. The first step is to note that it is now important, even at the most basic level, to distinguish individual human hosts, rather than aggregate all the schistosomes in the population, since it is the effect of schistosomes upon the individual hosts which is supposed to exert the moderating influence on the transmission cycle. One way of doing this is to keep track of the numbers of human hosts having various levels of infection – this is in fact the way that snails were treated previously, with just one level of infection being distinguished – and to use these as the basic variables in the equations. In a sweeping attempt at simplification, we shall take this approach, and consider only three classes of human host: those that are currently susceptible (Z_0) those that are infected (Z_1), and those that are immune (Z_2) – see also Lewis (1975a). Since only one level of infection is allowed for, the model effectively assumes that currently infected persons are immune to further infection. A period of infection in a host ends when the schistosomes he carries have all died, and it is followed by a further time during which he remains immune from re-infection, after which he becomes susceptible once again. No account is taken of human host mortality, with slightly less than the usual justification, since the average period of infection might be appreciably longer than the average lifetime of an individual schistosome pair, and may therefore be more comparable with a human lifetime, but this loss of realism is likely to be less than that implicit in some of the other assumptions. The snail host is treated as before, so that Macdonald's mechanism of snail moderation is retained, but now only infected humans contribute to the snail infection rate.

Much as with the basic model, suitable postulates are made about the rates of flow of infection. The rate at which susceptible human hosts are infected is taken to be $aY(Z_0/A)$, where Y is the current number of infected snails, A is the accessible water area $- Z_0/A$ thus replacing the constant σ previously used – and a is a constant analogous to, but not quite the same as, α. Individual infections are assumed to terminate at a rate g (to be compared with γ), so that there is an overall flow at rate gZ_1 between the infectious and immune classes. For similar reasons, there is a flow at rate cZ_2 between the immune and susceptible classes, where $1/c$ represents the average length of time that immunity subsists after infection has terminated. Finally, the rate of increase of infected snails is $bZ_1(1 - Y/N)$, where b is analogous to β, and it is compensated by a loss of infected snails through death at an overall rate δY.

These rates give rise to the following equations for the four populations:

$$dZ_1/dt = aYZ_0/A - gZ_1, \quad dZ_2/dt = gZ_1 - cZ_2$$

$$dZ_0/dt = cZ_2 - aYZ_0/A, \quad dY/dt = bZ_1(1 - Y/N) - \delta Y$$

(6.4)

The total human population $Z_1 + Z_2 + Z_0 = M$ is constant. The complete absence of infection, represented by $Z_0 = M$, $Z_1 = Z_2 = Y = 0$, is always an equilibrium of the equations, and is stable only if $R' = ab\sigma/g\delta \leqslant 1$ (compare with R). If $R' > 1$, there is another equilibrium, corresponding to endemic infection, at which, in particular, the proportions of infected human and snail hosts are given by:

$$\bar{Z}_1/M = \frac{(1 - 1/R')}{k(1 + g/k\rho a)}$$

$$\bar{Y}/N = \frac{(1 - 1/R')}{(1 + k\rho\delta/b\sigma)}$$

(6.5)

where $\rho = N/A$ is the snail density, and $k = 1 + g/c$. It is a stable equilibrium, and the solution to Equations (6.4) following any introduction of infection is eventually attracted to it. Thus the situation, as regards permanent eradication, is superficially very similar to that discussed in Section 6.2; R' has to be reduced below unity, and the factors influencing R' are very much those that influence R.

Estimating R' from field observations is rather more difficult than was the case for R, since it is no longer directly related to the easily observable quantities $\bar{Z}_1/M$ and $\bar{Y}/N$. There is, however, an analogous formula:

$$R' = 1/[(1 - \bar{Y}/N)(1 - k\bar{Z}_1/M)]$$

showing that an estimate of R' derived from observations of endemic transmission would now involve the proportion of infected hosts, as well as of infected snails. The factor $k = 1 + g/c$ can in principle be estimated. For instance, if longitudinal studies of the population were available, $1/g$, the mean length of an infected period, and $a\bar{Y}/A$, the rate of incidence of the disease among susceptibles, could be directly estimated. Then the equilibrium equation:

$$\bar{Z}_1/M = (1/g)\Big/\left(\frac{1}{g} + \frac{1}{c} + \frac{A}{a\bar{Y}}\right)$$

could be used to derive an estimate of c, and hence, combining it with the estimate of g, an estimate of k would be obtained.

Taking Bradley and McCullough's (1973) data for *S. haematobium* in Tanzania, and analysing their age–prevalence curves as indicated in the following section, one derives estimates $\bar{Z}_1/M = 0.5$, $a\bar{Y}/A = 0.2$ per year and $1/g = 10$ years, leading to values of 5 years for $1/c$ and 4 for $1/(1 - k\bar{Z}_1/M)$. Incorporating the value of 0.38 for the proportion of infected snails, derived from the Tanzania data of Sturrock and Webbe (1971) by allowing for the effects of snail latency and of the age structure of their snail sample, would then give an estimate of R' of around 6.5, whereas, if Webbe's (1962) proportion were used; R' would be evaluated at around 4.5. These estimates are based on assuming that the whole population is behaving as if over 37 years of age, which is the age at which Bradley and McCullough observed that it had apparently reached equilibrium with respect to the infection. The much greater prevalence and intensity of infection in the younger age groups indicate that the true value of threshold is probably considerably larger.

The age–prevalence curves for *S. japonicum* in Malirong, as recorded in Pesigan *et al.* (1958a), suggest the estimates $\bar{Z}_1/M = 0.7$ and $a\bar{Y}/A = 0.14$, which, for any value of $1/g$ less than 17 years, would suggest that $1/c = 0$, or, equivalently, that immunity to further infection lasts no longer than the current infection. Under these circumstances, $k = 1$, and $R' = 3.3/(1 - \bar{Y}/N)$, or between 3.5 and 6.0, depending on which of the estimates of the previous section is taken for $\bar{Y}/N$. However, the shape of the age–prevalence curve, which shows a small decline from its peak at around age 20, suggests that $1/c$ may in fact be positive, even if rather small when compared with $1/g$. A further interesting piece of evidence is the pattern of response to an intradermal antigen test also carried out at Malirong, which gave higher rates of prevalence than stool examination. If the steady-state proportions registered by this test were assumed, as is tempting, to be measuring $(\bar{Z}_1 + \bar{Z}_2)/M$, a direct estimate of k would be obtained, since:

$$[(\bar{Z}_1 + \bar{Z}_2)/M]/[\bar{Z}_1/M] = k$$

This would suggest a value of 25/21 for k at Malirong, giving the estimates $R' = 6/(1 - \bar{Y}/N)$ or between 6.5 and 12, $1/c = 6$ years and $1/g = 30$ years. Even though 20–30 years seems much too long a time for a single infection to last, it is encouraging to see that the estimates of R' are very much larger than those previously obtained for R. The explanation for the long periods of infection may be that, in practice, concomitant immunity is not total, and that the period of infection is effectively lengthened by intermittent reinfection. Clearly, a more sophisticated model would be needed to properly describe this.

It should be noted that, whereas the incidence rate $a\bar{Y}/A$ was estimated as 0.14 per year from the age–prevalence curves in Pesigan *et al.* (1958a), the same study also included direct measurements of the rate of incidence in children. Between the ages of 5 and 10, the rate of incidence was apparently between 45% and 50% per year. Such a rate appears to be quite incompatible with their age–prevalence curves.

Equations (6.5) can be used to predict the qualitative effects of modifying the parameters of the model by amounts insufficient to reduce R' below 1. Any reduction in R' reduces $\bar{Z}_1/M$ through the factor $1 - 1/R'$, which, however, is relatively insensitive to changes in R' if R' is at all large. For instance, reducing R' from 12 to 6 would only reduce $1 - 1/R'$ by around 10%. The parameters which influence $\bar{Z}_1/M$ other than through $1 - 1/R'$ are g, ρ, a and c. If $g/k\rho a$ is much larger than one, $\bar{Z}_1/M$ is reduced more or less in proportion to reductions in ρ, a and $1/g$, and is insensitive to changes in c. In this case, the dependence of $\bar{Z}_1$ on the parameters is essentially the same as that of X in the basic model. If, at the other extreme, $g/k\rho a$ is much smaller than one, $\bar{Z}_1/M$ is insensitive to ρ and a, and is approximately inversely proportional to $k = 1 + g/c$, k itself being insensitive to changes in g and c if g/c is much smaller than one. Thus, of all the parameters, the prevalence $\bar{Z}_1/M$ is most consistently sensitive to changes in g.

If the lack of uninfected snails exerted no moderating influence at all upon the transmission cycle, the equilibrium value of Z_1/M would be $(1 - 1/R')/k$, and so a small value of $g/k\rho a$ shows that human immunity is effective in controlling transmission. Similar consideration of the value of $\bar{Y}/N$ shows that moderation through the snail host is effective if $k\rho\delta/b\sigma$ is small. The quantities $g/k\rho a$ and $k\rho\delta/b\sigma$ are linked by the fact that their product is equal to $1/R'$, giving some feeling for the relative importance of the two mechanisms in controlling transmission. Now it follows from Equations (6.4) that, at equilibrium:

$$\frac{\bar{Y}}{N}\left(\frac{M}{k\bar{Z}_1} - 1\right) = g/k\rho a \quad \text{and} \quad \frac{k\bar{Z}_1}{M}\left(\frac{N}{\bar{Y}} - 1\right) = k\rho\delta/b\sigma$$

enabling one to estimate $g/k\rho a$ and $k\rho\delta/b\sigma$ in terms of $\bar{Y}/N$, $\bar{Z}_1/M$ and k. It is interesting to note that, on the above figures for Malirong, $g/k\rho a$ is estimated to lie between 0.1 and 0.2 and $k\rho\delta/b\sigma$ between 0.65 and 0.85, if the value of 0.5 from Section 6.3 is taken for $\bar{Y}/N$, and the grand average estimate of 0.1 for $\bar{Y}/N$ would yield values of the order of $1/35$ and 8 respectively. In other words, the level of transmission is apparently limited mostly by the effects of immunity in the human host. Since also g/c is estimated to lie between 0 and 0.2, the situation is precisely the one in which, for a given value of R', the prevalence $\bar{Z}_1/M$ is least sensitive to changes in the parameters of the model. The corresponding estimates of $g/k\rho a$ and $k\rho\delta/b\sigma$ for *S. haematobium* in Tanzania are 0.13 and 1.22, if Sturrock and Webbe's snail infection rate is used, and 0.02 and 14 if Webbe's is taken, with g/c around 0.5; in either case, human immunity appears to be much the more important.

There are two main drawbacks to estimates such as these. The first is the tentative nature of the model on which they are based. It would require a certain stretch of the imagination to discount the possibility of superinfection in the human host. It would require a rather larger effort to believe that the human population was immortal, and had reached equilibrium with the infection to the extent that age–prevalence curves were effectively flat. Finally, the discussion in Section 6.3 shows the dangers of supposing that the host population and its environment are to any degree homogeneous. Despite all these criticisms, it would be surprising if the qualitative picture were different from that outlined here, even if the quantitative estimates were considerably altered.

The second drawback lies in making estimates on the basis of the curves of age against prevalence and egg output. The simple model is, as it stands, too rough and ready to make good predictions of the shape of the age–prevalence curves, with the result that it is difficult to know quite how estimates from the curves should be translated into the terms of the simple model – just as, to allow for field data, Macdonald's model had to be variously adapted. The method adopted here, as already remarked, is likely to underestimate the true value of R. Then, as has widely been observed, prevalence ought naturally to be related to degree of exposure, and age–prevalence curves can therefore be expected, at least in part, to derive their shape from the way that exposure varies with age. Thus, for instance, the equilibrium prevalence $\bar{Z}_1/M$ was estimated by referring to the almost steady prevalence achieved in later life, whereas the rate of incidence $a\bar{Y}/A$ among susceptibles was estimated from the earlier part of the curve. Since exposure is often found to decline in later life, an inconsistency in the estimates may be being introduced by supposing a constant level of water contact. The same considerations also apply if $1/g$ is estimated by assuming that the age–prevalence curve declines from its peak because of loss of infection due to immunity.

However, with regard to the argument that the shape of the age–prevalence curve is a consequence only of variations in the amount of water contact with age, and that immunity is unimportant, there is more to be said. The evidence of Kloetzel and da Silva (1967) has already been mentioned. It is supplemented by that of Bradley and McCullough (1973), who, whilst observing a very decided pattern of variation in both prevalence and egg output over the first 20 years of life, were unable to detect any marked change in water-contact rates during this period. To explain their age–prevalence curves in terms of varying exposure alone would require a reduction in exposure of at least half between early and late childhood. However, there is a further, more serious problem: variable patterns of exposure do not in themselves exert any controlling influence on the transmission cycle. Thus, if immunity were not an effect significant enough to show up on age–prevalence curves, one would essentially be back to Macdonald's model, and all the problems of its lack of stability that are removed by admitting an immunological response. It might be possible to argue for some other mechanism of moderation through the human host, but any other explanation which accounted for the age–prevalence and egg output data in Bradley and McCullough (1973) would seem to have to be rather contrived. It therefore seems very likely that acquired immunity in the human host is the most important natural factor in limiting the transmission of schistosomiasis.

It has been noted earlier that, under these circumstances, the level of infection in the human population is relatively insensitive to variations in the transmission parameters, but may be somewhat more responsive to variations in $1/g$, the average duration of an infectious period, this advantage, however, being minimal if $1/g \gg 1/c$, where $1/c$ is the mean duration of immunity beyond the end of an infectious period. The most natural way of reducing $1/g$ is by regular screening and chemotherapy. However, in applying such a policy, the development of residual immunity might be impeded, and $1/c$ reduced as well, thus eliminating the extra sensitivity that could have been hoped for. In any case, the evidence of the data considered above suggests that $1/c$ is likely in practice to be smaller than $1/g$, and one must probably accept that evolution has succeeded in finding the most stable arrangements for transmission that were available to it.

6.5 STOCHASTIC MODELS

In the previous sections, not much has been done to incorporate into the models any element reflecting the part that chance plays in transmission. The treatment of events with random outcomes has so far been to decide on an 'average outcome', and to suppose that it always occurs. For example, a miracidium, which may or may not succeed in infecting a hitherto uninfected snail, is taken always to have infected a certain small fraction of a snail. Yet it is clear that, in reality, transmission depends upon the outcome of a succession of random events, and it is logical to try to assess the extent to which this is important.

Macdonald (1965), in his pioneering work, was very concerned with the effects of randomness, for the following reason. Adult schistosomes, being dioecious, cannot reproduce unless they mate. Hence they must share a human host with at least one schistosome of the opposite sex, making the distribution of male and female schistosomes among the human population important when calculating egg output. In order to discover what this distribution might be, it is necessary to build a stochastic model. Macdonald supposed that the cercariae of each sex made successful penetrations individually and at random, with no preference for any particular host. These assumptions give rise to a specified distribution of adult schistosomes among hosts for any given overall level of parasitization, and, in particular, imply that, to a good approximation, each host carries independent numbers of male and female schistosomes, each distributed according to a Poisson distribution. If one supposes also that, within a given human host, schistosomes pair off if they possibly can, one can deduce the average egg output for each overall level of parasitization.

This was as far as Macdonald took his stochastic argument. He incorporated the average egg output, as a function of overall worm burden, into a model similar to that described in Section 6.2, and thereafter argued deterministically. But the contribution of the random model was important, because it raised an interesting possibility. Suppose that $2m$ schistosomes, which may be of either sex, are distributed at random among a population of M human hosts, as implied by Macdonald's model. Then, if $m \ll M$, the chance of a given female schistosome being mated is of the order of m/M, and hence the overall reproductive rate of the parasite population is, on average, proportional to m^2/M. On the other hand, the overall death rate of parasites is proportional to m. Comparing these two expressions, it follows that the ratio of reproductive rate to death rate is proportional to m, and hence that, if m is reduced far enough, the parasite population may fail to reproduce itself, and ultimately die out. Put another way, the net reproductive rate of schistosomes is proportional to the chance that a female schistosome is mated, and this chance declines as m/M is reduced. The critical value of m, below which the population is no longer viable, is called the breakpoint (see Chapter 2).

The above formulation has to be examined in the light of observation. The main conflict with experimental evidence is that, in most parasitic diseases, the distribution of parasites among hosts is not usually found to follow the Poisson distribution. Instead, it is usually the case that most parasites are aggregated among a few very heavily infected hosts, the rest being lightly infected or uninfected. Such a pattern was observed by Bradley and McCullough (1973) in egg output from human schistosomiasis. In May (1977b), the effect of a range of different distributions on Macdonald's model was explored. The most important conclusion to be drawn was that, if aggregation is sufficiently intense, there may be no breakpoint, because the chance of a given female being mated may not be reduced to zero by reducing m. Since there are quite plausible mechanisms for transmission which would lead to high aggregation (Barbour, 1978b), the significance of Macdonald's break-point remains in doubt.

These models, though based on certain stochastic arguments, are still treated deterministically when the whole transmission cycle is considered, and are therefore little different in this respect from the earlier models. However, Nåsell and Hirsch (1973) went further, building a model in which the transmission mechanism explicitly included the randomness of events, and whose solution yielded a probability distribution for the level of infection and its distribution among the hosts. This was an important advance upon the previous models, and led, directly or indirectly, to much of the subsequent interest in theoretical models for schistosomiasis. Their model is more difficult to analyse than Macdonald's, as is to be expected with a stochastic formulation, but gives broadly the same picture, thereby lending some justification to the policy of approximating the stochastic by the deterministic. However, it too is not really a stochastic model, since, in order to facilitate the analysis, a number of random events were again replaced by 'average outcomes'. Unfortunately, predictions of quantities of an essentially random nature are inclined to be very sensitive to this sort of approximation, and so the stochastic information, which might have been expected from it as a supplement to Macdonald's findings, has to be treated with caution. In particular, their model predicts a Poisson distribution of parasites among hosts, and is unable to give any extra information on what is perhaps the most interesting question of a genuinely stochastic nature: in a community in which there is currently no infection, but where infection could potentially become established, what is the chance of an imported infection taking hold?

This question was addressed by Lewis (1976), and also in Barbour (1978b), where a simple fully stochastic model was proposed based on Macdonald's assumption of moderation via the snail host. As before, analysis of the stochastic model confirmed the view that a deterministic model gives an adequate description of endemic transmission. A formula for the chance of an imported infection becoming established was also derived, and it was shown that, in order to protect against such a possibility in an uninfected locality, the parameters β and γ of the model in Section 6.2 – in practice, improved sanitation, and screening and treatment of immigrants – appeared to give the best response for a given percentage change. However, information relating to genuinely stochastic effects still appeared to be much more vulnerable to perturbations in the model than was the information derived from the deterministic models, and so the results of simplified models ought perhaps to be treated with circumspection.

Constructing more realistic stochastic models requires much finer detail than that required for a deterministic model. This is principally because, in a deterministic model, it is enough to specify rates of flow, whereas, in a stochastic model, more information is required about how the flow takes place. As an illustration of the extra effort that is entailed, as well as of the greater insight that can be obtained, we shall conclude the section with a deeper analysis of the flow of infection between snail and man, using the data of Bradley and McCullough (1973) to provide the evidence on which to base our model.

In the models of the earlier sections, an expression was derived for the average rate of flow of infection into the human host population. However, many different random mechanisms could lead to the same average rate of flow. Both Hairston and Macdonald assumed, as is natural, that a human host was subject to regular invasions by individual cercariae, arriving according to a Poisson process. This assumption implies that the proportion of uninfected hosts should decline exponentially during childhood except for an initially slower phase which comes about because cercariae of both sexes are needed to cause overt infection. Bradley and McCullough's data confirm an exponential decline over time in the proportion of uninfected hosts, with about 20% succumbing each year, but apparently without the deviation predicted by Macdonald's analysis. This leads to the question: why is it that, despite constant exposure to hazardous water, children do not become infected more rapidly than is observed? It could be the case that the pattern of incidence merely reflects the times at which children first start to expose themselves to infection, or has to do with differential susceptibility, but it would be difficult from such hypotheses to account for the observed age–prevalence curves. It seems more likely that, as suggested by Warren (1973), the low rate of infection is the result of low cercarial densities, conditions less ideal for infection than those found in the laboratory, and some form of defence in the human host against minor challenge infections; this is the explanation that we shall accept hereafter.

On this hypothesis, the data of Bradley and McCullough actually imply a mechanism very different from Macdonald's. They record peak egg output at around age 9, and peak prevalence some 4 or 5 years later, which, with an incidence of 20% per year, would mean that, at the most important ages for transmission, the schistosomes harboured by a human host would on average have been delivered at only two successful infections. This suggests that cercarial penetrations do not necessarily occur singly, but in groups, as envisaged in some of Tallis and Leyton's (1969) models, and that the aggregated distribution among hosts indicated by egg output data can be explained, at least in part, by the random distribution of the numbers of cercariae in each infecting group. Of course differing amounts of water contact may also have their effect, as may differences in the efficiency of defensive mechanisms in the human host.

Group infection would also have other consequences. It may keep the chance of a female schistosome being mated large enough (even at low infection rates) to make the existence of a breakpoint unlikely and the precise degree of aggregation qualitatively unimportant. It would also render the detail of the mating mechanism less important, since it is likely to be enough to suppose that pairs are only formed from among a single infecting group. This is because schistosomes are thought unlikely to be able to survive unmated for more than a few months, whereas the above data indicate an average period of five years between infections.

In view of these considerations, the following modification of the infection process in the model described in Section 6.4 is proposed, to account for Bradley and McCullough's data on *S. haematobium* in Tanzania. Each human host is assumed, as before, to be susceptible, from around the age of 1, to infection by groups of cercariae arriving as a Poisson process of rate $a\bar{Y}/A$, the numbers of worm pairs successfully delivered at each infection being independent and identically distributed. However, after receiving two such infections, a human host becomes immune to further infection until all the worm pairs that he has so far acquired have died. The subsequent pattern of infection is then taken to be similar to that of the model of Section 6.4, with each single infection again conferring immunity and with susceptibility between periods of infection being reduced relative to that during childhood, in that the rate of incidence is lower and the number of worms acquired at an infection is smaller. The model gives a very good fit to both the prevalence and the egg output curves of Bradley and McCullough, if 1. the initial rate of incidence is taken to be 0.2 per year, 2. the productive lifetime of a worm pair to be 7.5 years, 3. the duration of infection resulting from either of the first two large groups of worm pairs to be 13–15 years, and 4. that from any subsequent invasion to be 10 years, 5. the final rate of incidence to be 0.1 per year and 6. the ratio of the sizes of the larger initial and smaller subsequent groups of worm pairs to be 4.5:1. The duration of infection resulting from a group of worm pairs arriving simultaneously is likely to be longer than that of a single pair, because the productive lifetime of a worm pair is not a fixed quantity, and because overt infection lasts until the last pair ceases laying. Rather curiously, Bradley and McCullough's data suggest that the productive life of a worm pair may span a relatively definite length of time, in that the coefficient of variation is smaller than that of, say, an exponential distribution. Naturally enough, the duration of an infectious period seems rather more variable. The figures for worm lifetimes are also rather larger than those usually quoted in the literature, though Bradley and McCullough themselves suggested a similar value.

It can, of course, quite reasonably be argued that, with a model as complicated and as tailored to a particular set of data as this, it is hardly surprising that a reasonable fit is obtained, and that there may be many other models of equal complexity which would explain the data equally well. Variation in water contact has already been discussed, and the reasons against its being the only explanation for the age–prevalence curves have been clearly explained; but it may well contribute in part to the peaks of intensity and prevalence, making the above estimates less reliable. Bradley and McCullough themselves favoured an immunity which took several years to develop. Although superficially similar to the above formulation, it differs in one important respect: it would not exercise any moderating influence on transmission through children of less than ten years of age, whatever the intensity of transmission. This means that if, as seems plausible in view of their egg output, children under ten could alone maintain transmission in Mwanza, the transmission intensity must be being limited by the lack of uninfected snails, and one is again returned to the problems of Section 6.3. However, time could still, with exposure, be a contributory element in the development of immunity. And there may be other possibilities. But it is interesting that it is much more difficult than one might suppose to concoct a satisfactory model for the mechanism of infection.

The curves relating egg output to age, to which the model has been fitted, are based on the sample averages of the egg counts of the members of each age group. However, the variability of the counts between one person and another is very striking, and average values only give a poor picture of the real situation. May (1977b) considered the effect on Macdonald's mating probability of distributions to be more dispersed than the Poisson, by assuming a negative binomial distribution of parasites in a host. The empirical conclusion of Bradley and McCullough's (1973) study was that the positive egg counts followed a log-normal distribution, implying rather fatter tails, and therefore even more irregular behaviour, than that obtainable from the negative binomial family. Their estimates indicate that, for the people in their study aged over 35, the number of eggs passed in 10 ml of urine was on average 27, with standard deviation 170. Yet, in a sense, even a ratio of 6.5 of standard deviation to mean understates the true variability they observed, since, assuming their estimated log-normal distribution, the largest egg counts they recorded came from a part of the distribution where the tail probabilities, although very small, were falling off very slowly indeed – locally, like a distribution with infinite mean and variance.

The effect of this is that, even in large populations, the values of sample averages tend to be unstable, depending to a noticeable extent on the large values obtained from a few individuals, and hence admitting considerable random variation. In Bradley and McCullough's data, 2 % of the populace in any age group typically contributed 25 % of the overall average output. This leads to the question of how, in constructing a model which is based on 'average' transmission rates, one should estimate the required averages. One way of deriving a more stable estimate of a typical count is to use the geometric mean of the egg counts, instead of the arithmetic mean. This procedure has its descriptive virtues, in that, if the logarithms of the egg counts are indeed normally distributed, the logarithm of their geometric mean is the best estimator of the mean of this normal distribution. However, transmission depends on the total number of eggs excreted per unit time, and not on a sum of logarithms, and if there is, in any practical sense, an average rate of output, it is estimated by the arithmetic mean of egg output, and underestimated by the geometric mean by a factor which, for Bradley and McCullough's data, is around 5. Thus one has really to accept that, even in populations of an appreciable size, the random fluctuations in overall transmission remain significant, and that the unstable estimates of average rates obtained in practice are no more than a faithful reflection of this.

6.6 CONCLUSIONS

In the preceding sections, an attempt has been made to describe the transmission of schistosomiasis in mathematical terms. The results illustrate the way in which a mathematical description is able to draw attention to critical aspects of the assumptions being made, and to provide a framework within which to compare alternative hypotheses. Even the simple model of Section 6.2 proved useful in evaluating the effects of different methods of control; in particular, it was possible to show that the effectiveness of molluscicide for the purposes of eradication is very sensitive to the reductions in snail densities achieved, and to the searching ability of miracidia. Naturally enough, when making policy decisions between one control strategy and another, much more must be taken into account, not only in respect of the cost and feasibility of each strategy, but also with regard to their effects on other diseases and on the general level of amenity. Nevertheless, without the basic information provided by a model about what is attained or attainable by particular methods, it is much more difficult to come to good decisions.

The model of Section 6.2 was not only useful for evaluating the merits of control strategies, it also had its uses in clarifying how transmission is actually maintained. Its instability with respect to changes in its parameters, apparent even after the modifications of Section 6.3, was the reason for considering acquired immunity in the human host as possibly an important feature of the cycle. The subsequent analysis in Section 6.4 indicated that, both at Mwanza, Tanzania (*S. haematobium*) and at Malirong, Philippines (*S. japonicum*), human immunity was the most important natural factor in limiting the level of transmission.

Deterministic models were, by and large, found to be the most useful of the tools available, mainly because of their simplicity. However, many of the rate constants appearing in them were explained in terms of, or estimated by means of, an underlying stochastic model describing in detail a particular part of the transmission cycle. Two points of practical interest arose in the course of one such detailed analysis of the infection process. First, human hosts seemed to get infected rather more rarely than one would expect, and, second, there was empirical support for supposing that, in *S. haematobium*, immunity to further cercarial penetration became effective in the human host after two infections, and not just one. Finally, it was observed that assuming homogeneity of almost any kind has the effect of making transmission appear more marginally stable than in fact it really is, and that it is therefore necessary to take careful account of heterogeneity when assessing the values of the parameters of a model.

This discussion of mathematical models for schistosomiasis is not intended as a survey of the subject; a recent review can be found in Cohen (1977). Instead, it gives a personal view of a particular case history in mathematical modelling, designed principally to illustrate how simple models can be used effectively. As is inevitable with a large and complicated system such as the transmission of schistosomiasis, the argument has evolved out of the vast corpus of knowledge and ideas built up by previous work. But it is precisely when faced with such complexity that mathematical models are at their most powerful; they clarify the effects of, and relationships between the different elements of the system.

ACKNOWLEDGEMENTS.

I would like to thank many people for the help and encouragement they have given me over the years: especially D. J. Bradley and W. Haas, for freely sharing their wide knowledge of schistosomiasis, and N. T. J. Bailey, for liaison with the World Health Organization.

7 The population dynamics of onchocerciasis

K. Dietz

7.1 INTRODUCTION

This chapter describes an attempt to fit a mathematical model to epidemiological data relating to onchocerciasis. In the first section I present a brief survey of the life cycle of *Onchocerca volvulus* and discuss the biological evidence for its regulation. On the basis of this I draw some general conclusions about the structure of the model. Before specifying in detail the model's assumptions and the definition of the model's parameters I present the data which have been used for the model construction. The observations come from seven Sudan savanna villages which cover a wide range of endemicity levels. For each of the seven villages entomological observations have been collected for several years such that a direct estimate of the 'Annual Biting Rate' and the 'Annual Transmission Potential' is available. A cross-sectional survey of the total population gives the age-specific densities of microfilariae and the prevalence of eye lesions and blindness caused by the parasite. Assuming that the measured biting rates have been at this level for a long time, the observed parasitological situation can be considered to represent an equilibrium state. The model constructed allows us to specify in numerical terms a critical level of the rate at which men are bitten; below this rate the infection cannot maintain itself at an endemic level. This critical level will of course depend on the particular characteristics of the vector population, i.e. longevity and rate of feeding on man. For each of the seven villages I shall specify the factor by which the man biting rate would have to be reduced in order to reach this critical level. This would be relevant for an attempt to eradicate the parasite. The model also allows us to make projections of the effects of reductions in the man biting rate to a level which is above the critical level required for eradication. These projections allow us to estimate the time required for a new equilibrium to establish itself. They also allow us to identify equilibria where the parasite is present but the prevalence of blindness is negligible. So far these dynamic projections cannot be tested against observations but the ongoing Onchocerciasis Control Project (OCP) in seven West African countries is collecting data with which the present projections could be compared.

The model tries to describe microfilarial densities, prevalence of eye lesions, prevalence of blindness in the human population and average number of infective larvae in the vector population as a function of a single variable describing vector–man contact. The special feature of the present model is its ability to describe age-specific variables in a dynamic way for non-equilibrium situations. Usually in modelling infectious diseases one looks either at the values averaged over age for time-dependent situations or at age-specific variables for situations with constant incidence. Since the model has been developed on the basis of equilibrium situations only, it cannot be claimed that it can also describe, in a realistic way, the rate of transition between different equilibrium states. Thus, as more information on the effects of vector control becomes available, the model parameters, or even its structure, may have to be modified.

7.2 LIFE CYCLE OF *ONCHOCERCA VOLVULUS* AND ITS REGULATION

Onchocerciasis or river blindness is caused by *Onchocerca volvulus*, a filaria (thread-like) worm. The infection is transmitted from person to person by black flies belonging to the genus *Simulium*. It is estimated that more than 20 million people are affected by this disease which is particularly prevalent in tropical Africa and in parts of tropical America.

The transmission cycle is shown schematically in Fig. 7.1. When a female *Simulium* fly bites man, infective-stage larvae of *Onchocerca volvulus* enter the skin through the wound caused by the bite of the fly. From there they migrate to subcutaneous tissues and mature. Fertilized female worms produce microfilariae which can then be picked up from the skin by the vector flies during their blood-meal. Most of the microfilariae thus ingested die or are digested together with the blood-meal but a few are successful in penetrating the wall of the fly's stomach and these settle in the thoracic muscles. After passing through three larval stages they finally become free larvae capable of infecting a human host.

The following discussion of the density-dependent regulating factors of the parasite population is partly based on an unpublished working paper by Molineaux (1975) which gives a survey of the relevant literature. For all arthropod-borne infections the concept of vectorial capacity, as developed for malaria by Garrett–Jones (1964), is applicable. It specifies the contact rate and is determined by the product of the following factors: the biting density on man, the proportion surviving for a period equal to the incubation period of the parasite in the vector, the expectation of residual life and the rate at which the individual vector feeds on man. If one would like to determine the relationship between vectorial capacity and the endemic level, one has to estimate these factors in the field. The biting density on man varies considerably by hour and season. A yearly total is estimated from a sample of whole days distributed over the year. Usually a small number of fixed stations distributed around a village are used. Human baits catch all flies trying to feed.

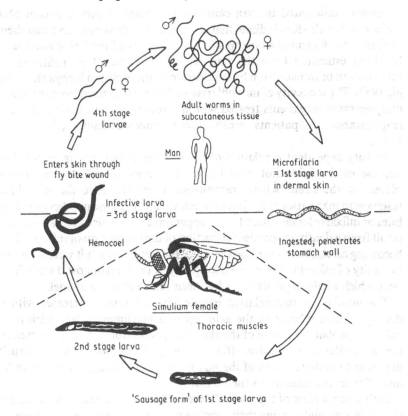

Figure 7.1   Life cycle of *O. volvulus*.

The estimate obtained is probably higher than the biting rate of an average individual in the population and the bias of the estimate of the Annual Biting Rate (hereafter called the ABR) may vary from place to place.

The age-dependent dispersal of *Simulium* (Duke, 1975) affects the estimation of the proportion surviving the extrinsic cycle and of the expectation of life. The frequency at which the individual vector feeds on man is the product of the frequency of feeding multiplied by the proportion of meals taken on man. This proportion cannot be estimated directly. An indication of the anthropophilic behaviour of a vector is the low proportion of infective larvae of non-human filariae.

A vector population may be composed of several species which can only be reliably diagnosed by examining larval polytene chromosomes. Recently, for example, *Simulium damnosum* has been split into several species. Their relative importance as vectors of *O. volvulus* is not yet completely known. The probability of successful development and mating of the infective larvae of

O. volvulus inoculated in man cannot be estimated directly. Recent observations by Schulz–Key indicate that the species is polygamous and that there is probably an efficient chemotropism. The longevity of the fertile adult female has been estimated from the rate of disappearance of microfilariae after interruption of transmission by eradication of the vector in Kenya (Roberts *et al.*, 1967). The longevity of microfilariae in the skin is derived from their rate of disappearance in patients treated with macrofilaricides or from their rate of reappearance in patients treated with microfilaricides (Duke, 1957, 1968).

Density-dependent regulation of the parasite population in man is likely because of the epidemiological finding that microfilarial densities reach a plateau in the adults where transmission is intense. Also the microfilarial reservoir in man varies much less between villages than the number of infective bites or infective larvae offered. This upper limit to the microfilarial load could result from a density-dependent reduction of the proportion of infective larvae becoming adults, or of the longevity, or of the fertility of adult worms, or of the longevity of microfilariae, or even longevity of the human host. I shall discuss later which of these possibilities has been included in the model.

The number of microfilariae ingested by the vector increases with the density of microfilariae in the skin, up to a maximum, after which it may decrease, probably because of the skin changes resulting from the presence of the microfilariae themselves (Duke, 1962). There seems to be density-dependent regulation both of the number of microfilariae in the human host and of their accessibility to the vector.

Only a proportion of the microfilariae ingested are successful in penetrating the haemocele and starting their development. The proportion is independent of the number ingested in the Cameroon forest (Duke and Lewis, 1964), while in the West African savanna the proportion decreases as the number ingested increases (Philippon and Bain, 1972). There seems to be no density-dependent mortality of the larvae while developing in the vector in the Cameroon forest (Duke, 1962a). Mortality of the vector at high intakes increases with the number of microfilariae ingested in the Cameroon forest but the increase is relatively small (Duke, 1962b).

By the comparison of flies caught immediately before feeding with flies caught immediately after completing their blood-meal it was estimated that in the Cameroon forest during the meal 80 % of infective larvae escape and 40 % of the infective flies become non-infective (Duke, 1973). The proportion of escaping larvae entering into man and maturing is not known.

The rate at which eye lesions and blindness appear as a function of the microfilarial density depend on the strain of the parasite and on the sex of the host. The lower prevalence of eye lesions and blindness in females has sometimes been attributed both to lower exposure and to intrinsic host factors (Anderson *et al.*, 1974).

7.3   GENERAL ASPECTS OF MODELLING THE TRANSMISSION OF FILARIAL DISEASES

Most epidemiological models describe the prevalence of infection in man and disregard the density of the infection. This approach is justified if the infectivity of an individual and the probability of developing disease is practically the same for all the infected individuals. This is, however, not true for infestations caused by helminths, where the worm load varies considerably from host to host. In the case of onchocerciasis there may be villages where practically everybody above a certain age is infected such that the prevalence of the infection is identical in the two villages but the average worm load and the average prevalence of the disease differ considerably. For this reason we have to take into account the actual parasite density. Macdonald (1965) was the first to construct a model for the transmission of helminth infections which takes into account the average worm load in the human host. With respect to the intermediate host he only considered the prevalence of infection. He also took into account the probability of pairing of worms in the human host. This aspect leads to the concept of a so-called 'breakpoint', i.e. a critical worm load which represents an unstable equilibrium. May (1977b) and Bradley and May (1978) showed that for aggregated transmission this breakpoint is so low that it can be neglected (Anderson, 1980). I shall therefore disregard the problem of pairing of worms (see Chapters 3 and 6). On the other hand I shall take into account not only the worm load in the human host but also the number of infective larvae in the intermediate host, because these are usually counted by entomologists when they dissect the vectors.

I introduce the following notation. Let w and l be the number of parasites in the human and the intermediate host respectively. Parasite in the human host, refers to adult worms, parasite in the intermediate host, means infective larvae. Special equations for the dynamics of microfilariae are not written, since their life expectancy is relatively short compared to the life expectancy of adult worms and they are assumed to be always at their equilibrium level for a given number of adult worms. For the following general considerations the human and intermediate host are treated in a symmetrical way. I shall discuss the effects of density-dependent regulation on the basis of the following integro-differential equations (representing changes in w and l with respect to time, t, and host age, a):

$$\frac{\partial w}{\partial t} + \frac{\partial w}{\partial a} = \{\lambda_1 \bar{l}/[1 + f_1(\lambda_1 \bar{l})]\} - \sigma_1 w[1 + g_1(w)]$$

$$\frac{\partial l}{\partial t} + \frac{\partial l}{\partial a} = \{\lambda_2 \bar{w}/[1 + f_2(\lambda_2 \bar{w})]\} - \sigma_2 l[1 + g_2(l)] \qquad (7.1)$$

Here $\bar{w}$ and $\bar{l}$ represent average values of the parasite densities where the averages are taken with respect to the age distributions of the human and the intermediate host populations. The rates λ_1 and λ_2 denote the effective contact rates from vector to man and man to vector respectively. The rates σ_1 and σ_2 are the basic death rates in the human and the intermediate host respectively, if there is no density-dependence. The functions f_1 and f_2 represent density-dependent regulation of the input of parasites into the human and the intermediate host respectively. The functions g_1 and g_2 represent the relative density-dependent increase in the death rate of the human and the intermediate host respectively. In order to study equilibrium relations the partial derivatives are set equal to zero with respect to time. I assume that there is a stable exponential age distribution with parameter μ for the human population and parameter v for the vector population. Then the average values $\bar{w}$ and $\bar{l}$ can be represented as follows:

$$\bar{w} = \mu \int_0^\infty w(a)e^{-\mu a}\,\mathrm{d}a, \qquad \bar{l} = v \int_0^\infty l(a)e^{-v a}\,\mathrm{d}a \tag{7.2}$$

With this exponential age distribution the following relationship holds:

$$\mu \int_0^\infty \frac{\mathrm{d}w}{\mathrm{d}a}e^{-\mu a}\,\mathrm{d}a = \mu^2 \int_0^\infty w(a)e^{-\mu a}\,\mathrm{d}a = \mu\bar{w} \tag{7.3}$$

and similarly for $\bar{l}$. Hence we obtain the following equilibrium equations after some simple rearrangements:

$$\begin{aligned}\lambda_1\bar{l}/[1+f_1(\lambda_1\bar{l})] &= (\mu+\sigma_1)\bar{w}\{1+[\sigma_1/(\mu+\sigma_1)]\overline{wg_1(w)}/\bar{w}\}\\ \lambda_2\bar{w}/[1+f_2(\lambda_2\bar{w})] &= (v+\sigma_2)\bar{l}\{1+[\sigma_2/(v+\sigma_2)]\overline{lg_2(l)}/\bar{l}\}\end{aligned} \tag{7.4}$$

Here the bar above the function denotes the averages with respect to the corresponding age distribution:

$$\overline{wg_1(w)} = \mu \int_0^\infty w(a)g_1[w(a)]e^{-\mu a}\,\mathrm{d}a, \qquad \overline{lg_2(l)} = v \int_0^\infty l(a)g_2[l(a)]e^{-v a}\,\mathrm{d}a \tag{7.5}$$

If we multiply the two Equations (7.4) with each other we obtain the following expression:

$$R = \frac{\lambda_1\lambda_2}{(\mu+\sigma_1)(v+\sigma_2)} = \tag{7.6}$$

$$[1+f_1(\lambda_1\bar{l})]\,[1+f_2(\lambda_2\bar{w})]\left[1+\frac{\sigma_1}{\mu+\sigma_1}\frac{\overline{wg_1(w)}}{\bar{w}}\right]\left[1+\frac{\sigma_2}{v+\sigma_2}\frac{\overline{lg_2(l)}}{\bar{l}}\right]$$

The quantity R can be interpreted as the net reproduction rate of the parasite population, i.e. the number of parasites per host which one parasite per host can produce during its lifetime. In order to see this more clearly the transmission rates λ_1 and λ_2 can be broken down into their main components. Let m denote the density of vectors with respect to man. The vectors take blood-meals at the rate ϕ. The proportion of blood-meals taken from a human host is h. Then λ_1 can be written as follows: $\lambda_1 = m\phi h b_1$, where b_1 denotes the number of worms which reach maturity resulting from the number of infective larvae ingested during one blood-meal on man. Similarly, $\lambda_2 = \phi h b_2$, where b_2 is the number of infective larvae which one worm can generate during one blood-meal on man. The product $m\phi h$ is the rate at which human hosts are bitten by vectors. With this notation the parameter R can be rewritten as follows:

$$R = \left(\frac{1}{\mu + \sigma_1} \times m\phi h\right) b_2 \left(\frac{1}{\nu + \sigma_2} \times \phi h\right) b_1$$

$$= B_1 b_2 B_2 b_1 \tag{7.7}$$

During the lifetime of a parasite in the human host $(1/(\mu + \sigma_1))$ the human host is bitten at a rate $m\phi h$, hence $B_1 = m\phi h/(\mu + \sigma_1)$ is the number of blood-meals which are taken on one human host during the lifetime of one parasite. This is multiplied by b_2 to give the number of infective larvae which one worm can induce in the vector population during its lifetime. The factor B_2 is the number of blood-meals which one vector takes on human hosts during the average lifetime of an infective larva. If we multiply this by b_1 we obtain the number of worms which one infective larva can generate during its lifetime. The total product is dimensionless. I shall later assign numerical values to the individual parameters. No attempt will be made to break down the factors b_1 and b_2 into further components, such as the probability of an infective larvae leaving the vector during a human blood-meal, the probability of an infective larva penetrating the skin, the probability of reaching maturity in the human host etc.

I shall now investigate the relationship between the average worm load and the average number of infective larvae as a function of R and h. For the existence of a stable equilibrium at least one of the four functions describing density-dependent regulation has to be different from zero. There are 15 different models which are determined by the combination of density-dependent factors included. I shall examine only three of them:

$$\text{Model I}\ :\ g_1 \neq 0, f_1 = f_2 = g_2 = 0$$
$$\text{Model II}\ :\ g_2 \neq 0, f_1 = f_2 = g_1 = 0 \tag{7.8}$$
$$\text{Model III:}\ f_1 \neq 0, f_2 \neq 0, g_1 = g_2 = 0$$

In models I and II density-dependent regulation is restricted to differential mortality in the human or the vector host respectively. In model III we assume that the input is regulated for the human and the vector host, but there is no differential mortality.

For model I , Equation (7.6) reduces to:

$$R = 1 + \left(\frac{\sigma_1}{\mu + \sigma_1}\right)\left(\frac{\overline{wg_1(w)}}{\bar{w}}\right) \tag{7.9}$$

From this we infer that the average parasite load in the human host depends only on the product $\lambda_1\lambda_2 = m\phi^2 h^2 b_1 b_2$. The average number of infective larvae per vector is given by:

$$\bar{\Gamma} = \lambda_2\bar{w}/(v + \sigma_2) = \phi h b_2 \bar{w}/(v + \sigma_2) \tag{7.10}$$

i.e. it is proportional to the probability h of choosing man as a host.

For model II we obtain the opposite result: the average number of infective larvae per vector is a function of R and the average number of parasites per human host is inversely proportional to the human host choice probability h:

$$\bar{w} = R\bar{\Gamma}(v + \sigma_2)/(\phi h b_2) \tag{7.11}$$

Finally for model III Equation (7.6) reduces to the following expression:

$$R = \left\{1 + f_1\left(\frac{\lambda_1\lambda_2\bar{w}}{(v + \sigma_2)(1 + f_2(\lambda_2\bar{w}))}\right)\right\}\{1 + f_2(\lambda_2\bar{w})\} \tag{7.12}$$

In order to obtain an explicit formula for $\bar{w}$ and $\bar{\Gamma}$ we take into account only the first-order terms of f_1 and f_2:

$$f_1(x) = \alpha_1 x; \qquad f_2(x) = \alpha_2 x \tag{7.13}$$

where α_1 and α_2 are parameters which determine the density-dependent regulation of the input of parasites into the human and the intermediate host, respectively. With these assumptions we can deduce the following expressions for the average parasite load and the average number of infective larvae:

$$\bar{w} = (R-1)/[\alpha_1 R(\mu + \sigma_1) + \alpha_2\lambda_2]$$
$$\bar{\Gamma} = (R-1)/[\alpha_1\lambda_1 + \alpha_2 R(v + \sigma_2)] \tag{7.14}$$

Figure 7.2 shows the following relationships which determine the equilibrium values:

$$\bar{w} = m\phi h b_1\bar{\Gamma}/[(\mu + \sigma_1)(1 + \alpha_1 m\phi h b_1\bar{\Gamma})]$$
$$\bar{\Gamma} = \phi h b_2\bar{w}/[(v + \sigma_2)(1 + \alpha_2\phi h b_2\bar{w})] \tag{7.15}$$

I have chosen two values for h and two values for m. When h is changed m is also changed, such that the product mh^2 remains constant. Notice that the average number of infective larvae $\bar{\Gamma}$ decreases nearly proportionally to h. The average parasite load $\bar{w}$ increases slightly, but the increase is smaller for higher m. Table 7.1 gives the numerical values for the four equilibrium points. Figure 7.3(a) and (b) shows Equations (7.14) for two values of h. Note that $\bar{w}$ is practically independent of h, therefore only one curve is drawn. However, $\bar{\Gamma}$ is approximately proportional to h. We shall see later that such a relationship exists in the data.

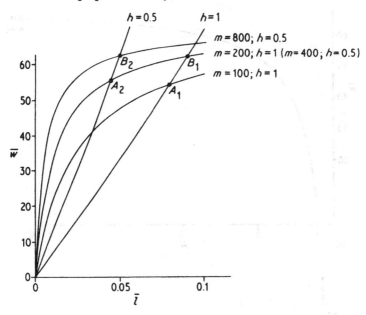

Figure 7.2 Relationships between average worm load and average number of infective larvae which determine the equilibrium levels of both variables. Parameter values used: $\alpha_1 = 0.143$; $\alpha_2 = 0.040$; $\varphi b_1 = 3$; $\varphi b_2 = 0.09$; $(\mu + \sigma_1)^{-1} = 10$; $(\mu + \sigma_2)^{-1} = 0.02$; $mh^2 = 100$ and 200. These values yield the reproductive rates $R = 5.4$ and $R = 10.8$ respectively.

Table 7.1 Equilibrium points for model III (see Fig. 7.2).

Point	Worm load, $\bar{w}$	Infective larvae/fly, $\bar{\iota}$	Vector density, m	Human host choice probability, h	Reproductive rate R
A_1	54.5	0.082	100	1.0	5.4
A_2	55.7	0.046	400	0.5	5.4
B_1	62.1	0.091	200	1.0	10.8
B_2	62.8	0.051	800	0.5	10.8

7.4 THE DATA BASE FOR THE MODELLING OF ONCHOCERCIASIS

In the absence of longitudinal data which show the rate of change of microfilarial densities and prevalence of eye lesions as a function of monitored and controlled Annual Biting Rates (ABR), we have to restrict ourselves to

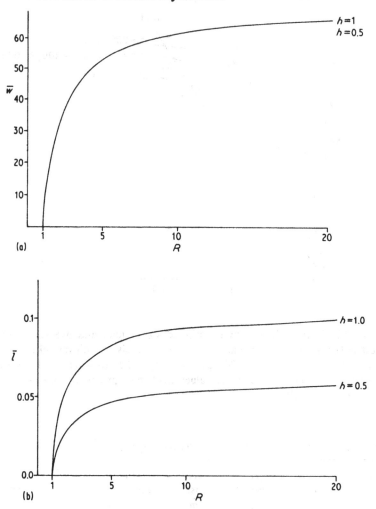

Figure 7.3 (a) The average worm load as a function of the reproductive rate R. Only values $R > 1$ yield positive values of $\bar{w}$. The two curves for $h = 1$ and $h = 0.5$ are nearly indistinguishable within drawing accuracy. Therefore only one curve is shown. For large values of R, the worm load approaches the asymptotic value $1/[\alpha_1(\mu + \sigma_1)] = 70$. (b) The average number of infective larvae/fly as a function of the reproductive rate R. For large values of R, the variable $\bar{l}$ approaches the asymptote $\phi h b_2/[(v + \sigma_2)(1/\bar{w}_\infty + \alpha_2\phi h b_2)]$, i.e. 0.101 and 0.056 respectively.

equilibrium situations covering a wide range of ABR. In order to be able to relate the parasitological measurements in man to the vector densities, one needs at least one cross-sectional survey of a total population and an estimate of the ABR and the average number of infective larvae per vector which covers at least 1 year because of marked seasonal variations. Since the estimation of the ABR requires visits to selected catching stations for 1 year or more, there are very few places for which this estimate is available. The present study is based on the data from seven villages for which Table 7.2 gives the location, size and times when the observations were made. The data for the four villages outside Cameroon are taken from Thylefors, Philippon and Prost (1978). The data for the three villages in Cameroon are published here for the first time. The parasitological and ophthalmological examinations were performed by Fuglsang and Anderson respectively. The entomological observations were collected by Renz.

Table 7.2   Characteristics of the seven villages forming the data base of the present study.

Name	Country	No. examined parasitol- ogically	Parasitological observations, Calendar year and month	Entomological observations, Calendar year
Rey Manga	Cameroon	88	1976–10	1976–78
Douffing	Cameroon	93	1976–10	1976–78
Nasso	Upper Volta	508	1977–05	1964–72
Péndié	Upper Volta	234	1975–05	1970
Mayo Galké	Cameroon	114	1976–10	1976–78
Dangouadougou	Upper Volta	205	1975–02	1963–68
Fétékro	Ivory Coast	154	1977–04	1973–76

Since the measurements were not standardized between the two sets of villages, certain scaling factors have to be applied in order to compare results. The parasitological examination method is described by Thylefors *et al.* as follows: 'Two skin snips were taken at the iliac crests, using a Holth punch. The snips were examined under a microscope with × 30 magnification after 30 minutes in distilled water. Negative snips were incubated for another 24 hours in normal saline solution and then verified again.' Fuglsang took all snips with the same type of corneo-scleral punch between 7.00 and 11.00 a.m. The snips were placed immediately in the same model of microtitration plates in separate wells, each containing 2 drops of commercially bought normal saline, which had been put into the wells at the village immediately before the start of the morning's work. The snips were left in the wells till about 2.30 p.m. when they were removed by a pin from one plate at a time. The contents of each well were then transferred one after the other to a microscope slide for immediate counting under the same microscope and using the same magnification. There is evidence that microfilariae emerge from the snip at a lower rate if they are put in distilled water rather than saline. The weight of the snips was not measured. Renz estimated the average weight of one snip on a small sample to be 2 mg. Therefore the figures reported for Cameroon in the following tables and graphs are obtained by dividing the actual counts of microfilariae by 2. In contrast, the figures for the West African villages have been multiplied by 2 in order to maintain the same relationship between average microfilarial density and prevalence of eye lesions for the two sets of villages. Since the eye lesions were recorded in a comparable way the other alternative would have been to assume a difference in the pathogenecity of the strain in West Africa from that in Northern Cameroon. Since both sets of villages belong to the savanna this was considered unlikely. In the paper by Thylefors *et al.* (1978) the average values of the microfilarial densities represent geometric means of the positive values. In the following I use arithmetic means including the zero values. The parasitological and ophthalmological data of the four West African villages were made available for the present study from the data file of the Onchocerciasis Control Project.

The entomological examinations in the West African villages were performed as follows: One catching boy exposed his two legs up to the knee, or two catching boys working alternatively one hour each, from 7 a.m. to 6 p.m. The flies were collected in individual tubes kept humid and cool, brought back to the laboratory in the evening and placed in the refrigerator for the night. Dissections took place the following morning. The flies were dissected to determine physiological age (parous or nulli-parous) and the infection rates by *Onchocerca volvulus*; they were assumed to be infective when they showed infective larvae morphologically indistinguishable from *O. volvulus* in any part of the body; infective larvae are third stage larvae moving outside the thoratic muscles and have an empty hind-gut and a functional anus (Bain, 1969); they were counted in head, thorax and abdomen of the flies.

Renz describes his methods as follow: '*Simulium* flies were caught in hourly samples by fly-collectors exposing their legs in a sitting position to the flies and catching them with a sucking tube as they came to land. A team of two collectors worked simultaneously at a distance of 20–50 m from each other at one catching station from 6 a.m. to 12 a.m. and a second team took their place from 12 to 6.30 p.m. Care was taken to assemble teams of comparable efficiency by pairing collectors with different skill and degree of attractivity to the flies . . . The flies brought to the laboratory were kept in a refrigerator and dissected as soon as possible either on the same or on the following day(s). If the flies could not be dissected immediately they were kept frozen.' Renz also recorded the number of infective larvae separately in head, thorax and abdomen and in this chapter the average number of infective larvae per fly refers to all three components.

For the four West African villages either one or two catching stations close to the river were selected. For each of the three villages in Cameroon four catching stations were selected according to the following criteria:

'at places where the biting density was supposed to be the highest, i.e. near the *S. damnosum* breeding sites along the perennial rivers, at places where the biting density was supposed to be the lowest, i.e. in the open field inland away from the river, at rainy season tributaries, which form the routes of fly-migration during the dry season and which may provide suitable *S. damnosum* breeding sites at their lower reaches, at the village well or waterhole often situated near a rainy season tributary which was frequently visited by the village populations and which was attractive to the flies too, due to the high humidity and dense vegetation of the place.'

Renz estimated the sojourn times of the human population at the four catching stations around each of the three villages in order to calculate weighted average ABR for each village. Since the ratio between the ABR at the most productive catching site to the average ABR is about 2.5 we can assume that the estimates for the ABR for the four West African villages have to be reduced by this factor.

Table 7.3 presents a summary of all the average values for the seven villages. The recorded ABR varies between 2200 and 48 000. The Annual Transmission Potential (ATP) is the product of the ABR times the average number of infective larvae per fly. In order to explain how the reproductive rate R has been estimated we first look at Fig. 7.4 which shows the relationship between the average microfilarial density and the average number of infective larvae per fly. Notice that the two sets of points lie approximately on two curves whose slopes at zero differ by a factor of 2.5. This discrepancy can either be explained by a different human host choice probability or by different vector survival or both. The proportion of larvae of non-human origin in the vector of the West African villages is about 1 % as compared to 50 % in the Cameroon villages.

Table 7.3 Observed average values used for fitting the model.

Village name	Annual Biting Rate ABR × 1000	Annual Transmission Potential ATP	Average no of infective larvae/fly	Average microfil- arial density	Prevalence of eye lesions (%)	Prevalence of blindness (%)	Estimated reproductive rate, R
Rey Manga	2.2	47	0.016	12.3†	2.4	0.0	3.1§
Douffing	2.5	55	0.022	23.3†	4.8	0.0	3.5§
Nasso	2.6	222	0.085*	28.0‡	8.3	0.2	9.0‖
Péndié	9.7	959	0.099*	41.5‡	14.7	2.1	33.7‖
Mayo Galké	36.2	1.318	0.039	46.3†	15.2	2.6	50.3§
Dangouadougou	21.3	1.601	0.075*	54.3‡	20.9	4.5	74.0‖
Fétékro	48.0	1.948	0.041*	66.0‡	25.0	7.6	166.7‖

* Estimated by ATP/ABR.
† Arithmetic mean, microfilariae/mg.
‡ Arithmetic mean of microfilariae/snip, multiplied by 2 (see the text).
§ ABR/720.
‖ ABR/288.

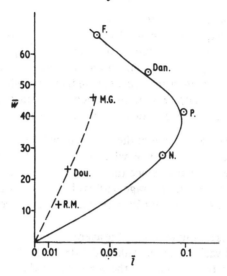

Figure 7.4   The observed relationship between the average microfilarial density $\bar{w}$ and the average number of infective larvae/fly $\bar{l}$, based on three villages in Cameroon (Rey Manga = R.M.; Douffing = Dou.; Mayo Galké = M.G.) and four villages in the area of the Onchocerciasis Control Programme (Nasso = N.; Péndié = P.; Dangouadougou = Dan.; Fétékro = F.) The hypothetical curves linking the points go through the point $(\bar{w}, \bar{l}) = (0, 0)$ since this corresponds to a trivial equilibrium.

This suggests that the vector in West Africa is more anthropophilic. If the human host choice probability of the two sets of villages differs by a factor of 2.5, then the reproductive rate will differ by a factor of $2.5^2 = 6.25$. Since the ABR in the West African villages has been over-estimated by a factor of 2.5 we only have to divide the ABRs of the Cameroon villages by a factor of 2.5 in order to obtain a common scale which is proportional to the reproductive rate. Figure 7.5 shows the average number of infective larvae, the average microfilarial density and the percentage of eye lesions as a function of this common scale. Notice that the seven points for the eye lesions can be linked by a curve which approaches zero at an ABR of 720 for the Cameroon villages, corresponding to 288 for the West African villages. If we take these values as the critical ABRs for a non-zero endemic level we can calculate the reproductive rates as ratios of the observed values to the corresponding critical value. The result of this calculation is given in the last column of Table 7.3. Notice that the estimated reproductive rates vary between about 3 and 167.

These considerations show that it is possible to specify an absolute critical level for the man biting rate below which onchocerciasis cannot maintain itself, if one takes into account the local characteristics of the vector and the relative bias of the sampling procedures.

Figure 7.6 shows the relationship between the prevalence of blindness due to

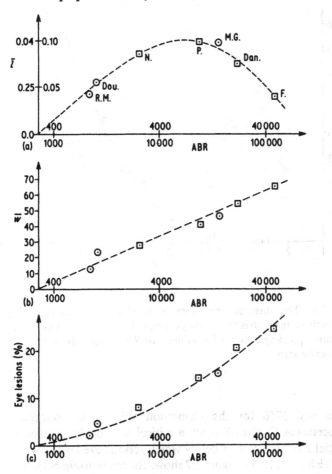

Figure 7.5 The Annual Biting Rate (ABR) is the common abscissa to (a)–(c). The upper scale refers to the OCP villages, the lower scale to the Cameroon villages. (a) Shows the average number of infective larvae/fly on a different scale for the two sets of villages; the scale on the left hand side of the ordinate refers to the Cameroon villages (⊙), the scale on the right hand side refers to the OCP villages (▢). The hypothetical curve linking the points is extrapolated for lower values of ABR until $\bar{l} = 0$. The corresponding critical values for ABR are 720 for the Cameroon villages and 288 for the OCP villages. The same critical values are obtained by extrapolating the curves for the average microfilarial density ($\bar{w}$) and the prevalence of eye lesions until they reach the zero level. (see Fig. 7.4 legend for full names of villages.)

onchocerciasis and the reproductive rate. Here it appears to be justified to identify a critical level of R below which blindness does not occur. An acceptable estimate seems to be $R = 8$. This corresponds to a critical ABR of about 2300 for a vector with the characteristics found in the four West African

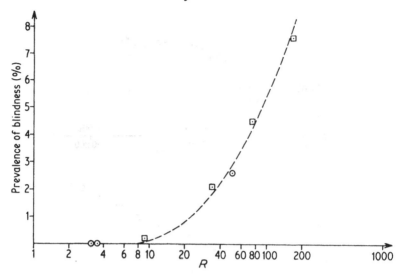

Figure 7.6 The observed prevalence of blindness as a function of the observed reproductive rate which is obtained by expressing the observed ABR values as multiples of the corresponding critical ABR values. For R less than 8 the prevalence of blindness is practically zero.

villages and 5750 for the Cameroon villages. In connection with the Onchocerciasis Control Project, a critical level of the Annual Transmission Potential has been sought below which serious eye lesions would not occur (see Walsh *et al.*, 1979). Figure 7.7 shows the relationship between ATP and R. For R below 35 the ATP is simply proportional to $R - 1$. For $R = 8$, i.e. the critical value for zero blindness, we get ATP = 203.

We shall now look at the average microfilarial density, the prevalence of eye lesions and blindness as a function of the ATP (Fig. 7.8). There is no critical level for the ATP below which the prevalence of eye lesions is zero. The average microfilarial density approaches an asymptote with a very small (if not zero) slope. On the contrary, the slope of the prevalence of blindness increases for large values of the ATP.

Finally the age- and sex-specific microfilarial densities for two Cameroon villages are presented in Table 7.4. There is a marked sex difference. The microfilarial densities in Mayo Galké reach a maximum value between 40 and 50 years after which they decline. A satisfactory model should not only describe the average values for varying values of R, but also the different shapes of the age-specific prevalence curves.

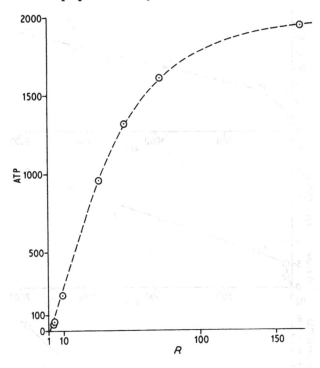

Figure 7.7   The relationship between the Annual Transmission Potential (ATP) and the reproductive rate *R*. For *R* up to 35 corresponding to ATP of 1000 the relationship can be described by a straight line passing through zero for *R* = 1 with a slope of about 29.

7.5   THE MODEL

A preliminary version of the present model has been published in the proceedings of the *Vito Volterra Symposium on Mathematical Models in Biology* (Dietz, 1980). That model, however, was only concerned with the transmission dynamics of the parasites without taking into account the prevalence of eye lesions and blindness. It predicts a monotonically increasing microfilarial density as a function of age of the human host. This is in contrast to the observations at high endemic levels. In the present model we assume that this decline of the microfilarial density in higher age groups is due to differential survival rates of blind individuals. There is some evidence that villages with a high endemic level, and therefore a higher rate of blindness, also have higher death rates. Other explanations of this decline in higher age groups are also conceivable: increased death rate of the worms due to increased reactions of the host, decrease of input of new worms due to immunological

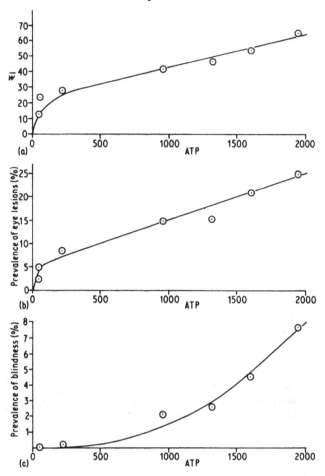

Figure 7.8 The average microfilarial density $\bar{w}$ (a), the prevelance of eye lesions (b) and the prevalence of blindness (c) as a function of the Annual Transmission Potential (ATP). There is no positive critical level of the ATP for which the prevalence of eye lesions is zero. A zero prevalence of blindness corresponds to an ATP of approximately 200.

effects and, finally, atrophy of the skin in old individuals due to the presence of large numbers of microfilariae. If one tries to fit models with any one of these assumptions to data, then the age at which the peak microfilarial density is reached is predicted much earlier than is observed. Therefore I adopted the assumption of differential survival due to blindness. Since blindness occurs relatively late in life the differential survival will only affect the higher age groups. In the following I list the assumptions of the model and define the parameters.

Table 7.4   Age- and sex-specific arithmetical mean microfilarial densities/mg.

Age (years)	Mayo Galké			Rey Manga		
	Male	Female	Total	Male	Female	Total
0–4	2.7	4.7	3.8	0.0	0.0	0.0
5–9	18.0	27.7	22.3	0.5	0.0	0.1
10–14	79.2	17.7	45.9	2.2	0.3	0.9
15–19	59.5	39.5	42.9	1.9	0.0	1.4
20–29	102.4	17.6	56.8	24.3	0.0	7.0
30–39	108.8	71.2	83.7	29.0	6.0	16.7
40–49	129.2	77.5	117.7	32.8	10.1	17.2
50–59	4.0	53.5	46.5	19.4	19.5	19.4
60+	62.5	53.5*	62.5	19.4*	17.4	12.3

* Extrapolated value (no person examined in age group).

In order to take into account differential exposure of male and female individuals we assume that the population is composed of two subpopulations of relative size p and $1 - p$ such that the ratio of the exposure rates is r. The value for p has been set *a priori* at 0.5.

The probability $c(\lambda)$ that an infective larva turns into a mature worm is described by the expression $c(\lambda) = (b_0\delta + b_\infty\lambda)/(\delta + \lambda)$, where b_0 and b_∞ determine $c(0)$ and $c(\infty)$, respectively, and δ is the Annual Transmission level for which $c(\delta) = (b_0 + b_\infty)/2$. This expression has been chosen on the basis of Fig. 7.8 where the average microfilarial density behaves asymptotically as a linear function of the Annual Transmission Potential.

The age-specific microfilarial densities show a small rate of increase in low age classes which is attributed to age-dependent exposure. If one assumes that the rate of exposure is roughly proportional to body surface, this is to be expected. In the model we assume a logistic function for the approach to full exposure as age increases. The age at which 50% of full exposure is reached is denoted by the letter A. The slope of the logistic function at A is proportional to β. The functional expression for the probability of exposure is as follows:

$$1/\{1 + \exp[-\beta(a - A)]\} \tag{7.16}$$

where a denotes age.

The death rate of worms is denoted by σ. The number of microfilariae per snip is assumed to be proportional to the number of worms at any age. This is certainly a great oversimplification but in the absence of more detailed information about the relationship between the worm load and the microfilarial density this seems to be justified. The rate of acquiring eye lesions is proportional to some power of the worm load. It is thought that a certain minimum number of worms is required for eye lesions to occur. The exponent is denoted by j and the factor of proportionality is φ. Similarly the rate of getting blind is proportional to the kth power of the number of eye lesions. The factor of proportionality is ψ. I assume that blind individuals have a differential death rate ρ.

In order to calculate average microfilarial densities, average prevalence of eye lesions and average prevalence of blindness, we use the age distribution which is adopted by the Onchocerciasis Control Programme for age standardization of measurements. Table 7.5 gives the corresponding weights $n(a)$ for the different age classes.

Table 7.5 The relative weights of the different age groups based on the standard population of the Onchocerciasis Control Project (OCP). (Proportions are obtained by adding together the corresponding values for males and females.)

Age group	Percentage
0–4	12.5
5–9	14.8
10–14	14.5
15–19	9.1
20–29	14.3
30–39	13.3
40–49	10.4
50–59	7.4
60+	3.7

No attempt has been made to model in detail the uptake of microfilariae by the vector or their development into infective larvae. We simply fitted the following relationship between the average number of infective larvae per fly and the average microfilarial density $\bar{w}$ of a village to the data:

$$\bar{l}(\bar{w}) = f\bar{w}/[1 + \exp\{q(\bar{w} - W)\}] \tag{7.17}$$

where f, q and W are three adjustable parameters. Since $[1 + \exp(-qW)]^{-1}$ is close to 1, f represents approximately the factor of proportionality between $\bar{l}$ and $\bar{w}$ for small average microfilarial densities. These assumptions lead to the following dynamic equations where the partial derivatives have been approximated by differences. As a time interval for the simulations, 1 year has been chosen since this was considered sufficient in view of the relatively small rates of change as hosts age.

The variables of the model are defined as follows: the index i refers to the subpopulations $i = 1$ and 2, which differ with respect to the exposure to bites by the vector. The index b or g is attached to the variables depending whether or not an individual is blind, respectively (whether he or she has blind or good eyes). The argument a refers to the age of an individual. The argument t denotes the time. Thus $w_{g1}(a, t)$ is the average worm load of an individual in exposure group 1, without blindness, of age a at time t; and $e_{b2}(a, t)$ is the average number of eye lesions of a blind individual in exposure group 2, of age a at time t. $s_{gi}(a, t)$ is the probability at time t that an individual of age a in exposure group i is not yet blind. $s_{bi}(a, t)$ is the probability at time t that a blind individual of age a in exposure group i is still alive. $s_i(a, t) = s_{gi}(a, t) + s_{bi}(a, t)$ is thus the probability at time t that an individual of age a has not died as a result of blindness. $B_i(a, t) = s_{bi}(a, t)/s_i(a, t)$ is the prevalence of blindness at time t in individuals of age a in exposure group i (see Appendix). $E_i(a, t)$ is the prevalence of eye lesions at time t in individuals of age a in exposure group i. We drop the index i if we take the average of the two exposure groups. An average with respect to age is denoted by a bar above the variable, e.g. $\bar{w}(t)$. The Annual Potential Transmission is denoted by λ, and the Annual Biting Rate by V.

With these definitions and the assumptions stated above we arrive at the following set of difference equations. They are listed here exactly as they are programmed to produce the equilibrium results and the dynamic projections to be discussed in the next section. Since we are working with a time interval of 1 year in these difference equations, we must take care that variables do not become negative for high transition rates. This problem was important only for $s_{gi}(a, t)$ in the exploratory phase, when parameter values in a wide range were tried out. First the equations describing the dynamics are listed:

$$
\begin{aligned}
w_{gi}(a+1, t+1) &= w_{gi}(a, t)(1 - \sigma) + b_0 \lambda_i(t)\gamma_i(t)/[1 + e^{-\beta(a-A)}] \\
w_{bi}(a+1, t+1) &= w_{bi}(a, t)[1 - (\sigma + \rho)] + b_0 \lambda_i(t)\gamma_i(t)/[1 + e^{-\beta(a-A)}] \\
e_{gi}(a+1, t+1) &= e_{gi}(a, t) + \varphi w_{gi}^j(a, t) \\
e_{bi}(a+1, t+1) &= e_{bi}(a, t)(1 - \rho) + \varphi w_{bi}^j(a, t) \\
s_{gi}(a+1, t+1) &= s_{gi}(a, t)\exp[-\psi e_{gi}^k(a, t)] \\
s_{bi}(a+1, t+1) &= s_{bi}(a, t)(1 - \rho) + s_{gi}\{1 - \exp[-\psi e_{gi}^k(a, t)]\}
\end{aligned}
\tag{7.18}
$$

Here $\gamma_i(t)$ is calculated according to the following steps: The expression

$$
w_i(a, t) = (1 - B_i(a, t))w_{gi}(a, t) + B_i(a, t)w_{bi}(a, t) \tag{7.19}
$$

is the average worm load in exposure group i. We get the average age-specific worm load by the following formula:

$$
w(a, t) = [pw_1(a, t)s_1(a, t) + (1 - p)w_2(a, t)s_2(a, t)]/s(a, t) \tag{7.20}
$$

In order to obtain the population average of the worm load we have to take as

weights the product of the standard population weights and the differential
survival probabilities:

$$\bar{w}(t) = \left[\sum_a w(a, t)n(a)s(a, t)\right]\bigg/\left[\sum_a n(a)s(a, t)\right] \qquad (7.21)$$

This population average determines the average number of infective larvae $\bar{l}$
according to (7.17). Finally we set

$$\lambda(t) = V(t)\bar{l}(t) \qquad (7.22)$$

This average ATP is distributed among the two exposure groups according to
the formulae

$$\lambda_1(t) = r\lambda(t)/[rp + (1-p)] \quad \lambda_2(t) = \lambda(t)/[rp + (1-p)] \qquad (7.23)$$

The input γ_i into the human host is regulated by the expression:

$$\gamma_i(t) = (c\lambda_i(t) + \delta)/(\lambda_i(t) + \delta) \qquad (7.24)$$

$V(t)$ is the time-dependent Annual Biting Rate, which can be specified in
order to simulate the effects of vector control programmes. The boundary
values for the variables in Equation (7.18) are obviously

$$w_{gi}(0, t) = w_{bi}(0, t) = e_{gi}(0, t) = e_{bi}(0, t) = s_{bi}(0, t) = 0$$
$$s_{gi}(0, t) = 1 \qquad (7.25)$$

The initial values for $t = 0$ and $a \geqslant 0$ are simply determined by one initial value
of $\lambda(0)$ using Equation (7.18) except that the argument t and $t + 1$, respectively,
is replaced by zero. This $\lambda(0)$ may be the equilibrium ATP corresponding to the
initial $V(0)$. Instead of calculating the equilibrium ATPs for given values of V,
it is easier to start with ATP values and to determine in a direct way the
corresponding V value according to the following steps:

1. Determine λ_1 and λ_2 by Equations (7.23).
2. Determine γ_1 and γ_2 by Equation (7.24).
3. Solve Equations (7.18) without the argument t, i.e. use Equations (7.18) to
   get a time-independent equilibrium age distribution.
4. Determine $\bar{w}$ by successively using Equations (7.19), (7.20) and (7.21).
5. Determine $\bar{l}$ by Equation (7.17).
6. Then V is given by $\lambda/\bar{l}$.

Table 7.6 lists the numerical values of the parameters which were determined
as follows. As mentioned above we consider two exposure groups of equal size,
i.e. $p = 0.5$. The ratio of high to low exposure is set equal to 5, i.e. $r = 0.2$. The
parameters b_∞ and δ were estimated on the basis of Fig. 7.8a, which shows an
asymptotically linear relationship between λ and $\bar{w}$. The parameter b_0 was
chosen such that the critical V^* corresponds roughly to the observed value in
the West African villages of 288. If there were no age-specific exposure, one

Table 7.6 Parameter values of the model used for fitting the data and for the projections of vector control effects.

Meaning of the parameter	Symbol	Numerical value
Proportion of the population with low exposure	p	0.5
Ratio low exposure rate/high exposure rate	r	0.2
Probability $c(\lambda)$ that an infective larva turns into a mature worm for $\lambda = 0$	b_0	0.16
$c(\infty)$	b_∞	0.00043
Annual Transmission Potential for which $c(\lambda) = (b_0 + b_\infty)/2$	δ	28.3
Parameters of the logistic function describing the approach to full exposure as a function of age	A β	10.0 0.55
Death rate of worms in the surviving host	σ	0.08
Differential death rate of blind individuals	ρ	0.04
Parameters describing the rate of appearance of eye lesions	φ j	0.5×10^{-9} 4
Parameters describing the rate of becoming blind as a consequence of eye lesions	ψ k	0.1×10^{-3} 3
Parameters describing the relationship between the average number of infective larvae/fly as a function of the average worm load (see eqn. 7.17)	f q W	0.0037 0.09 49

could determine b_0 from the relationship for the critical reproductive rate:

$$R = V^* f b_0/(\sigma + \mu) = 1 \qquad (7.26)$$

where μ denotes the average human death rate. The formula neglects the factor $[1 + \exp(-qW)]^{-1}$, since this is very close to 1. The value for f has been estimated from the relationship between $\bar{w}$ and Γ for low values of $\bar{w}$, and the life expectancy $(\sigma + \mu)^{-1}$ of the worm is set equal to 8.3 years ($\sigma = 0.08$, $\mu = 0.04$). For $f = 0.0037$ and $V = 288$, we get $b_0 = 0.11$. Since full exposure is only attained by adults, b_0 has to be increased to 0.16 to keep V^* at the desired level. The age A at which 50% of the maximum exposure is reached is set equal to 10 years. The slope β has been chosen such that at age 18 approximately 99% of full exposure is reached ($\beta = 0.55$). The parameters φ, j, ψ and k, which determine the prevalence of eye lesions and blindness were chosen such that the predicted values corresponded approximately to the observed values in the village with the highest ATP. The average residual length of life of a blind individual is set at 12.5 years, which is achieved by choosing $\rho = 0.04$. For the relationship (7.17) between $\bar{w}$ and Γ the parameters $q = 0.09$ and $W = 49$ were

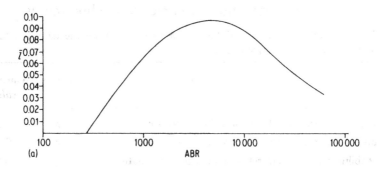

(a)

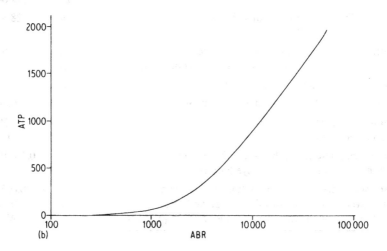

(b)

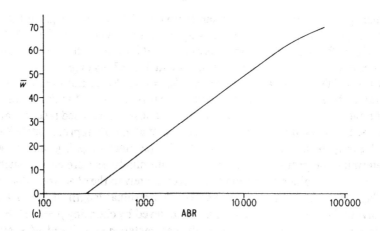

(c)

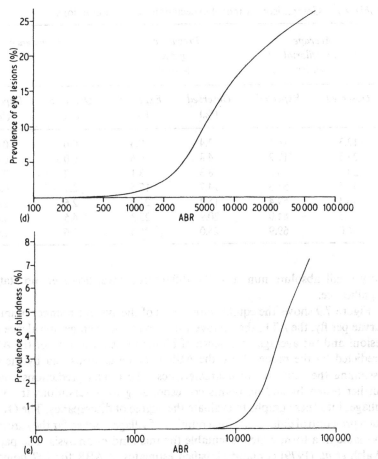

Figure 7.9   (a) Model prediction of the relationship between the average number of infective larvae/fly Γ and the Annual Biting Rate (ABR) as measured by the OCP, assuming the same vector characteristics. (b) Model prediction of the relationship between the Annual Transmission Potential (ATP) and the Annual Biting Rate (ABR). (c) Model prediction of relationship between the arithmetic average of the microfilarial density $\bar{w}$ and the Annual Biting Rate (ABR). (d) Model prediction of the relationship between the prevalence of eye lesions and the Annual Biting Rate (ABR). (e) Model prediction of the relationship between the prevalence of blindness and the Annual Biting Rate (ABR).

determined. A brief attempt to estimate parameters by a least-squares method has not been continued since the estimates depended too much on the relative weights attributed to the individual variables.

Table 7.7 shows the extent to which the model predictions agree with the observations. Note that the prevalence of eye lesions and blindness is systematically underestimated for low ATPs. Since we are dealing here with

Table 7.7   Comparison of model expectations with observations

Average microfilarial density		Prevalence of eye lesions		Prevalence of blindness	
Observed	*Expected*	*Observed* (%)	*Expected* (%)	*Observed* (%)	*Expected* (%)
12.3	16.1	2.4	0.5	0.0	0.0
23.3	17.2	4.8	0.6	0.0	0.0
28.0	28.5	8.3	3.1	0.2	0.0
41.5	51.3	14.7	17.5	2.1	0.4
46.3	59.4	15.2	21.3	2.6	2.4
54.3	64.0	20.9	23.3	4.5	4.8
66.0	69.9	25.0	25.4	7.6	7.0

very small absolute numbers, the differences have, however, no statistical significance.

Figure 7.9 shows the equilibrium values of the average number of infective larvae per fly, the ATP, the average worm load, the average prevalence of eye lesions and the average prevalence of blindness as a function of the ABR as predicted by the model. Here the ABR is taken as measured by the OCP, assuming the same vector characteristics. The model predictions could be further tested by adding points corresponding to observations from other villages into these graphs to evaluate the degree of discrepancy. The OCP has such pre-control data on file for a number of villages, but so far they are not yet available in a form which is suitable for this kind of analysis. The paper by Walsh *et al.* (1979) contains classified estimates of ABR for 127 points and Prost *et al.* (1979) show relationships between some average indicators of onchocerciasis, such as prevalence of the infection, prevalence of eye lesions and prevalence of blindness. It is hoped that there is a large proportion of villages for which both kinds of data are recorded such that the model can be further tested and revised if it turns out that the relationships found for the present seven villages are not representative.

7.6   DYNAMIC PROJECTIONS OF VECTOR CONTROL EFFECTS

I shall compare three different vector control strategies:

S_1: 100% vector control for 9 years starting in year 2. Then return of the vector density to its original level.

S_2: 100% vector control for 20 years, starting in year 2. Then return of the vector density to its original level.

S_3: Reduction of the original ABR of about 21 000 to the level 2000 in year 2
and maintenance of this level for 29 years.

If vector control operations are interrupted in the OCP area and reinvasion of
the vector is not prevented it can be assumed that the vector density reaches its
pre-control level within 1 year. Strategy S_3 is based on the hope of achieving
the maintenance of a non-zero endemic level but with practically zero
prevalence of blindness.

Figure 7.10 shows the average microfilarial densities, the prevalence of eye
lesions and of blindness, and the ATP for the three strategies as a function of
time.

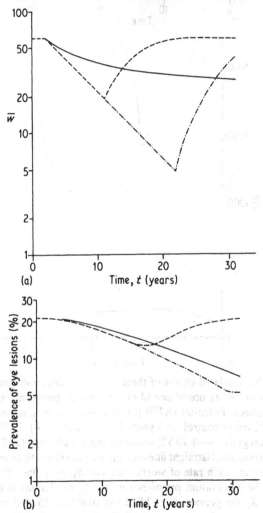

Figure 7.10 (for caption see overleaf)

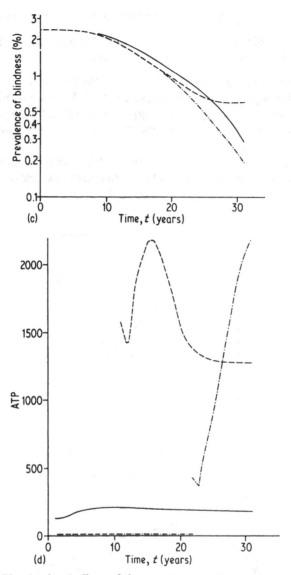

Figure 7.10 The simulated effects of three vector control strategies on the average microfilarial density $\bar{w}$ (a), prevalence of eye lesions (b), prevalence of blindness and Annual Transmission Potential (ATP) (d) as a function of time in years. Strategy S_1 (– – – –): 100% vector control for 9 years. Strategy S_2 (– · – · –): 100% vector control for 20 years. Strategy S_3 (——): 90.5% vector control for 29 years. (a) For S_1 and S_2 the decline of $\bar{w}$ is exponential (straight line on semi-log paper) due to an assumed age- and density-independent death rate of worms. (b) For S_3 even after 29 years of 90.5% vector control the equilibrium prevalence of 2.25% eye lesions is not yet reached. (c) For S_1 and S_2 the prevalence of blindness continues to decline for some time beyond the termination of vector control. (d) For S_1 and S_2, the ATP after termination of vector control is higher than before the beginning of vector control.

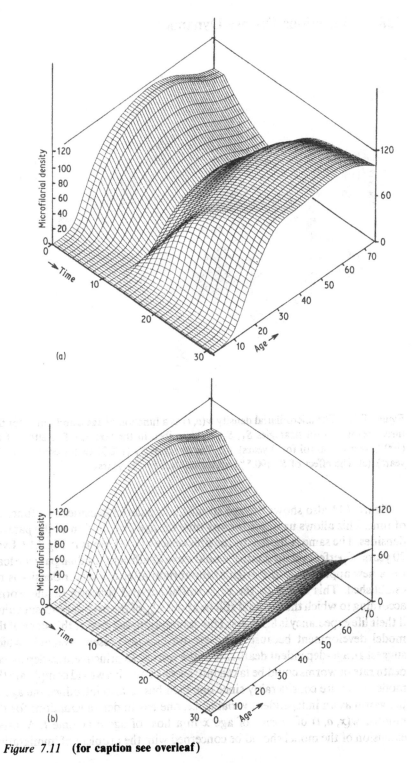

(a)

(b)

Figure 7.11 (for caption see overleaf)

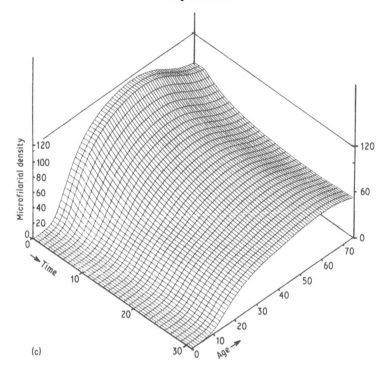

Microfilarial density

120
100
80
60
40
20
0
0

Time

10

20

30

120

60

0

70

60

50

40

30

20

10

0

Age

(c)

Figure 7.11 The microfilarial density $w(a, t)$ as a function of age a and time t for the three vector control strategies S_1, S_2, S_3 described in the text. (a) The effect of S_1 (100% vector control for 9 years). (b) The effect of S_2 (100% vector control for 20 years). (c) The effect of S_3 (90.5% vector control for 29 years).

Figure 7.11 also shows the age-specific microfilarial densities as a function of time. This allows us to see for any time the age distribution of the parasite densities. The same is shown for the prevalence of eye lesions in Fig.7.12. Even 20 years of perfect vector control would leave a sufficient residual parasite load for a new approach to the original equlibrium after the vector density is re-established. This is due to the exponential survival function of the worms according to which there would still be about 9% of the original parasites alive if their life expectancy is 8.3 years. This assumption was used at this stage of the model development because there are no data at present available which suggest an age-dependent death rate of the worms. In principle, age-dependent death rate of worms could be taken into account but this would complicate the model structure considerably since one then has to also introduce the age of the worm as an independent variable, i.e. one has to derive equations for the number $w(x, a, t)$ of worms of age x in a host of age a at time t. Another extension of the model should be concerned with the problem of immigration

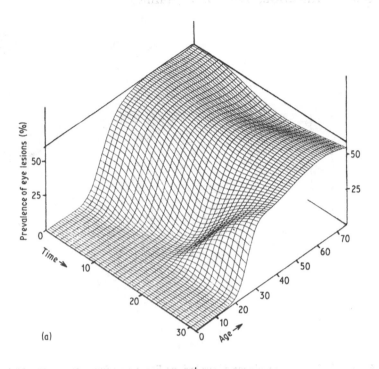

(a)

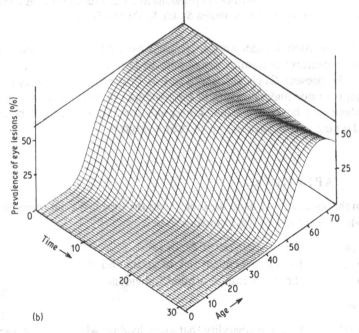

(b)

Figure 7.12 **(for caption see overleaf)**

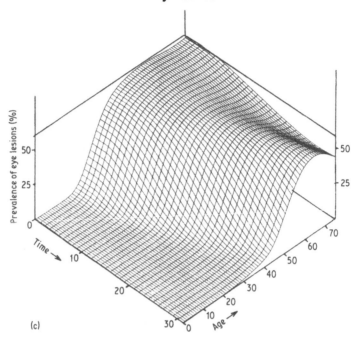

Figure 7.12 The prevalence of eye lesions $E(a, t)$ as a function of age a and time t for the three vector control strategies S_1 (a), S_2 (b) and S_3 (c).

of parasitized human and/or vector hosts. Also the application of mass chemotherapy or nodulectomy could be built into the model.

The present Onchocerciasis Control Project is a unique opportunity to improve our understanding of the dynamics of onchocerciasis transmission, which can be incorporated into predictive models for the benefit of the planning and the evaluation of future projects.

APPENDIX

In this appendix we drop the index i and the time t. We only consider a cohort which is subject to the following risks:

$\mu(a)$	the age-dependent death rate
$\eta(a)$	the age-dependent risk of getting blind
ρ	the death rate of a blind individual

Let

$n_g(a)$ be the probability that an individual who would be age a is alive and not blind, and let

$n_b(a)$ be the probability that an individual who would be age a is alive and blind.

Then these probabilities satisfy the following set of differential equations:

$$\frac{dn_g}{da} = -[\mu(a)+\eta(a)]n_g,$$

$$\frac{dn_b}{da} = \eta(a)n_g-[\mu(a)+\rho]n_b.$$

In the main text equations are given for the conditional probabilities under the condition $\mu(\alpha) \equiv 0$, i.e. death due to other causes except blindness are excluded. These conditional probabilities satisfy the equations

$$\frac{ds_g}{da} = -\eta(a)s_g,$$

$$\frac{ds_b}{da} = \eta(a)s_g-\rho s_b.$$

One easily verifies that

$$n_g(a) = \exp\left\{ -\int_0^a \mu(\tau)d\tau \right\}s_g(a),$$

$$n_b(a) = \exp\left\{ -\int_0^a \mu(\tau)d\tau \right\}s_b(a)$$

The survival probability $n_g(a)+n_b(a) = n(a)$ is given by

$$\exp\left\{ -\int_0^a \mu(\tau)d\tau \right\}[s_g(a)+s_b(a)],$$

and the prevalence of blindness $B(a)$ is simply the ratio

$$n_b(a)/n(a) = s_b(a)/[s_g(a)+s_g(a)].$$

ACKNOWLEDGEMENTS

I thank J. Anderson, H. Fuglsang, A. Renz for access to their data from Cameroon, M. L. Bazin, former Director of OCP, for the permission to use data from OCP, H. Federmutz and U. Thieszen for help in the analysis of the Cameroon data, H. Renner for programming the various versions of the model, P. Wenk for Fig. 7.1, B. O. L. Duke for stimulating discussions and Betty Kirkwood for constructive criticism. This investigation received support from the Filariasis component of the UNDP/World Bank/WHO Special Programme for Research and Training in Tropical Diseases.

8 Fox rabies

Roy M. Anderson

8.1 INTRODUCTION

Throughout the world rabies has been, and is still, regarded as one of the most terrifying diseases known to man. It is a directly transmitted viral infection of the central nervous system, to which all mammals are thought susceptible although not equally so. The most highly susceptible animals are foxes, coyotes, jackals, wolves, kangaroo rats, cotton rats and field voles. Dogs, although only regarded as moderately susceptible, are of major importance as transmitters of the infection to man. The disease is usually transmitted by the bite of an infected animal, the saliva of which contains virus particles (Kaplan, 1977; Baer, 1975).

The incidence of rabies within human populations is generally very low. The number of people dying from rabies in Europe, for example, is around four per annum in recent years, and even the global total, which is estimated as 15 000 per annum, is dwarfed by other infectious diseases. The nature of the clinical symptoms, however, which are distressing and often hideous, plus the knowledge that death is virtually inevitable once they appear makes rabies a continuing cause for concern.

The disease remains endemic throughout many regions of the world as a consequence of the reservoir of infection in wild animals. Rabies is largely maintained by species belonging to the orders *Chiroptera* and *Carnivora*, although the epidemiological role of rodents and other small mammals is also thought to be important. Infection in man plays no part in the endemic persistence of rabies in the world today.

This chapter examines the recent epidemic of rabies in Europe and, in contrast to the preceding chapters (which are concerned with disease behaviour within human communities), focuses on the impact of infection within fox populations. The reason for doing so is that the current European epidemic is characterized by a high incidence of rabies in the red fox, *Vulpes vulpes* (Nikolitsch, 1965). Of the 16 820 cases of animal rabies reported in Europe in 1979, over 70% were in this host species. Throughout Europe, and to a lesser extent in Canada and the United States, foxes (red, grey and arctic species) play a dominant role in the transmission and maintenance of the disease. The current European epidemic was thought to have originated in Poland in 1939 and has spread outwards at an annual rate of 30–60 km, with the present front in France being less than 40 km from the Channel coastline (Fig. 8.1).

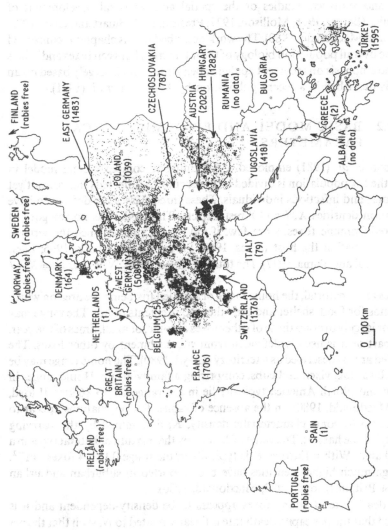

Figure 8.1 Geographical distribution of reported European cases of rabies, both in wildlife and domestic animals, during 1979 (number of cases in parentheses). Each dot denotes one reported case, except for a few dots in northern Switzerland and southern Germany which represent between one and four cases.

FINLAND
(rabies free)

EAST GERMANY
(1483)

CZECHOSLOVAKIA
(787)

AUSTRIA
(2020) HUNGARY
(1282)

RUMANIA
(no data)

BULGARIA
(0)

TURKEY
(1595)

GREECE
(2)

ALBANIA
(no data)

YUGOSLAVIA
(418)

POLAND
(1039)

SWEDEN
(rabies free)

NORWAY
(rabies free)

DENMARK
(164)

NETHERLANDS
(1)

WEST
GERMANY
(5089)

BELGIUM (25)

ITALY
(79)

SWITZERLAND
(1376)

GREAT
BRITAIN
(rabies free)

IRELAND
(rabies free)

FRANCE
(1706)

SPAIN
(1)

PORTUGAL
(rabies free)

0   100 km

Over the past few decades there have been many studies of the epidemiology of rabies in fox populations. Attention has been focused on the characteristics of the viral infection within the host and on the ecology of the fox. Recent reviews of this literature have been published by Nagano and Davenport (1971), Baer (1975), Lloyd (1976), Andral and Toma (1977), Macdonald (1980) and Zimen (1980). Much less attention has been given to the dynamics of rabies within fox populations although recent work has included computer simulation and statistical studies of the spatial and temporal development of epidemics (Berger, 1976; Mollison, 1977; Preston, 1973; Smart and Giles, 1973; Bacon and Macdonald, 1980). The work described in this chapter is concerned with the overall population biology of the interaction between foxes and rabies with the emphasis on recurrent epidemic behaviour, and is largely based on an analysis described in a recent publication by Anderson et al. (1981).

8.2   BASIC MODEL AND EPIDEMIOLOGICAL PARAMETERS

Anderson et al. (1981) employed a deterministic compartmental model in which the fox population is divided into susceptibles, infecteds that are not yet infectious, and infectious individuals. These three classes are defined to have population densities X, I and Y respectively. The model has no category of recovered immune foxes, since few, if any, foxes recover once the virus is established within the host (Sikes, 1962; Parker and Wilsnack, 1966; Baer, 1975; Andral and Toma, 1977). The total density of foxes, N, is thus $N = X + I + Y$.

Foxes are territorial, the home range of a settled fox being the area on which it depends for food, shelter and the other requirements of life. The range may partly or largely overlap those of other foxes at some, or at all, times of the year, but a part of it is usually defended from encroachment by other foxes. The defended area is described as a territory (Lloyd, 1980). The home range may be shared by a dog, vixen and cubs, comprising a family group. Home ranges in Europe and North America typically lie in the range 2.5 to 16 km² (Lloyd, 1980; Macdonald, 1980). In the absence of rabies, fox populations appear to increase up to some characteristic density, K, determined by the 'carrying capacity' of the habitat. The value of K is set by the mixture of habitat types in a defined area. Within Europe, K is typically in the range 0.1 to 4 foxes km^{-2}, although much higher densities have been reported in suburban and urban areas of Britain (Lloyd, 1980; Macdonald, 1980).

The death rate of young foxes appears to be density-dependent and it is assumed that the per capita death rate is linearly related to N, such that the net rate is $(b + \gamma N)N$. The parameter $1/b$ denotes fox life expectancy in the absence of resource limitation and γ measures the severity of density-dependent constraints. As recorded in Table 8.1, life expectancy is typically in the range 1.5 to 2.7 years within Europe. Wandeler (1976) argues that the rate of

Table 8.1 Life expectancy ($1/b$) of the red fox.

Life expectancy (years)	Study area	References
1.5	Denmark	Lloyd (1976)
1.7	Wales	Lloyd (1980)
1.8	Scotland	Klob and Hewson (1980)
1.9	Suburban London	Harris (1977)
2.2	Germany	Bromel and Zettl (1974)
2.7	Netherlands	Van Haaften (1970)

reproduction is independent of population density for foxes in Europe although other reports suggest it may be limited by food availability (Zimen, 1980). For simplicity, it is assumed that the net effects of density-dependence are captured by the parameter γ (encompassing effects on reproduction and survival) and that the per capita birth rate in the absence of such constraints is a. The number of cubs in a litter ranges from 1 to 10 with, in Europe, a mean of 4.7 (Lloyd, 1976). Sex ratios are in general close to unity at birth, and the pregnancy rate is on average in the region of 90 % with a further 10 % of vixens failing to produce offspring (Englund, 1970; Wandeler, 1976; Lloyd, 1980; Macdonald, 1980). Combining these figures an average value of a of 1.0 per annum is arrived at. With a life expectancy of roughly 2 years this gives an intrinsic per capita population growth rate, r, where $r = a - b$, around 0.5 per annum. This value will tend to vary in different habitats depending on food availability and other factors (Zimen, 1980).

These assumptions about the population biology of the fox lead to the familiar logistic equation for the dynamics in the absence of rabies where:

$$dN/dt = rN(1 - N/K) \tag{8.1}$$

The carrying capacity K of the habitat at equilibrium is defined as r/γ.

Turning to the dynamics of the disease, Anderson *et al.* (1981) made the conventional assumption that the rate at which foxes acquire rabies is proportional to the number of encounters between susceptible and infectious foxes, βXY (Bailey, 1975). Here the parameter, β, is a transmission coefficient where $1/\beta$ is proportional to the average time interval between fox contacts. Behavioural studies suggest that individuals from adjacent family groups meet, on average, every 4 to 6 days (Macdonald, 1980). It is assumed that foxes pass from the latent or incubating class to the infectious state at a per capita rate σ, such that the average incubation period is $1/\sigma$. This period is known to be variable in foxes, ranging from 12 to 110 days, and depends on factors such as age, site of infection and nutritional state (Tierkel, 1959; Parker and Wilsnack, 1966; Andral and Toma, 1977; Winkler, 1975). On average, $1/\sigma$ appears to be around 28–30 days. Infectious, or 'rabid', foxes have a short life expectancy, varying from 3 to 10 days, with an average of about 5 days (Tierkel,

1959; Parker and Wilsnack, 1966; Winkler, 1975; Andral and Toma, 1977). It is assumed that rabid animals die at a constant per capita rate α where $1/\alpha$ is their life expectancy. Since the infection is severely debilitating, and of relatively short duration, infected foxes do not contribute to the reproductive effort of the population.

The biological assumptions outlined above enabled Anderson *et al.* (1981) to define a set of first-order differential equations to describe the dynamics of fox populations infected with rabies:

$$dX/dt = rX - \gamma XN - \beta XY \tag{8.2}$$

$$dI/dt = \beta XY - (\sigma + b + \gamma N)I \tag{8.3}$$

$$dY/dt = \sigma I - (\alpha + b + \gamma N)Y \tag{8.4}$$

By adding the above three equations together, an equation for the dynamics of the total fox population is obtained:

$$dN/dt = aX - (b + \gamma N)N - \alpha Y \tag{8.5}$$

A summary of the parameter estimates used to explore the dynamics of this model is given in Table 8.2.

Table 8.2 Values of epidemiological and other parameters (from Anderson *et al.*, 1981).

Symbol	Meaning	Value
b	Average per capita intrinsic death rate	0.5 year^{-1}
a	Average per capita birth rate of foxes	1 year^{-1}
r	Per capita population growth rate, $a - b$	0.5 year^{-1}
K	Fox carrying capacity, $K = r/\gamma$	Various
σ	$1/\sigma$ is the average latent period	13 year^{-1}
α	Death rate of 'rabid' foxes	73 year^{-1}
β	Transmission coefficient (estimated via Equation 8.7) for threshold density, $K_T = 1.0 \text{ fox/km}^2$)	$79.7 \text{ km}^2 \text{ year}^{-1}$

8.3 POPULATION DYNAMICS

The model described by Equations (8.2)–(8.5) differs from conventional epidemiological formulations, as discussed in other chapters within this text, in that the host population N is a dynamical variable affected by both the disease and density-dependent constraints imposed by resource limitation. Rabies will be maintained within the fox population provided that the basic reproductive rate, R, of the infection exceeds unity. As discussed in Chapter 1, R is the expected number of secondary cases produced during the life span of an infectious fox introduced into a population of K susceptible animals. For the model defined by Equations (8.2)–(8.5):

$$R = \sigma\beta K/[(\sigma+a)(\alpha+a)] \qquad (8.6)$$

The condition $R > 1$ for endemic maintenance of rabies may equivalently be expressed as the requirement that the fox population exceeds a critical threshold density K_T, with the definition:

$$K_T = [(\sigma+a)(\alpha+a)]/(\beta\sigma) \qquad (8.7)$$

If $R < 1$, or equivalently $K < K_T$, the fox population will settle to its disease-free equilibrium density K.

As usual in epidemiological studies, the most difficult parameter to estimate is the transmission coefficient β. However, a rough guide to the value of this parameter can be obtained from information concerning the minimum fox density in which rabies persists endemically. Available epidemiological evidence suggests that K_T lies in the range 0.25 to 1.0 fox km^{-2}, with the most frequently quoted value in Europe being around 1.0 fox km^{-2} (Lloyd, 1976; Andral and Toma, 1977). This observation can be used, in conjunction with Equation (8.7), along with the parameter estimates recorded in Table 8.2, to make a rough estimate of β. The value $\beta \approx 79.7$ km^2 year^{-1}, obtained in this manner agrees well with independently obtained behavioural observations in rabies-free populations concerning the average time interval between fox contacts in regions where the average density is roughly one fox km^{-2} (Anderson et al., 1981). Such agreement appears surprising in the light of the belief that rabid foxes have higher contact rates than healthy animals. It is probable, however, that altered host behaviour, as a consequence of infection, acts to compensate for the fact that only a certain proportion of contacts between healthy and rabid animals result in disease transmission.

When $R > 1$, rabies will regulate fox abundance below the disease-free level K to an equilibrium density N^* where:

$$N^* = \frac{(\sigma+a)(\alpha+a) - ar}{\alpha\beta - a\gamma} \qquad (8.8)$$

The degree of depression, d, from the disease-free state K, where $d = 1 - (N^*/K)$, rises as the density K increases (Fig. 8.2a). The regulated state, N^*, however, may be a stable constant value, or it may be a stable cycle. The cyclic solutions tend to arise when the carrying capacity of the fox habitat is relatively large (K significantly larger than K_T). More formally, cyclic solutions arise if:

$$(2b+\alpha+\sigma+3\gamma N^*)[(b+\sigma+\gamma N^*)N^* + \alpha(N^*-Y^*)+aN^*] - C < 0 \qquad (8.9)$$

Here N^* is as defined in Equation (8.8) and the equilibrium densities of susceptibles, X^*, and infectious foxes, Y^*, are given by:

$$Y^* = (r - \gamma N^*)/\beta \qquad (8.10)$$

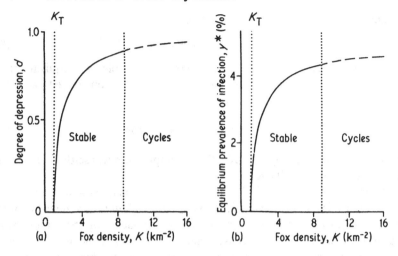

Figure 8.2 (a) The degree of population depression, d, induced by rabies where $d = 1 - (N^*/K)$, is plotted for various values of K. In the region denoted 'stable' the model exhibits damped oscillations to a stable state, and in the region labelled 'cycles' limit cycle behaviour occurs, and the dashed line denotes the average degree of depression throughout one cycle. Parameter values are as listed in Table 8.2. (b) This graph portrays the relationship between the equilibrium prevalence of infection y^* and K, where $y^* = (Y^* + I^*)/N^*$. The regions labelled 'stable' and 'cycles' are as defined in the legend to graph (a) and the dashed line in the cycles region denotes the average prevalence of rabies throughout one cycle. Parameter values are as listed in Table 8.2.

and

$$X^* = (b + \sigma + \gamma N^*)(b + \alpha + \gamma N^*)/(\sigma\beta) \qquad (8.11)$$

The quantity C is defined for notational convenience as:

$$C = X^*(K - N^*)(\sigma\beta - \gamma a) \qquad (8.12)$$

Figure 8.3 shows the types of dynamical behaviour which can occur, as functions of the latency interval $1/\sigma$ and the density of the disease-free fox population K, where the other population parameters are as defined in Table 8.2. The values of σ and K discussed above tend to suggest cycles with periods in the general range of 3–5 years. Such periods are precisely what is observed in Europe and North America, where a striking feature of rabies epidemiology is the regular 3, 4 or 5 year oscillations in fox density and in the prevalence of infection (Friend, 1968; Kauker and Zettl, 1963; Johnston and Beauregard, 1969; Steele, 1973; Lloyd, 1976). The cycles are most frequently observed in regions where fox densities were high before the introduction of rabies, and cyclic behaviour is often absent in low-density populations (Johnston and Beauregard, 1969). These observed patterns are in accord with the predictions of the model as shown in Fig. 8.3. The period of the cycle is to a large extent

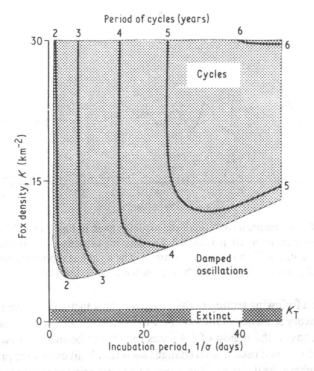

Figure 8.3 The three regimes of dynamical behaviour that can be exhibited by the model defined in Equations (8.2)–(8.5) are illustrated in the $K - (1/\sigma)$ parameter space. As discussed in the text these three regimes are: rabies unable to maintain itself within the fox population ($R < 1$), labelled 'extinct'; fox density controlled to a stable state, N^*, labelled 'damped oscillations' ($R > 1$); and limit cycle behaviour in fox abundance and disease prevalence ($R > 1$), labelled 'cycles'. In this cycle region, the contour lines correspond to specific periods of oscillation, labelled in years. All rate parameters are expressed in units of year^{-1} and have the values listed in Table 8.2.

determined by the intrinsic growth rate, r, of the fox population. Rabies acts as a form of time-delayed density-dependent regulator of fox population growth where the length of the time lag is determined by how long the fox density is below K_T. It is well understood that such mechanisms can induce oscillatory behaviour (May, 1976; Gurney, Blythe and Nisbet, 1980).

For the parameter values most relevant to the dynamics of rabies in Europe, namely, $1/\sigma \simeq 30$ days and K in the region 1 to 4 foxes km^{-2}, Fig. 8.3 shows the model to predict damped oscillations in fox density and disease prevalence with periods around 3 to 4 years. The dampling time, however, is long, being of the order of 40 years or more from the first appearance of the disease (Fig. 8.4). This propensity to prolonged oscillations, even in the region labelled 'damped oscillations' in Fig. 8.3, is further accentuated by seasonal changes in the values of pertinent parameters (Anderson, 1981a). This point will be developed

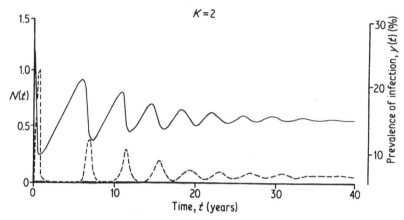

Figure 8.4 A numerical solution of the model defined in Equations (8.2)–(8.5) using the parameter values listed in Table 8.2. The carrying capacity of the fox habitat, K, is set at 2 animals km^{-2} and $K_T = 1$ fox km^{-2}. The solid line represents fox density at time t, $N(t)$, and the dashed line the prevalence of infection $y(t)$.

further in a following section in this chapter. Other factors can also accentuate the oscillatory tendency of the system. For example, if a lower estimate of K_T is accepted, say in the region of 0.4 foxes km^{-2}, the boundary between stable cycles and damped oscillations changes such that limit cycles are predicted in habitats where the density of foxes was fairly low prior to the introduction of the disease (Fig. 8.5).

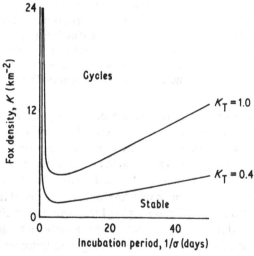

Figure 8.5 Similar to Fig. 8.3 but simply denoting the boundary between the regions in the $K - (1/\sigma)$ parameter space which separates the parameter values which give rise to stable cycles and a stable equilibrium point (damped oscillations). The boundary is denoted by the solid line and two such lines are shown, one for $K_T = 0.4$ and the other for $K_T = 1.0$.

As a direct consequence of its high pathogenicity, rabies will persist within fox populations only at very low levels of prevalence. This is an example of the commonly observed biological relationship between low 'standing crop' and high rate of turnover. Persistence is in part ensured by the high susceptibility of foxes to rabies. In regions with endemic disease, the prevalence (the proportion of the population infected, y, where $y = (Y+I)/N$) appears to lie in the range of 1–7% (Davis and Wood, 1959), although significant fluctuations are caused by seasonal effects and by the intrinsically oscillatory nature of the association between host and pathogen. As illustrated in Fig. 8.2(b), the model defined by Equations (8.2)–(8.5) predicts prevalence values in broad agreement with observed figures. In addition, the model predicts that the prevalence of rabies will be higher in favourable fox habitats (large K), which is again consistent with the available epidemiological evidence (Kauker and Zettl, 1963; Wandeler et al., 1974; Moegle et al., 1974).

8.4 SEASONAL PROCESSES

As noted earlier the oscillatory behaviour of the association between host and pathogen can be accentuated by seasonal changes in the value of any one of the population parameters contained within the model. Reproduction by foxes is clearly seasonal, the cubs usually being born around March to April in Europe (Lloyd, 1980; Macdonald, 1980). Other factors, however, are probably of greater significance to the transmission dynamics of rabies. These include seasonal changes in the behaviour of foxes which alter the rate of fox contact and hence the transmission of the disease. For example, the dispersal behaviour of young foxes in the autumn and the mating behaviour of adult foxes during December to March appear to enhance the rate of disease transmission such that a peak in disease prevalence is often observed in the winter and spring months of the year (Andral and Toma, 1977). An example of this trend is displayed in Fig. 8.6.

The impact of seasonal time-dependence in either the birth rate, a, or the transmission rate, β, can be examined by incorporating these parameters in the model as periodic functions of time, t. For instance, seasonal changes in β may be crudely captured by the function:

$$\beta(t) = A + B \sin\left[2\pi(t - \tau)\right] \tag{8.13}$$

where t is units of 1 year, τ is a phase angle, A is the average value of $\beta(t)$ and B is a constant determining the amplitude of the oscillations (Anderson, 1981a).

Two numerical simulations of the rabies model are shown in Fig. 8.7 in which either β or a are assumed to vary on a seasonal basis. In Fig. 8.7(a), the parameter β fluctuates on a seasonal basis with an average per capita value of $80 \, \text{km}^{-2} \, \text{year}^{-1}$ and a range of 30 to 130. In Fig. 8.7(b) the parameter a is a periodic function of time (of the form defined in Equation (8.13)) with an average value of 1.05 foxes km^{-2} and a range of 0.05 to 2.05. It can be seen from Fig. 8.7 that seasonality in transmission can act to increase the damping

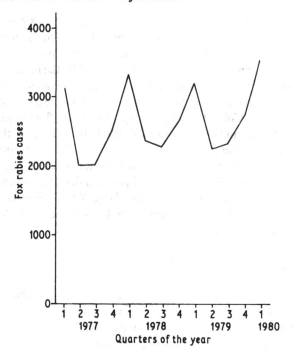

Figure 8.6   Reported cases of fox rabies in Europe in the four quarters of 1977, 1978, 1979 and in the first quarter of 1980 (WHO, 1980). The reported cases show a clear seasonal pattern.

time of the system (compare Fig. 8.7(a) with Fig. 8.4). As discussed in Chapter 1, seasonality in transmission may, under certain circumstances, generate undamped waves in host density and disease prevalence. Seasonality in host reproduction (Fig. 8.7(b)) does not appear to accentuate the non-seasonal oscillatory behaviour of the system; it simply imposes seasonal fluctuations on fox density and disease prevalence.

One obvious and important consequence of the oscillatory behaviour of the association between host and pathogen, whether induced by seasonal processes or the intrinsic dynamical properties of the interaction, concerns the probability of disease extinction during the periods when fox density is low ($N < K_T$ and $R < 1$). For example, in the trough of any one cycle both fox density and disease prevalence decline to very low levels (Fig. 8.4 and Fig. 8.7). This is particularly so when the disease-free carrying capacity, K, of the habitat is high, since the amplitude of the cycles are large in such circumstances. The likelihood of rabies becoming extinct in small areas of good habitat is therefore high due to stochastic effects. The persistence of rabies over large areas is probably ensured by the high spatial mobility of the fox host. Young males, for example, may disperse 13 km or more from their birth place, and

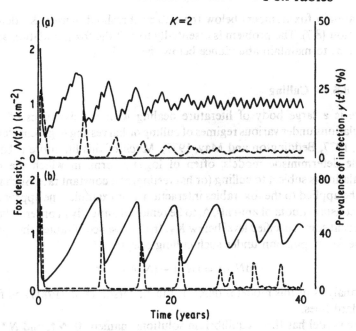

Figure 8.7 (a) Numerical solution of the model in which the fox birth rate, *a*, is assumed to vary on a regular seasonal basis. The periodic birth rate was of the following functional form: $a(t) = A + B \sin [2(t - \tau)]$. The parameter *t* is in units of 1 year and the constants *A*, *B* and τ have the values 1.05, 1.0 and -3.0 respectively. (b) Similar to graph (a) but showing a numerical solution of the model in which the transmission parameter, β, was assumed to vary on a regular seasonal basis. The functional form of $\beta(t)$ was as defined for $a(t)$ in the legend to graph (a). The constants *A*, *B* and τ have the values 80, 50 and -3.0 respectively.

adult foxes often travel 11–13 km each night (Lloyd, 1980; Macdonald, 1980). Empty territories created by deaths are rapidly occupied by itinerant and mobile male foxes. An additional factor in the maintenance of disease may be the involvement of other host species. In Europe, for example, badgers, rodents and deer are all known to be susceptible to rabies (Andral and Toma, 1977).

8.5 CONTROL

The broad agreement between model predictions and the observed epidemiology of rabies within fox populations provides encouragement to extend the model framework to examine the impact of control measures.

Attempts to control the spread of rabies in Europe and North America by hunting, gassing, poisoning or trapping foxes have in general met with little success (Zimen, 1980). Theory suggests the aim of such programmes should be to maintain fox numbers below the critical threshold density K_T defined in Equation (8.7). The problem is essentially to cull the fox population at a rate sufficient to maintain abundance below the level K_T.

8.5.1 Culling

There is a large body of literature dealing with the dynamics of natural populations under various regimes of culling or harvesting (e.g. Schaefer, 1954; May, 1977; Beddington and May, 1977). Much of this literature is based on simple deterministic models, often of logistic form, in which the natural population is subject to culling (or harvesting) at a constant rate. Such models may be applied to the fox–rabies interaction. For example, one approach is to set a constant quota of animals, Λ, to be removed annually in order to keep fox density at some specified level below K_T. In the absence of rabies, the dynamics of the fox population under such culling obeys:

$$dN/dt = rN[1 - (N/K)] - \Lambda \qquad (8.14)$$

The analysis of this model is described in Anderson et al. (1981) and follows standard lines.

The model has three equilibrium solutions; namely, 0, N_1^*, and N_2^* where $N_2^* > N_1^*$. These equilibria are portrayed diagrammatically in Fig. 8.8 where the relationship between the logistic population growth curve and the death rate Λ imposed by culling is plotted. It is well known that the equilibrium points 0 and N_2^* are locally stable while N_1^* is unstable (May, 1977). As the culling rate Λ increases toward the maximum growth rate, which occurs at a density $K/2$, the equilibrium points N_1^* and N_2^* draw closer together. Once Λ exceeds the growth rate at $K/2$, the dynamical trajectories of the system are attracted to the stable state $N^* = 0$; in other words the fox population is driven to extinction.

For the purpose of disease control we simply require that $N_2^* < K_T$. Two situations arise. If $K_T > K/2$, the threshold density lies above the point where the fox population growth curve has its maximum (in fisheries terminology, the 'maximum sustainable yield', MSY, point), and stable control to a density below K_T is possible provided that the culling rate Λ exceeds Λ_T where:

$$\Lambda_T = rK_T[1 - (K_T/K)] \qquad (8.15)$$

This situation applies to areas of poor fox habitat where the carrying capacity K is below 2 foxes km^{-2}, given that K_T is in the region of 1 fox km^{-2}. In such circumstances culling can maintain the fox population at a stable equilibrium density N^* which is less than K_T (Fig. 8.8).

If $K_T < \frac{1}{2}K$, two complications arise. First, the initial quota must exceed the MSY value, $\Lambda > rK/4$, in order to drive fox densities below the point at $\frac{1}{2}K$ where the population growth curve has its peak (Fig. 8.8). Second, the fox population cannot be stably maintained at a finite value below $\frac{1}{2}K$ by culling

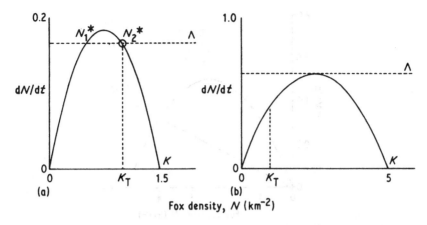

Fox density, N (km^{-2})

Figure 8.8   The relationship between the rate of population growth, dN/dt, of the disease-free fox population (solid line) and a constant-quota culling rate Λ (horizontal dotted line) for various population densities N. The dotted vertical line denotes the value of K_T which is set at 1 fox km^{-2}. In graph (a) the carrying capacity of the fox habitat, K, is set at 1.5 foxes km^{-2} and is thus less than $2K_T$ (i.e. $K_T > K/2$). The culling rate Λ shown in the graph results in a stable equilibrium fox density at the point labelled N_2^*. In this example culling at a rate Λ_T, where $rK/4 > \Lambda_T > rK_T[1 - (K_T/K)]$, will create a stable fox density below the threshold value K_T necessary for the maintenance of rabies. In graph (b), the carrying capacity K is set at $K = 5$ foxes km^{-2}. The culling rate Λ shown in the graph is greater than the maximum point on the population growth curve (the MSY point), and, as discussed in the text, under this regime the only stable point is $N^* = 0$. In this example it is not possible to create a non-zero equilibrium fox density which is less than K_T by a constant-quota culling regime ($r = 0.5$ year^{-1}).

since the equilibrium point at K_T, attained by culling at the rate Λ_T of Equation (8.15) is unstable. In principle, the population could be driven to extinction by operating at $\Lambda > rK/4$, but in practice a prohibitively large effort would be required to meet this quota when fox density was very low. This situation applies to areas of good fox habitat where $K > 2$ foxes km^{-2}.

Such populations will be difficult to control by culling because of the continually high effort needed to keep an area free of foxes in the face of their ability to disperse over large areas and rapidly to recolonize vacant territories.

An alternative approach to setting a constant quota is to devote some specified constant effort to killing foxes. For example, a constant number of man-hours per unit of time could be devoted to culling. This approach, in effect, changes the intrinsic per capita death rate of foxes from b to $b + \Delta b$, where Δb is the additional mortality imposed by constant effort culling. This regime, as illustrated in Fig. 8.9, generates a single stable equilibrium state, N^*, where:

$$N^* = K\left(1 - \frac{\Delta b}{r}\right) \qquad (8.16)$$

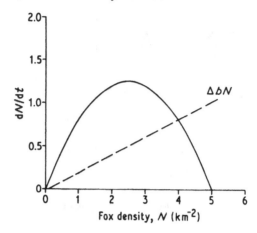

Figure 8.9 Similar to Fig. 8.8 but showing the constant-effort culling approach. As before the solid line denotes the rate of population growth dN/dt. The dashed line denotes the mortality rate, ΔbN, induced by a constant-effort regime. A stable equilibrium fox density, N^*, occurs at the point of intersect of the dashed and solid lines ($\Delta b = 0.2$ year^{-1}, $r = 1.0$ year^{-1}).

Fox density will be maintained below K_T, and rabies eradicated from the population, provided that:

$$\frac{\Delta b}{r} > 1 - (1/R) \tag{8.17}$$

where R is the basic reproductive rate as defined earlier (Equation (8.6)). If R is large, as it typically is in good fox habitats, Δb must essentially equal r itself, which implies a considerable level of effort. In practical terms these predictions require more detailed examination. It would be important, for example, to try to assess what a given value of Δb implies in terms of man-hours and cost. Similar considerations apply to culling regimes based on a constant quota design.

More elaborate culling regimes could be considered, but the broad theoretical conclusion remains that the control of rabies by culling foxes will be difficult to achieve except in poor habitats where the carrying capacity K is low. Even in these areas continual effort must be applied since fox populations have relatively high intrinsic growth rates for mammal species of their size and hence have the capacity to rapidly replenish their numbers. In Britain, for example, in the region of 100 000 foxes are killed annually but this pressure has had little effect on the overall fox population since there is no evidence of declining numbers (MacDonald, 1980).

Theoretical predictions concerning the difficulty of controlling rabies by the culling of fox populations are strongly supported by recent experience in Europe and North America. Intensive efforts to reduce fox densities by gassing and poisoning have, in general, had little impact on the persistance and spread of rabies (Macdonald, 1980; Lloyd et al., 1976; Winkler, McLean and Cowart, 1975; Wandeler et al., 1974; Bogel et al., 1976).

The use of pathogens such as canine distemper or canine hepatitis as suppressors of fox numbers may be a feasible alternative to culling. This approach, however, will only be successful provided that the threshold density for the maintenance of the introduced pathogen is lower than that for rabies. Field observations in North America suggest that a more detailed appraisal of this approach is warranted (Winkler, 1975).

8.5.2 Vaccination

The feasability of immunizing wild foxes against rabies has attracted a great deal of attention in recent years. This is in part due to the failure to control the spread of rabies in Europe by culling fox populations. Many problems surround the approach of immunization, not the least of which is the danger that an attenuated live vaccine which effectively immunizes foxes might introduce a mild form of the disease into other host species (Winkler and Baer, 1976).

Despite these difficulties, however, considerable progress has been made in the development of oral vaccines and in techniques for delivering them in baits (Winkler and Baer, 1976; Blancou, 1979; Dubreuil et al., 1979). Field trials have been carried out in Canada, Germany and Switzerland and preliminary results suggests that this approach may be a feasible alternative to culling provided a 'safe' vaccine can be developed.

In the design of these trials there has been much discussion about the level of protection needed within the fox population to eliminate rabies (Berger, 1976; Bacon and Macdonald, 1980).

The model defined in Equations (8.2)–(8.5) can be modifed to explore this problem (Anderson et al., 1981) by the inclusion of an immune category of foxes of density $Z(t)$ at time t. If susceptible animals are vaccinated at a per capita rate ϕ and immune animals lose immunity at a per capita rate δ then the new model is:

$$dX/dt = a(X + Z) - (b + \gamma N)X - \beta X Y - \phi X + \delta Z \qquad (8.18)$$

$$dI/dt = \beta XY - (\sigma + b + \gamma N)I \qquad (8.19)$$

$$d Y/dt = \sigma I - (\alpha + b + \gamma N) Y \qquad (8.20)$$

$$dZ/dt = \phi X - (\delta + b + \gamma N)Z \qquad (8.21)$$

For disease eradication the equilibrium solution of interest, obtained by setting $dX/dt = dI/dt = dY/dt = dZ/dt = 0$, is the disease-free state defined by $Y^* = I^* = 0$ and $N^* = K$. This state is locally stable provided:

$$\phi > (a + \delta)(R - 1) \qquad (8.22)$$

At this equilibrium the proportion of vaccinated foxes, p, where $p = Z^*/(Z^* + X^*)$ is given by:

$$p = \phi/(\phi + a + \delta) \tag{8.23}$$

Alternatively, this equation may be expressed as the proportion of the population, p, that must be protected at any one time to eradicate rabies where:

$$p > [1 - (1/R)] \tag{8.24}$$

Here R is the basic reproductive rate as defined in Equation (8.6). This expression is identical to that derived in an earlier chapter which was concerned with the control of directly transmitted viral and bacterial infections of man (see Chapter 1).

In the case of fox rabies, of major interest is the relationship between p and the carrying capacity of the fox habitat, K. Since R may equivalently be written as $R = K/K_T$ (see Equations (8.6) and (8.7)), then relationship Equation (8.24) may be expressed as:

$$p > [1 - (K_T/K)] \tag{8.25}$$

This general relation is illustrated graphically in Fig. 8.10. This figure also displays the results of an elaborate numerical simulation by Berger (1976) in which the model involved a detailed statistical description of dispersal by, and contact between, foxes on a large two-dimensional grid, along with statistical distributions for the duration of latent and infectious states in individual foxes. Berger also took K_T to be around 1 fox km^{-2}. The agreement between the results of this complicated simulation and the simple deterministic model defined in Equations (8.18)–(8.21) is extremely encouraging (Anderson *et al.*, 1981). It provides a good example of the basic understanding that can be gained from simple models.

Figure 8.10 shows clearly that the required degree of protection is greater in dense fox populations than in sparse ones. For example, a K value of around 2 foxes km^{-2} requires a 50% protection coverage. In the light of field evidence that bait acceptance levels by natural fox populations may approach 60–80%, immunization appears to be a feasible, and probably better, alternative to culling (Macdonald, 1980; MacInnes and Johnston, 1975). This conclusion, however, only holds in low-density fox habitats. In good habitats the required level of protection approaches 100% (Fig. 8.10) and will be very difficult to achieve. In these circumstances, in practical terms, immunization and culling are equally ineffective. A further point to note concerning immunization, is that, just as for culling, continual effort must be applied to maintain the level of protection, p, at the desired level (relationship (8.24)). New susceptibles will be introduced into the population each year by births and, in addition, unless the vaccine provides life-long protection, vaccinated foxes will lose immunity and have to be revaccinated. The degree of effort required to maintain a high level of herd immunity will probably be prohibitively large in all but low-density fox habitats.

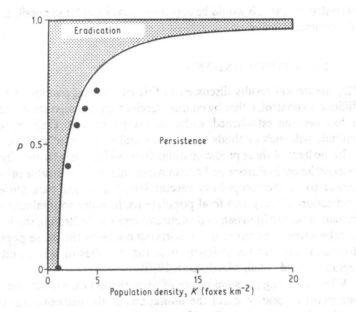

Figure 8.10   This figure depicts the relationship between the proportion of the fox population, p, protected by vaccination, and the disease-free carrying capacity of the fox habitat, K. The threshold density is taken to be $K_T = 1.0$. In the shaded region labelled 'eradication' rabies cannot persist (relationship (8.25) satisfied) while in the unshaded region labelled 'persistence' the disease is able to maintain itself (relationship (8.25) not satisfied). The four solid circles denote the boundary, as discussed in the text, predicted by Berger's simulation model, between levels of immunization which result in either disease persistence or eradication (Berger, 1976).

8.5.3   Vaccination and culling

Clearly, it is also possible to put into operation a combined control strategy based on culling and vaccination. If a proportion p of the fox population are immunized, combined with constant-effort culling which adds Δb to the fox death rate, the criterion for rabies eradication becomes:

$$p + (\Delta b/r)\,(1 - p) > 1 - (1/R) \tag{8.26}$$

For example, if $R = 4$ it would be necessary to immunize 75 % of the foxes, or kill at a rate $\Delta b/r = 75\%$ under a pure strategy. With a combined strategy it would be necessary to immunize 50 % of the population and cull at a rate $\Delta b/r = 50\%$. In the absence of any estimates of relative costs, it would appear likely that the expenses of vaccination or culling will rise faster than linearly with increasing p or Δb. In such circumstances a combined strategy may be the more cost-effective. However, it is important to note that many problems surround this approach not least of which is the operational timing of the two methods of control. Clearly, it would be desirable to avoid, as far as possible, the culling of immunized foxes.

8.6 CONCLUSIONS

The theoretical results discussed in this chapter suggest that rabies will be difficult to control, either by culling, vaccination or a mixture of the two, once it has become established within a fox population. Only in low-density habitats will such methods of control stand a chance of success.

In the light of these predicted difficulties (which are substantially borne out by experiences in Europe and North America) the most sensible priority would appear to be the compulsory vaccination of dogs and cats, along with the eradication of stray and feral populations, in order to minimize the risk of human exposure in urban and suburban regions. In Britain, the introduction of rabies would be particularly worrying owing to the dense populations of dogs and cats and the uniquely high fox densities in urban and suburban regions (Lloyd, 1980; Macdonald, 1980).

When assessing the significance of these theoretical predictions it is clearly important to bear in mind the limitations of the mathematical framework employed in the analysis. Specifically the model developed by Anderson *et al.* (1981) is deterministic in nature and is based on assumptions of homogeneous mixing. In addition, it ignores spatial and stochastic effects. The power of such simple formulations lies in the relative ease with which relationships can be established between important variables (such as p and K as illustrated in Fig. 8.10). This facility is rarely provided for by complex simulation models. The danger in trusting predictions based on simple formulations is naturally related to the fact that a simple model may fail to incorporate an important feature of the interaction between host and pathogen. It is important to note, however, that the deterministic model discussed in this chapter predicts patterns of population behaviour in good agreement with observed epidemiological trends. Specifically it faithfully mirrors the observed cyclic behaviour of rabies epidemics within fox populations and, in addition, predicts prevalence levels in good agreement with reported figures (Anderson *et al.*, 1981). This suggests that, by the specification of a few easily measurable parameters, the model captures the major features of the association between fox and pathogen, and, is thus of practical value to the design and implementation of control measures.

Aside from these issues, however, there clearly is a need for improvement in the biological accuracy of the mathematical framework described in Equations (8.2)–(8.5). The fact that the model predicts important features which conform to reality simply implies that it is worthy of further study and elaboration. Specifically, it would be desirable in future work to consider spatial elements in the dynamics of the association, by, for example, including an immigration term to mirror the arrival of new susceptibles and infecteds into the fox population. Aside from such additions to the deterministic framework, there is also a need to carry out Monte Carlo simulations in order to introduce stochastic elements. In particular, it is necessary to assess the frequency of disease 'fade out' in low-density fox populations when deterministic predictions suggest that the infection will persist at very low prevalence levels. There would be some advantage to such studies in changing the continuous time structure of the model to a discrete time formulation in order more faithfully to mirror descrete events such as the latent period of infection.

Finally, a major role of theoretical work in epidemiology is to help identify areas in which the data base is inadequate. The work of Anderson *et al.* (1981) suggests that additional information is required with respect to the threshold density, K_T, the demography of fox populations in Europe and the dispersal plus contact rates of rabid foxes.

9 Fascioliasis

R. A. Wilson, G. Smith and M. R. Thomas

9.1 INTRODUCTION

When cattle, sheep and other livestock are infected with the common liver fluke, *Fasciola hepatica*, they suffer from the debilitating condition termed fascioliasis. The clinical symptoms of the disease are manifestations of the progressive disruption of liver function that accompanies the establishment of mature flukes in the host bile ducts. The parasite has an indirect life cycle, the intermediate host in the UK and Western Europe being a small (1–12 mm) pulmonate snail, *Lymnaea truncatula*. In this chapter we shall examine the biology of this life cycle in terms of the dynamics of the interacting host and parasite populations.

The life cycles of the liver fluke and its intermediate host are illustrated in Fig. 9.1. The parasite exists in five distinct populations: mature flukes in the bile ducts of the mammal host, eggs in the external environment, free-swimming miracidium larvae, intramolluscan stages, and infective cysts on the herbage. The flow of parasites through the system, between one subpopulation and the next, is governed by a series of rate parameters indicated by the symbols μ, λ and β for mortality, birth and transmission respectively. (Transmission can be considered as simultaneously an emigration from one subpopulation and an immigration into another.) The rates are defined per parasite per unit time. In later sections we shall examine in detail the factors which influence these rates and the ways in which this knowledge may be used to achieve more complete control of the disease.

9.2 THE EXTENT OF FASCIOLIASIS

9.2.1 World distribution

The production of cattle and sheep is an important component of the economies of most countries in the world (Cole and Ronning, 1974). In only a few of these countries are the stock entirely free from the risk of infection by *Fasciola hepatica*. It occurs throughout N. America for example, though mainly in Florida and the western states. It is found in Cuba, Puerto Rico and Mexico, and extends southwards into Colombia, Venezuela, Brazil, Peru, Chile and Uruguay. In Africa and parts of the Middle and Far East it is largely replaced by *F. gigantica* but elsewhere in the Old World, and also in Australia and New Zealand, it is the cause of serious economic losses.

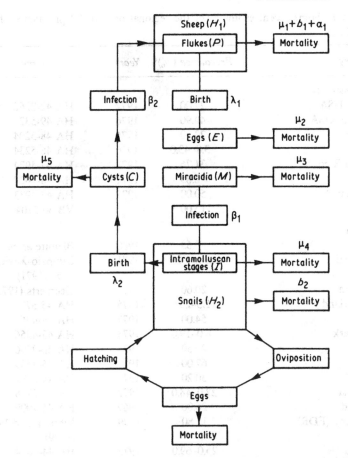

Figure 9.1 A flow chart of the life cycles of *Fasciola hepatica* and *Lymnaea truncatula*. The symbols designating the subpopulations and rate parameters are the same as those used in the analytical model in Section 9.6 (see text). Note that sporocysts, rediae, daughter rediae and cercariae are grouped together as a single intramolluscan population. Similarly the very brief free-living cercarial stage is subsumed in the cyst population.

Some recent estimates of the prevalence of *bovine* fascioliasis are given in Table 9.1. For any given region, the prevalence of infection in cattle is generally higher than in sheep (Boray, 1977; Blamire *et al.*, 1980) although locally it can approach 100 % in both species (Nansen and Midtgaard, 1977). It should not be inferred from Table 9.1 that the prevalence of disease in any particular region stays the same through time. In Puerto Rico, for example, bovine fascioliasis has increased from 7.55 % prevalence in 1948 to 31.76 % prevalence in 1976 (Frame *et al.*, 1979) whereas in the UK the prevalence of fascioliasis in cattle decreased from 26.83 % in 1960 to 5.63 % in 1978 (Blamire *et al.*, 1970,

Table 9.1 Some recent estimates of the regional or national prevalence of bovine fascioliasis.

Country	Prevalence (%)*	Year†	Source‡
The Americas			
Texas, USA	77.00	1972	HA 42-2262
Oregon, USA	44.90	1976	HA 49-532
Mexico	73.90	1976	HA 48-3204
Cuba	3.8–43.0	1976	HA 46-5234
Puerto Rico	31.76	1978	HA 47-4974
Brazil	2.85	1971	HA 48-1627
Uruguay	50.00	1977	HA 47-4983
Chile	13.00	–	VB 50-2104
Europe			
UK	5.63	1980	Blamire *et al.* (1980)
Portugal	up to 60.0	1971	Sampaio-Xavier *et al.* (1971)
Belgium	20.60	1971	Geeraerts (1971)
Switzerland	11.5–23.0	1975	HA 45-577
	54.00	1977	HA 49-436
Denmark	8.0–19.0	1973	HA 43-4356
Italy	20.50	1974	HA 48-2296
	67.00	1975	HA 45-4459
	30.20	1973	HA 44-5682
Sardinia	27.0–48.0	1972	HA 43-2778
Finland	26.00	1969	HA 41-1009
Germany (FDR)	11.80	1979	Ribbeck and Witzel (1979)
Poland	25.0–69.0	1973	HA 44-3674
Yugoslavia	34.9–62.8	1977	HA 47-3983
USSR	65.00	1977	HA 48-3195
	37.60	1975	HA 48-1005
Australasia and Asia			
China	10.17	1976	HA 46-2646
Taiwan	30.90	1976	HA 47-363
Australia	13.0–30.0	1977	Boray (1977)
New Zealand	6.00	1972	HA 42-848
West Timor	12.00	1979	HA 48-4324
West Sumatra	86.00	1979	HA 48-4070

* Figures obtained from slaughterhouse surveys.
† The 'year' is the year of publication.
‡ HA, Helminthological Abstracts; VB, Veterinary Bulletin.

1980). In fact, annual and seasonal variations in the proportion of animals infected are a prominent feature of the epidemiology of the disease (Honer and Vink, 1963; Evans and Pratt, 1978).

9.2.2 Temporal variations in the prevalence of fascioliasis in the UK

There are few reliable data on the precise prevalence (the proportion of sheep or cattle infected) of fascioliasis. Ideally, longitudinal studies over a period of 10 or more years, with a consistent sampling programme and positive identification of infection by examination of livers or faecal sampling, would be needed. A major factor making such studies difficult to undertake is the impact of the observer on the husbandry of the farmer. Regular visits to a farm or locality almost always result in extra dosing of stock, the fencing off or drainage of snail habitats, and other measures which drastically alter the course of disease transmission. It is, nevertheless, possible to reconstruct a reasonable picture of the changing prevalence of fascioliasis over the last 20 years in the UK using other less rigorous data.

Slaughterhouse condemnations provide the most extensive information (e.g. Ross, 1966; Blamire et al., 1970, 1980). The accuracy of the data is dependent on the skills of individual meat inspectors, and its interpretation is subject to several caveats. Crossland et al. (1969) have shown that the chance of a sheep liver being condemned increases directly with the intensity of infection (Fig. 9.2); thus, light infections of one or two flukes are frequently overlooked. On the other hand, a condemned liver need not be harbouring flukes. Its fibrotic state may have arisen as the result of an infection acquired some years ago and long since terminated either naturally (cattle only) or by drug treatment (cattle and sheep). It is also worth noting that the practice of grouping lambs with ewes and young beef cattle with old cows in the UK

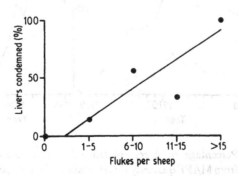

Figure 9.2 A comparison of the percentage of sheep livers condemned at slaughter by meat inspectors with the actual fluke burden per liver reproduced with permission from Crossland et al., 1969).

condemnation reports removes a potentially useful source of information on variations in the annual incidence of disease. (Annual incidence is defined as the proportion of previously uninfected animals acquiring an infection over a 12 month period.)

The percentage of livers condemned in the UK, 1960–1979, due to fascioliasis is illustrated in Fig. 9.3. The percentage of livers condemned is not precisely the same as prevalence since the ratio of young to old animals slaughtered is not identical with the ratio of young to old animals in the national flock or herd. The most obvious feature of condemnations in sheep and cattle is the gradual rise to peak values in 1969 followed by a marked and continuing decline to the present day. Although farmers have long considered fascioliasis to be more important in sheep (Ollerenshaw and Rowcliffe, 1961), it is noteworthy that over the period of the survey the condemnations in sheep were about one-third those in cattle. A partial explanation for the contrast between cattle and sheep lies in the fact that cattle are grazed for relatively longer before being slaughtered. Differences in actual grazing behaviour are probably also important. The observation by Peters and Clapham (1942) of 17.7% condemnation of cattle livers indicates that fascioliasis has prevailed at mid-sixties levels in the more distant past.

In a few slaughterhouse surveys, data on steers and heifers have been sepapated from data on cows, and similarly for lambs and ewes (Table 9.2). As might be expected the condemnations in old stock (both sheep and cattle) are considerably higher than in young animals. The average annual incidence

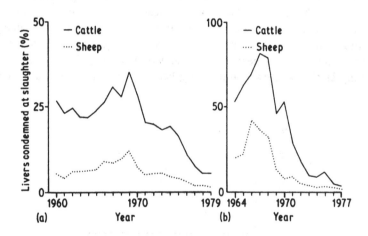

Figure 9.3 (a) Percentage of livers condemned due to fascioliasis in the UK, 1960–1979. Data from MAFF quarterly survey of approximately sixty slaughterhouses. Sample size currently represents about 11% of all animals slaughtered annually. (b) Percentage of livers condemned at Kirkwall slaughterhouse, Orkneys, 1964–1977. Data supplied by Mr. J. Walker.

Table 9.2 Slaughterhouse surveys (UK) in which data on young and old livestock were collected separately.

Location	Date	Sample size	Proportion of livers condemned (P)	Adjusted[§,‖] annual incidence (%)
UK*	1942	Cows 14464	0.30	5.0
		Steers 56013	0.15	10.0
UK†	1973–74	Ewes 77951	0.13	3.2
		Lambs 299288	0.05	6.7
		Cows 37338	0.40	7.0
		Steers 160113	0.17	11.3
Ribble Valley‡	1978	Ewes 830	0.14	3.0
Lancashire		Lambs 12128	0	0
		Cows 2383	0.52	10.0
		Steers 10089	0.03	2.0

* Peters and Clapham (1942).
† Froyd (1975) and personal communication.
‡ Wilson (unpublished data).
§ Assumes a grazing period prior to slaughter of 1.5 years for steers and 0.75 years for lambs.
‖ Calculated using equation (9.1).

required to produce observed percentage condemnation of livers can be estimated using the formula:

$$I = [1 - (1 - P)^{1/L}] \times 100 \qquad (9.1)$$

where I is incidence, P is proportion of livers condemned and L is the age at death. Estimates of annual incidence given in Table 9.2, range from 0 to 6.7% in sheep and 2 to 11.3% in cattle. Peak condemnations of both sheep and cattle livers occurred in the UK in 1969 (Fig. 9.3) and it would be instructive to know what levels of annual incidence these represented. Ewes and cows have formed an approximately constant proportion of stock slaughtered over the last 20 years (0.107 and 0.276 respectively). A rough estimate of the proportion of steers' livers (S) condemned in 1969 can be obtained (assuming a ratio of 3:1 for condemnations of livers in old stock: young) from the formula:

$$S = \frac{P}{3c + s} \qquad (9.2)$$

where P is the proportion of total cattle livers condemned, c and s are the proportions of cows and steers in the total cattle slaughtered respectively. The value for P in 1969 was 0.355 giving an estimate for S of 0.23 which, using Equation (9.1) above and an average age at slaughter of 1.5 years, is equivalent to an annual incidence of 16% for the steers.

Performing the same exercise for sheep liver condemnations in 1969

(P = 0.12) and inserting appropriate values for lambs and ewes in place of steers and cows in Equations (9.1) and (9.2) gives an estimate of 0.1 for the proportion of lambs livers condemned, equivalent to an annual incidence of 13.1 % assuming an average age at slaughter of 0.75 years. These estimates of incidence in steers and lambs should be taken only as a rough guide to the maximum magnitude for the annual rate of infection at a national level, required to produce observed levels of liver condemnations. Obviously, regional and local values of incidence could be much higher.

9.2.3   Regional variations in prevalence in the UK

The assessment of regional differences in the prevalence of fascioliasis is difficult because many of the larger slaughterhouses draw their livestock from a very wide area. Often, it is impossible to trace the infected animal back to its farm of origin and given also the frequent movement of stock between farms there may be no way of knowing where the infection was acquired. Nevertheless, the national abattoir survey of Froyd (1975) confirmed the traditional view that the disease is characteristic of the western and upland parts of the country (Fig. 9.4). This distribution reflects the annual distribution of precipitation (Ollerenshaw, 1966) rather than the distribution and density of livestock (Smith, 1982).

A number of short-term local surveys highlight the regional differences revealed in the national survey. For example, in Northern Ireland, Ross (1966) recorded 76% of cattle livers condemned at a Belfast slaughterhouse in 1964–1965.

Our own data collected from three small slaughterhouses in the Craven district of Yorkshire (an area once noted for fascioliasis) in 1976–1979 showed annual condemnations ranging from 0.4 to 1.2% for sheep and 3.9 to 11.8% for cattle. The best set of regional data we have obtained are for liver condemnations in sheep and cattle at Kirkwall slaughterhouse in the Orkneys in 1964–1977 (Walker, personal communication) (Fig. 9.3(b)). The animals in this survey came almost exclusively from the mainland of Orkney and neighbouring islands. The pattern of changes in condemnations for both sheep and cattle mirrors the national figures except that peak values are triple the national average for sheep and double for cattle. The decline in condemnations began earlier in the Orkneys (1966–1967), and by 1977 the figures were approximately equal to the national average for sheep and half the national average for cattle.

Finally, it should be noted that the estimate of average prevalence for any given region conceals considerable differences in the distribution of *Fasciola* between neighbouring farms. Table 9.3 illustrates the results of a survey of 38 farms in the North of England between the years 1975 and 1978 using faecal sampling to identify *Fasciola* infections in stock. Of the 38 farms visited, 29 were positive for fluke, 16 in both sheep and cattle, 8 for sheep only and 5 for

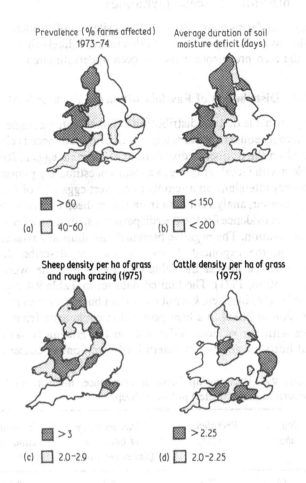

Prevalence (% farms affected)
1973-74

Average duration of soil
moisture deficit (days)

■ >60
(a) ☐ 40-60

■ <150
(b) ☐ <200

Sheep density per ha of grass
and rough grazing (1975)

Cattle density per ha of grass
(1975)

■ >3
(c) ☐ 2.0-2.9

■ >2.25
(d) ☐ 2.0-2.25

Figure 9.4 The pattern of disease prevalence in England and Wales (a) (Froyd, 1975) compared with the density and distribution of the primary hosts (c) and (d) (MAFF, 1975) and with regional variations in the duration of soil moisture deficit (b) (MAFF, 1976). Note that the prevalence of fascioliasis may be low even in places where the hosts are abundant.

Table 9.3 Frequency distribution of prevalence on 38 farms in the Peak District and Yorkshire Dales, 1975–1978.

Percentage stock positive for *F. hepatica*

	0	1–10	11–20	21–30	31–40	41–50	51–60	61–70	71–80	81–90	*Mean*
Sheep	10	15	3	1	3	0	0	1	1	0	9.2
Cattle	10	11	6	4	0	0	0	0	0	0	7.1

cattle only. The farms were visited at the invitation of farmers who thought they might have a fluke problem, and this makes it likely that the number of farms in the zero prevalence class has been underestimated.

9.2.4 Distribution of Fasciola within the flock or herd

It is highly probable that the distribution of flukes within a single flock or herd is also heterogeneous. Unfortunately, much of the evidence is circumstantial, being based on the frequency distribution of *Fasciola* eggs in faecal samples. The problem with faecal sampling as a means of estimating parasite burdens is the inaccuracy attendant on attempts to convert eggs g^{-1} of faeces to flukes per host. However, analysis of data from tracer sheep experiments (Table 9.4) provides direct evidence for the overdispersed distribution of parasites within the host population. The negative binomial distribution characterized by the mean, μ, and the exponent, k, can be used to describe the degree of overdispersion; the smaller the value of k the greater the overdispersion of parasites (Crofton, 1971). The limited data set in Table 9.4 suggests that in *Fasciola* infections in sheep, k is not a constant but varies with prevalence. The overdispersion of flukes in a host population could arise from e.g. increased prevalence with age of host, differences in the grazing behaviour between individual hosts, or genetically determined variations in susceptibility.

Table 9.4 Relationship between prevalence, intensity and over-dispersion (k parameter) in tracer sheep.

No. of sheep	Prevalence (%)	Mean intensity of infection (flukes per sheep)	Estimated value of k
15	53.3	2.47	0.43 ⎫ *
14	92.9	5.36	0.18 ⎪
15	41.4	12.20	0.54 ⎬
16	100.0	28.63	2.56 ⎪
12	100.0	157.25	2.77 ⎭
40	100.0	163.40	4.00 ⎬ †

* Crossland *et al.* (1977) and Crossland (personal communication).
† Hope-Cawdery and Moran (1971).

9.2.5 Economic losses associated with fascioliasis

Fascioliasis reduces the productivity of livestock. In sheep, unthriftiness and a shortened life expectancy are characteristic symptoms. There is a reduced live weight gain and a reduction in the quality and quantity of the wool crop (Crossland *et al.*, 1977; Sinclair, 1962; Sykes *et al.*, 1980; Edwards *et al.*, 1976;

Hawkins and Morris, 1978). Fewer lambs are born to infected ewes (Hope–Cawdery, 1976) and they gain weight less quickly than those born to uninfected animals (Crossland *et al.*, 1977). In cattle, there is a similar reduction in liveweight gain (Hope–Cawdery *et al.*, 1977; Oakley *et al.*, 1979). Milk yield and quality fall (Ross, 1970; Black and Froyd, 1972) and the number of artificial inseminations required for successful conception increases (Oakley *et al.*, 1979). The disease also renders both cattle and sheep more susceptible to serious bacterial infections, i.e. *Salmonella dublin* in cattle (Aitken *et al.*, 1976) and *Clostridium oedematiens* in sheep (Boray, 1977).

The severity of the symptoms depends upon four factors.

(1) The intensity of infection.
(2) The degree of host resistance.
(3) The nutritional status of the host.
(4) The presence of other gastrointestinal parasites.

Within this framework two forms of disease are recognized: acute fascioliasis and chronic fascioliasis. The acute form arises when a non-resistant host receives a massive infection over a short period of time. Death, due to anaemia or autointoxication as a result of gross liver dysfunction, occurs after some 6 to 10 weeks (Boray, 1977; Pullan *et al.*, 1970). The more common chronic form arises when moderate numbers of cysts are ingested over an extended period. Inappetence, poor efficiency of food conversion, increased catabolism of body protein and haemorrhage into the gut via the bile are all concomitants of chronic infection and result in the unthriftiness that characterizes the disease (Dargie *et al.*, 1979; Hawkins and Morris, 1978; Sykes *et al.*, 1980). The expression of these symptoms and their effect upon stock productivity depends upon the number of flukes that become established in the bile ducts. Some quantitative estimates of the effect of fluke burden on the mortality and productivity of sheep are illustrated in Fig. 9.5. Even with burdens of less than 100 flukes/sheep significant reductions in liveweight gain and fleece weight can be detected. Unfortunately no sophisticated cost analysis appears to have been carried out, incorporating such quantitative relationships between fluke burden and productivity, and taking account of the overdispersed distribution of flukes in livestock.

Chronic fascioliasis afflicts cattle and sheep of all ages though in cattle the symptoms are ameliorated by an acquired resistance to infection. A primary infection in cattle is met by a marked hepatic fibrosis which impedes the progress of the immature flukes across the parenchyma of the liver. The extent of this fibrotic reaction appears to be determined by the number of cysts ingested (Ross, 1965). The flukes that do become established in the bile ducts are eventually expelled (Doyle, 1972, 1973) and subsequent infections encounter cell-mediated and humoral immunological mechanisms in addition to the fibrotic reaction mentioned earlier (Armour and Dargie, 1975). Sheep do not develop any resistance to infection (Boray, 1977); consequently the burden

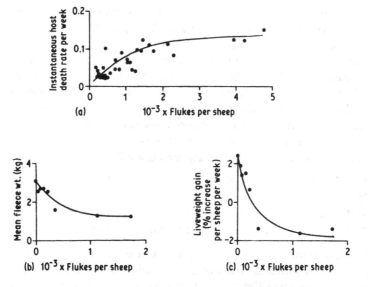

Figure 9.5 The relationship between intensity of infection and the loss of productivity in sheep. (a) Mortality of sheep (Sinclair, 1962; Ross, 1967; Boray, 1969; Pullan *et al.*, 1970; Hawkins and Morris, 1978). (b) and (c) Loss in wool production and liveweight gain respectively (Hawkins and Morris, 1978).

of flukes in an infected ewe is directly proportional to the number of viable cysts ingested, and the manifestations of chronic disease are correspondingly more severe. It also follows that sheep are susceptible to acute fascioliasis even as mature animals whereas cattle, usually, are not. The susceptibility of mature breeding sheep to infection is of particular significance since the incidence of fascioliasis in Europe is highest in the period immediately prior to and during pregnancy when ewes are under the severest nutritional stress (Sinclair, 1972). In the case of inwintered dairy cattle, where the food supply is adjusted for maximum milk yields, the effect of fascioliasis may go entirely unnoticed except for an increase in feeding costs (Vink, 1971) but sheep, unlike cattle, are generally outwintered and unless there are adequate food resources, particularly those rich in protein (Dargie, 1975; Dargie *et al.*, 1979; Berry and Dargie, 1976), productivity of the flock inevitably falls.

In most years it is the reduction in productivity due to chronic disease rather than deaths due to acute fascioliasis which constitutes the major economic loss. Ribbeck and Witzel (1979) investigated the losses due to chronic disease in an area of East Germany in which fascioliasis is not considered a major problem. Between 1969 and 1972, they estimated that the annual loss due to bovine fascioliasis alone in this area was nearly 2 million Marks. More than 80% of this was due to reduced milk production, 15% was due to reduced meat production and less than 5% was due to liver condemnations. In the UK,

Blamire *et al.* (1980) suggested that the current decline in the prevalence of bovine fascioliasis has resulted in the availability of an extra 2.4 million pounds worth of liver. It is interesting to speculate in the light of Ribbeck and Witzels' results on how much more has been saved in terms of milk and meat production.

World-wide the economic damage attributable to fascioliasis reaches prodigious levels. Ribbeck and Witzel (1979) and Euzeby and Jolivet (1972) have reviewed the situation in Europe. Liver condemnations, for example, amounted to losses of 3 million Marks per year in East Germany (1959 prices), 23.8 million Deutsch Marks in West Germany (1965 prices) and 3.6 million Guilders in Holland (1967 prices). To these figures we might add the 20 million Dollars suggested by Boray (1977) for bovine fascioliasis in Australia, and the 30 million Dollars suggested by Foreyt and Todd (1976) for bovine fascioliasis in the USA.

9.3 METHODS OF CONTROL

Several approaches to the control of fascioliasis are available but in practice they have not all found equal favour with farmers.

9.3.1 Habitat management

The presence of a population of *Lymnaea truncatula* on a farm is an absolute prerequisite for continuing transmission of *F. hepatica*. It follows that measures designed to diminish the snail population, either by reducing habitat area or directly killing snails, should reduce or eliminate transmission of the disease.

(a) *Drainage*

The annual rate of drainage of farmland in the UK has doubled since 1968 but most of the actvity has been concentrated in the arable areas of Eastern England (Armstrong, 1978). Drainage is an expensive solution (£350 per ha in 1977–1978) (Armstrong, 1978); despite the fact that 50 % government grants are available and since the annual income from an arable farm may be twice that of a livestock enterprise (MAFF, 1976–1977) it is not surprising that drainage as a means of improving productivity appeals more to the arable farmer than the owner of livestock. Even so, Edwards (1968) argued that though the initial investment in a system of drainage might be high it would be recouped after only 5–10 years as a result of improved stock performance.

In practice the areas of habitat occupied by *L. truncatula* may not be large (an average of 0.22ha/100ha on ten farms surveyed in 1978). In situations where prevalence and intensity of infection in stock are high (with consequent high probability of acute fascioliasis) drainage may be a commercially viable proposition. However, where fascioliasis has been controlled by other methods, usually chemotherapy, a drainage scheme is unlikely to be economically worthwhile for control of fascioliasis alone.

(b) Snail killing

The anecdotal, though probably little used, method of reducing snail populations was to keep a flock of domestic ducks on wet pasture land. Ducks are efficient predators of *L. truncatula* and wild mallard (*Anas platyrhyncos*), often seen feeding on snail habitats, probably represent one of the main natural agents limiting snail population density (Wilson, unpublished data). Other candidates include dipteran and caddis fly larvae. The use of more rigorous methods of snail control via molluscicides has not been taken up with much enthusiasm by the farming community (Wilson, unpublished data). Sales of molluscicide for control of *L. truncatula* can probably be measured in tens, or at most hundreds, of litres per annum in the UK (1980).

The objective of molluscicide application is either to reduce snail populations to low levels by spraying habitats in the Spring before snail breeding is underway, or by later spraying to kill snails before the infections they carry reach maturity (e.g. Crossland *et al.*, 1977). A number of studies have demonstrated the efficacy of the measures in reducing transmission (Urquhart *et al.*, 1970; Crossland, 1976). In at least one case the cost-effectiveness of antihelminthics and molluscicides in controlling fascioliasis were compared (Urquhart *et al.*, 1970) and the molluscicide application was shown to be marginally more economical.

The reduction in snail density resulting from a single treatment with Frescon (n-tritylmorpholine) can be as high as 90 % (Crossland, 1976), and 98 to 99 % of snails may be killed if a single application is made under favourable conditions (Heppleston, personal communication) or with several applications (Crossland *et al.*, 1977). Unfortunately the reproductive potential of the snail is enormous. Under favourable conditions in the laboratory a single snail is capable of producing 25 000 offspring in 12 weeks (Kendall, 1949b), an instantaneous rate of natural increase (r) of 0.84 per snail per week (a value which may approach the *intrinsic* rate of natural increase). Under field conditions r is much smaller but we have observed an increase in snail density from 2.24 to 193.7 snails m^{-2} on one habitat over a period of 90 days between July and October, 1978, an r of 0.35 per snail per week. Clearly under these conditions the effects of molluscicide treatment in depressing transmission rate cannot be expected to persist for more than 4 to 6 months. Although it is not necessary to kill all of the snails in order to eradicate fascioliasis, the effort required to reduce the snail numbers to below the transmission threshold level and *to maintain that situation* is probably prohibitive. The optimum strategy using molluscicides alone would be to reduce snail numbers such that the prevalence and intensity of infection in the primary host falls to acceptable levels but, clearly, this requires that molluscicides are applied every year for as long as the cattle and sheep are infected with mature flukes, or there is a chance of infected stock being brought on to the farm.

The technique of molluscicide application is difficult and its efficacy uncertain. For example, the kill rate depends on the density of vegetation cover and the amount of standing water on the habitat (Pearson, 1970). Snail habitats are not always easy to identify; not all wet areas harbour snails whilst, conversely, small patches of wet ground are often overlooked. *L. truncatula* is often confused with other snail species, particularly *Potamopyrgus jenkinsi* or the juveniles of *L. stagnalis* and *L. pereger*. If snail habitats are extensive, the labour involved in spraying can be excessive, particularly since access by tractor is impossible (Crossland, 1976).

In conclusion, molluscicides appear to be a viable means of controlling fascioliasis (or other digenetic trematodes) only under special circumstances. They might also be applied where no suitable anthelminthic has been licenced for use.

9.3.2 Stock management

Two options are available to the farmer in controlling fascioliasis by stock management. The simplest tactic is to prevent access of stock, particularly cattle, to boggy areas with snail populations. The method is cheap, the cost of a few fence posts and a strand of barbed wire, and semi-permanent. Sheep are more difficult to exclude from habitats. Fencing off snail habitats is carried out sporadically by many farmers particularly where a bog is small and well defined but it is doubtful whether it has much overall impact on fluke transmission.

The second and by far the commonest practice is the dosing of stock with flukicides (Armour, 1975). Its psychological appeal is obvious: the improved performance of treated stock is soon apparent (Reuss, 1973). Flukicides can be administered conveniently when stock are gathered together for some other purpose, and, combined in a single dose with nematocides, their routine use becomes part of 'an integrated worming programme'. Several cheap and effective flukicides are available (Table 9.5) sold under such trade names as Coriban, Ranide and Zanil. The manufacturers recommend routine dosing of stock at 6–8 week intervals between August and February. In practice farmers who suspect they have a 'fluke problem' appear to dose stock once, twice or at most three times a year. (The difficulty for the farmer lies in deciding, in the absence of acute fascioliasis, whether his stock is seriously infected.) Both serological tests and faecal examination can be used to identify infected stock but the cost of diagnosis to the farmer is as great or greater than the cost of routine mass chemotherapy. Dosing stock becomes an act of faith on the part of the farmer best viewed as a form of insurance against disease. The trend in recent years has been to combine dosing of stock for fluke with that for roundworm (Fig. 9.6). But treatment for roundworms in sheep and cattle is

Table 9.5 Cost of dosing stock using some currently available flukicides (figures are all up to date (3rd July, 1980).

	Cost per dose (£)				Routine recommendation (doses per animal per year)
	Sheep		*Cattle*		
Flukicide	50lb	125lb	200lb	600lb	
Diamphenethide*	0.14	0.27	–	–	
Nitroxynil	0.03	0.08	0.08	0.25	3–6
Oxyclozanide	0.03	0.05	0.08	0.19	
Rafoxanide	0.04	0.12	0.16	0.49	

* Diamphenethide (Coriban) is expensive because it is based on paracetamol, which is itself expensive!

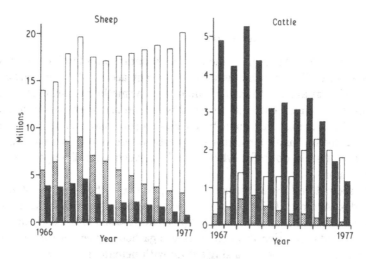

Figure 9.6 Doses of flukicide sold per annum in the UK (estimated from market research) compared with number of infected animals (estimated by adjusting slaughterhouse condemnations to reflect the age composition of the national sheep flock and cattle herd).□, Flukicide + wormicide;▨, flukicide alone; ■, no. of infected animals.

recommended between March and July, whereas for fluke it is between August and February.

It is difficult to obtain reliable information on the total number of doses of flukicide sold in the UK per annum but estimates based on market research are illustrated in Fig. 9.6, together with data on the total stock infected in each year. It is interesting to note that prior to 1970 the total number of infected sheep and cattle were similar (the sheep population of the UK outnumbers the cattle by a factor of 3 to 1). The level of dosing in sheep in 1966 exceeded the number of infected animals by a factor of 3 or 4 to 1. By 1977 the number of doses exceeded infection by a factor of 20 to 1 and at the time of writing (1980) the number of infected sheep has fallen to such a low level that even allowing for some decline in sales of flukicides, the number of doses used probably exceeds the number of infections by a factor of 50:1.

The pattern in cattle is quite different and also more difficult to interpret. The estimates for number of infected animals do not take account of the development of immunity in older stock. However, it seems highly likely that for at least half the decade 1966–1977 the number of infected animals exceeded the doses of flukicide sold. Only post-1975 does the number of doses exceed the number of infected animals. It is also apparent that doses of flukicide sold for sheep exceed those for cattle by a factor of ten.

It is obvious that the use of flukicides on such a scale must have consequences for the epidemiology of fascioliasis. Indeed, it is possible that chemotherapy of stock has been the dominant factor in the marked decline in prevalence observed over the last decade. The other major contender is summer rainfall which will influence the mortality of the extramammalian stages. The chief feature of temperate summers is the unpredictability of rainfall from year to year so that one might expect its impact on fascioliasis over a decade or more to average out around a mean level. The decline in fascioliasis since 1970 has been so consistent that it is tempting to conclude that chemotherapy is the major cause of declining prevalence.

The relative costs of various control measures are illustrated in Table 9.6.

Table 9.6 Summary of the comparative cost of various control measures at 1980 prices (UK).

Farm profile /100 ha	Treatment	Frequency of application	Unit cost (£)	Estimated cost per annum (£)
2 ha of snail habitat	Drainage	Once/10 years	500/ha	100
	Molluscicide	Once/year	27/ha	50*
100 ewes			0.1/dose	
150 lambs	Chemotherapy	Twice/year	0.05/dose	54*
25 cows			0.25/dose	
30 steers			0.1/dose	

* Excludes labour costs.

9.3.3 Forecasting incidence

The Ministry of Agriculture, Fisheries and Food (MAFF) publish an annual forecast in early September of the likely incidence of fascioliasis in an effort to minimize overdosing in years of low incidence and to ensure that adequate control measures are taken in years of high incidence. This 'fluke forecast' (Ollerenshaw and Rowlands, 1959) was one of the first of a whole battery of predictive systems ranged against the diseases of economically important plants and animals (Krause and Massie, 1975).

Ollerenshaw and Rowlands derived an index of climate, the M_t index, based on the difference between monthly evapotranspiration and rainfall. They correlated this index with estimates of *Fasciola* infections obtained from veterinary investigation centre records, and found a significant association. Ollerenshaw (1974) states that although the index is based on soil moisture parameters ' . . . in practice, some allowance is made for unusual temperature deviations'. He does not describe these allowances.

Ollerenshaw and Rowlands' index is essentially a convenient summary of practical wisdom. It gives no insight into the dynamics of transmission, and despite the mathematical notation of their original paper it is in no sense a model. Since each year is considered independently of every other, it would predict high incidence in a wet year even if a preceding 10 years drought had eradicated every source of infection. Ollerenshaw (1974) has reviewed the operation of this forecasting system over a period of years.

In practice the fluke forecasts made by MAFF appear to provide a balanced assessment of likely disease incidence each year. However, it is difficult to discern the extent to which the forecast is based on the M_t index relative to disease monitoring in stock and snails. At the time of writing (1980) the prevalence of fascioliasis in the UK is very low and it must be assumed that disease monitoring is the dominant element in the forecast, the climate-based M_t index being relegated to a very subordinate role.

9.4 CLIMATE AND SNAIL HABITATS

L. truncatula habitats are the foci on which transmission is centred but only those habitats which stay wet and warm for a period sufficiently long to permit the completion of the parasite life cycle present any risk to stock. The mere coincidence of both mammalian and molluscan hosts is not enough to ensure the transmission of fascioliasis.

In Section 9.2 we noted that regional variations in disease prevalence were associated with regional differences in the amount of precipitation. The life cycle of *F. hepatica* is extremely sensitive to climatic variation. Seasonal, annual and regional differences can be accounted for largely in terms of the effect of weather on the conditions that prevail at the surface of the snail habitats.

In temperate regions there is a consistent annual pattern of climatic variation but meteorological records show that in the long term there may be considerable deviations from the mean values. For example, the total number of day-degrees above 10°C (an index of the potential for growth and development of *L. truncatula* and the larval stages of *F. hepatica*) may vary

Table 9.7 Regional and annual variation in climate and climate-derived statistics in areas prone to fascioliasis in the UK (MAFF, 1976).

	Day degrees above 10°C		Excess winter rain (mm)		Mean annual rainfall (mm)	Duration of the soil moisture defect (days)
	Mean	10 year extreme	Mean	10 year extreme		
Lowland dairy areas						
N.W. England	550	454–688	550	435–650	1045	122
N. Wales	765	650–918	305	220–385	786	176
S.W. England	880	770–1021	175	105–230	630	238
Upland livestock areas						
N. England	425	351–531	1200	1000–1400	1663	37
N. Wales	550	467–660	675	550–800	1184	109
S.W. England	640	560–742	725	565–900	1265	98

from one year to the next, even at the same location, by as much as 25 % (Smith, 1978). Regional differences may be much greater (Table 9.7). Similarly, the estimated soil moisture deficit calculated after the method of Penman (1948) can be used as a crude index of inter-year variations in snail habitat wetness. Data from the Cumbrian region for the 3 years 1972–1974 (Fig. 9.7) illustrate that the onset of the deficit, its maximum extent, and the autumn return to field capacity vary considerably. The differences in pattern are primarily a reflection of the distribution and intensity of rainfall through the summer months.

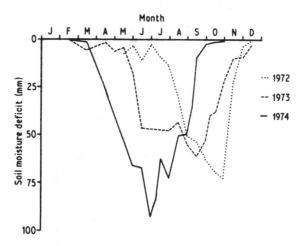

Figure 9.7 The estimated soil moisture deficit in the Cumbrian region of the UK 1972–1974 showing the variations in time of onset, severity and return to field capacity (Meteorological Office, Bracknell).

The annual cycle of climate generates a similar cyclical fluctuation in the transmission of fascioliasis, and deviations from the usual climatic pattern are manifested in the magnitude of transmission. However, variations in macroclimatic parameters like rainfall and air temperature are significant only in the extent to which they affect conditions at the surface of the snail habitats. We shall discuss the relationship between macroclimate and microclimate in following sections, but first, since the character of the relationship is determined by the nature of snail habitats, we shall describe the kinds of situation where *L. truncatula* is typically found.

9.4.1 Soil and vegetation

L. truncatula can inhabit a variety of situations whose common characteristic is to remain wet for 10 or more months of the year but nevertheless would not be considered ponds. In this context, there is some overlap between the habitats of *L. truncatula* and *L. pereger*, a more truly aquatic species. Ditches, seepages, flushes and springs are typical sites, almost always fed by ground water (Styczynska–Jurewicz, 1965; Smith, 1978, 1981). In such diverse conditions it is difficult to generalize about habitats but some features appear to be common throughout the UK and W. Europe.

Habitats are distinguished by associations of helophytic plants, the combination of *Alopecurus geniculatus, Glyceria* sp. and *Ranunculus repens* being typical (Over, 1962; Ghestem *et al.*, 1974; Greer, 1976; Smith, 1978). The snails are more often found on smooth mud than on soils with a gritty texture. In an analysis of 20 bogs in the Peak District, Greer (1976) found that the presence or absence of snails was determined by the proportion of organic matter in the soil. Bogs with an organic content of less than 15 % of dry matter supported snails, those with more did not. The concentration of minerals such as calcium and iron, and the pH of the soil, appeared to be without influence. High organic content is an indicator of anaerobic conditions and probably explains why sometimes extensive areas of bog, particularly on poorly drained land, do not support snails. A continuous water throughput, however slow, is needed to maintain snail populations.

9.4.2 Temperature

Standardized recordings of temperature are readily available at national or regional level in the U.K. but in any simulation study of fascioliasis it is essential to be able to reinterpret these recordings in terms of the microclimate which exists at the soil surface of *L. truncatula* habitats. The first point to make is that there is no general, consistent quantitative relationship between temperature at the soil surface of a habitat and the prevailing weather (Smith and Wilson, 1980). Topographical, pedological and vegetational features unique to each habitat preclude such a relationship. Nevertheless, the differences between habitat microclimate and regional macroclimate are sufficiently great to warrant the use of approximations which may not describe habitat microclimate exactly but do so at least *more precisely* than standard meteorological measurements.

Smith and Wilson (1980) found that monthly mean temperatures at the soil surface of a habitat were always *higher* than the corresponding air temperatures between April and October; for the remainder of the year monthly mean temperatures at the soil surface were *lower* than the corresponding air temperatures. The difference was sometimes as great as 4°C. In addition the daily temperature range at the soil surface was always less than that experienced at screen height especially during the autumn and winter. A detailed analysis of these relationships is beyond the scope of this chapter (see Smith, 1978, and Smith and Wilson, 1980, for a full discussion) but we suggest that the following model provides reasonable estimates of the average temperature regime at the soil surface of any group of habitats:

	Period I	Period II
Temperature maxima	$y = 0.93x + 2.34$	$y = 0.94x - 0.85$
Temperature minima	$y = 1.12x + 1.34$	$y = 1.08x + 0.74$

where y is soil surface temperature and x is temperature at screen height. Period I is the end of capacity date to mid-August and Period II is mid-August to end of capacity date in following year.

In a more detailed analysis involving additional meteorological factors (Trippick, personal communication) it was found that inclusion of solar radiation improves the accuracy with which temperatures at the habitat surface can be predicted during the summer months.

It is pertinent at this point to include a note on how measurements of daily maximum and minimum temperature are used in the simple simulations described in the following sections. It is Meteorological Office practice to estimate daily mean temperature from the average of daily maximum and minimum. Hope–Cawdery et al. (1978) extended this approach to estimate the mean daily temperature and the proportion of the day above a cut-off of $10\,°C$. This procedure can be adopted for any cut-off (Table 9.8). Thomas (1979) has tested these formulae with temperature cut-offs of $4\,°C$ and $10\,°C$, corresponding respectively to the temperatures at which snail and fluke eggs cease development, against hourly temperature records. He found an excellent agreement and demonstrated that they could be used in simulations to predict the timing of events in the snail and parasite life cycles with remarkable precision.

Table 9.8   The use of daily maximum and minimum temperatures in simulation.

	Equation	Condition
Mean temperature above cut-off	$(Mx* + Mn\dagger)/2$	$Mx \geqslant Mn \geqslant C\ddagger$
	$(Mx + C)/2$	$Mx \geqslant C \geqslant Mn$
	0	$C \geqslant Mx \geqslant Mn$
Proportion of day above cut-off	$\begin{smallmatrix}1\\(Mx - C)/(Mx\ Mn)\\0\end{smallmatrix}$	$Mx \geqslant Mn \geqslant C$
		$Mx \geqslant C \geqslant Mn$
		$C \geqslant Mx \geqslant Mn$

* Mx is daily maximum temperature.
† Mn is daily minimum temperature.
‡ C is cut-off temperature.

9.4.3 Habitat wetness

The various components of the hydrological cycle determine the soil moisture conditions at the surface of L. truncatula habitats. The various forms of precipitation are the input, not just over the summer months in the immediate vicinity of a habitat, but over preceding seasons via effects on ground water, and over the surrounding land which comprises the catchment area of the habitat. The fate of precipitation is complex. A considerable proportion may pass rapidly into streams as surface run-off. The remainder infiltrates the soil where it is 'stored' and contributes to ground water flow or is removed by evaporation back to the atmosphere. As already noted habitats are almost always maintained by a seepage of ground water which together with evapotranspiration will determine their wetness.

The problem facing the epidemiologist is how to measure habitat wetness. Direct gravimetric estimates of water content can be made using superficial soil cores 1–2 cm deep. However, water content is dependent on soil type. Soil suction pressure (pF) is independent of type and so should overcome this limitation. Unfortunately measurements are tedious to make and the technique is not suited to routine use. The best that is possible is to calibrate the suction pressure of a given soil against gravimetric water content. As a simple alternative, Smith (1978) and Smith and Wilson (1980) proposed that the moisture conditions at the soil surface should be rated visually on a four-point ordinal scale which ranged from 'standing water' through 'wet' and 'damp' to 'dry'. The method dealt directly with the moisture regime actually experienced by the organisms on the soil surface of the habitat and each of the four categories was chosen so as to correspond to conditions for which the responses of the snails and larval flukes had already been established (Smith, 1978; Nice, 1979). The proportions of a habitat in each category can be estimated by quadrat sampling the entire habitat if it is small or taking a transect if it is large (Fig. 9.8). The index of habitat wetness obtained can be used in the analysis of snail and parasite population data. It can also be used directly to drive simulation models of various parts of the life cycle (Section 9.5) in conjunction with temperature.

In order to make such simulations more generally applicable it is necessary to find an index of habitat wetness analogous to the standard meteorological data used to predict soil surface temperature. There are a variety of possibilites. Ground water levels were suggested by Hope–Cawdery et al. (1978). The MAFF liver fluke forecast is based upon a cumulative index of soil moisture deficit (the M_t index) which is in turn determined from rainfall, and evapotranspiration calculated according to the method of Penman (1948). The Meteorological Office now provides weekly estimates of soil moisture deficits for 40 km grid squares in the UK via its MORECS service (Fig. 9.8). A third possibility is the use of river-flow records collected by regional water authorities. These can be expected to correlate well with run-off and ground water flow in individual river catchments (Fig. 9.8).

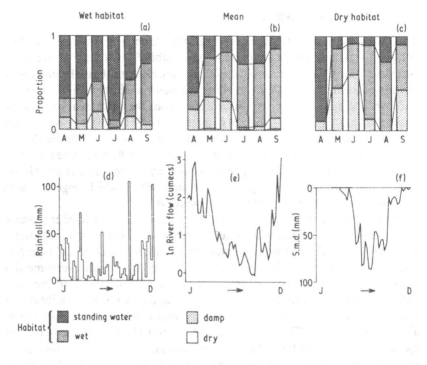

Figure 9.8 (a)–(c) The proportions of snail habitats under standing water, wet, damp and dry conditions during the summer months, Peak District, 1978. (d) Annual rainfall in the vicinity of the farms (courtesy of Portland–Blue Circle Cement). (e) River flow on the River Derwent (Severn–Trent Water Authority). (f) Estimated soil moisture deficit (s.m.d.) (Meteorological Office, MORECS).

Trippick (personal communication) has analysed the correlation of habitat wetness with ln (river flow) and soil moisture deficit in three river catchments in the North of England. In all three areas he found that ln (river flow) was a significantly better predictor of the proportions of habitat wet and under standing water than soil moisture deficit. This is not surprising in view of the fact that soil moisture deficit estimated using the Penman formula describes the moisture characteristics of the average well-drained field: the very reverse of a snail habitat. The formula for predicting habitat wetness in the River Derwent catchment of the Peak District is:

$$\text{probit } \hat{y}_i = a_1 + a_2 x_i \qquad (9.3)$$

where $\hat{y}_i$ is the estimated proportion of habitat with a particular state of wetness, a_1 is a constant, a_2 is the slope of regression and x_i is ln (river flow) (cumecs). For the proportion of habitat under standing water the values of a_1 and a_2 were -0.851 and 0.426 respectively. For the proportion of habitat wet they were 0.638 and 0.219 respectively.

9.5   POPULATION BIOLOGY OF THE PARASITE AND ITS HOSTS

Natural populations are characterized by age-specific rates of mortality and fecundity. Summarized in a life table, these can be used to estimate the expected reproductive success of an average individual in the population. This statistic, the net reproductive rate (R_0), governs the changes in population size that occur between one generation and the next (Krebs, 1972). In the case of parasites like the liver fluke, which pass through several distinct life-cycle stages that overlap in time, it is more convenient to deal with *stage*-specific rates of mortality and fecundity rather than with age-specific rates. Thus, the net reproductive rate of *F. hepatica* depends on:

(1) Stage development time;
(2) Stage mortality;
(3) Transmission success;
(4) Fecundity of the reproductive stages.

   Taken together, stage development time and stage mortality define the stage survival probability. Transmission success determines the proportion of parasites that reaches an environment in which reproduction is possible.

   The net reproductive rate of any particular population varies in time and space as a result of the action of density-dependent and density-independent processes which exert their influence on population numbers through the effect they have on the stage-specific rates listed above.

9.5.1   The biology of *Lymnaea truncatula*

The hydrology of the snail habitats was considered in detail in Section 9.4 but their chief feature is a very variable annual cycle of wetting and drying. Accordingly the snail is an *r* strategist (McArthur and Wilson, 1967) capable of a rapid increase in numbers during the brief periods when the habitat is warm and wet enough (Smith, 1982).

(a) *Fecundity*

The very high fecundity of *L. truncatula* was noted in Section 9.3. The snails mature and commence egg laying when 3–5 mm long and after maturation fecundity can be considered time (age)-independent (Thomas, 1979). Under conditions of excess moisture fecundity is optimal around 20°C, tending to zero above and below this point (Fig. 9.9) (Nice, 1979). Drying of the habitat markedly reduces fecundity and over a very small range of soil moisture content (pF 1.9 to 2.2) the fecundity declines to zero (Fig. 9.9(b)) (Nice, 1979). Thomas (1979) has described these relationships empirically:

$$F = \exp\,(\alpha_0 + \alpha_1 T + \alpha_2 T^2) \quad \text{when pF} < 2 \qquad (9.4)$$
$$F = 0 \quad \text{when pF} > 2$$

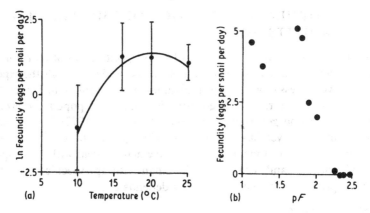

Figure 9.9 The fecundity of *Lymnaea truncatula*. (a) The relationship between fecundity and environmental temperature. (b) The relationship between fecundity and soil suction pressure (pF) at a constant temperature of 20 °C. (Reproduced with permission from Nice, 1979, and Thomas, 1979.)

where F is fecundity in eggs per snail per day and T is temperature in °C. Parameter values for α_0, α_1 and α_2 ($\pm$ s.e.) were $-7.915 \pm 1.194, 0.910 \pm 0.151$ and -0.022 ± 0.0045 respectively (Thomas, 1979). These relationships form the basis of the simulation model described in Section 9.6.

Snail eggs are not resistent to desiccation, requiring a surface film of moisture to survive. Thus as soon as the habitat surface drops below saturation eggs will be killed. The rate of egg development (defined as the reciprocal of the time to hatching; Varley, Gradwell and Hassell, 1973) is linearly related to environmental temperature (Fig. 9.10(a)). The low temperature cut-off for development is around 3.5°C. The combined effects of environmental temperature and moisture result in a marked seasonality of egg production (Fig. 9.10) and hatching in the field. There appears to be no information on the density-dependent processes such as competition for food or predation which might be expected to regulate both snail fecundity and egg mortality.

(b)   *Growth*

Snail growth following hatching is dependent on temperature and soil moisture. Thomas (1979) has fitted a logistic equation to laboratory-derived data relating growth rate to temperature when moisture is in excess:

$$l_t = A/(1 + K\mathrm{e}^{-Act}) \qquad (9.5)$$

where A is maximum length, c is a rate constant, K is a constant fixed by initial shell length and l_t is shell length at time t. Only parameter c varied significantly with temperature (Fig. 9.11(a)). In biological terms *L. truncatula* grows to the same maximum size independent of temperature, only the rate at which it approaches this maximum varies.

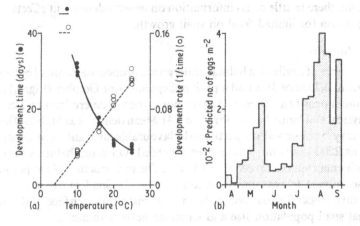

Figure 9.10   Eggs of *Lymnaea truncatula*. (a) The effect of environmental temperature on the rate of egg development. (Linear regression of development rate, *R*, on Temperature, *T*. $R = 0.00506 \times T - 0.0175$; Data from Nice, 1979; Thomas, 1979.) (b) The pattern of egg deposition on snail habitats predicted from a simulation model incorporating Equation (9.4), the above regression and daily maximum and minimum temperatures for the Peak District, 1978 (Wilson, unpublished data).

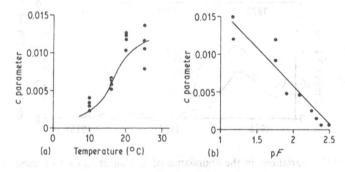

Figure 9.11   Growth of *Lymnaea truncatula*. Growth is defined by the parameter *c* of the logistic Equation (9.5). (a) The growth rate at different constant temperatures, moisture and food not limiting. (b) Growth rate at 20 °C with different soil suction pressures (pF). (Data from Nice, 1979, and Thomas, 1979.)

When soil moisture is limiting both parameters *c* and *A* are affected (Fig. 9.11(b)). The rate of growth diminishes as soil moisture content (pF) is reduced and a lower maximum length is attained (Thomas, 1979). The analysis of snail growth carried out by Thomas suggests that during the summer months under field conditions in the UK with optimum soil moisture, a snail can grow from hatching to egg laying in about 6 weeks.

Again, there is little or no information on density-dependent effects such as competition for limited food on snail growth.

(c) *Mortality*

The number of snails on a habitat undergoes a pronounced annual cycle with a low around June or July and a peak in September or October (Fig. 9.12). The maximum density attained by a given population is determined by a complex of physical and biotic factors (Section 9.4). Mean densities as high as 200 snails m^{-2} may be observed on particularly favourable sites and spot densities as high as 2500 snails m^{-2} have been recorded. On other habitats maximum densities may seldom exceed snails 5 m^{-2}. The size structure of the population is also subject to seasonal variation (Fig. 9.13). Snail mortality, like snail fecundity, tracks fluctuations in the microclimate at the surface of the habitat so that snail population size and structure never stabilize.

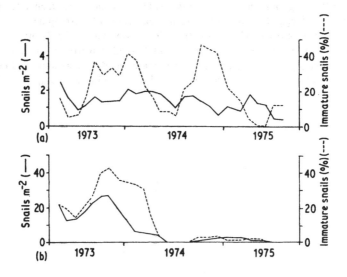

Figure 9.12 Variations in the abundance of *L. truncatula* on two habitats, one in Cumbria (a) and one in N. Wales (b). The decline in abundance at the Welsh site in 1974 was due to a prolonged summer drought extending into August. Data from Smith, 1978.

Under laboratory conditions, in the absence of stress, snails routinely reach a much larger size at death (9–12 mm) than is observed in the field. Empty snail shells collected in quadrat samples provide data on size at death (Fig. 9.14). Maximum densities, expressed as a proportion of live snails, are observed in June and July. Between size classes 3 and 8 mm, the numbers of shells found are an approximately constant proportion of live snails in those classes, suggesting that mortality is size-independent.

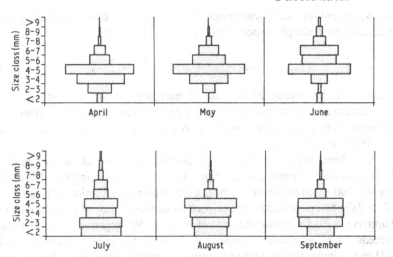

Figure 9.13 The size-class structure of natural populations of *L. truncatula* in the summer months, 1975–1979, North of England (pooled observations on more than 10 000 snails). The build-up in numbers of juvenile snails in July and August is evident, even allowing for the underestimates of numbers in lower size classes by quadrat sampling. Wilson, unpublished data.

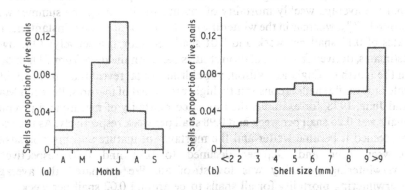

Figure 9.14 Mortality of *L. truncatula* in the field as indicated by data on empty shells collected. (a) Mortality by month as a proportion of total live snails found. (b) Mortality by size class as a proportion of the live snails found in each class.

Shells less than 3 mm are under-represented – more likely a reflection of sampling than of reduced mortality of juveniles. Shells greater than 9 mm are over-represented, relative to the proportion of live snails in that class, suggesting a greater than average mortality for very large snails. The mean size of all empty shells collected was approximately 5 mm. Thomas (1979) showed that senescent mortality was temperature-dependent and could be adequately described by a simple exponential model of the form:

$$r_{t+\delta t} = r_t \times \exp\left[(\alpha + \beta T)\delta t\right] \qquad (9.6)$$

where r_t is the instantaneous rate of mortality at time t, and $r_{t+\delta t}$ is the instantaneous rate of mortality at $t+\delta t$. T is temperature, assumed to be constant during the time interval t to $t+\delta t$. α and β are fitted constants (-0.0077 and 0.00162 respectively).

There have been numerous and conflicting accounts of the ability of *L. truncatula* to withstand drought. Laboratory experiments (Nice, 1979) suggest that when moisture is limiting (equivalent to a suction pressure deficit, $pF > 2.0$) snail populations experience an increased mortality due to drought. Thomas (1979) discussing the data of Nice (1979) suggested that when the pF exceeds 2.0 this additional component of mortality can be modelled by adding 0.03 to the instantaneous rate of senescent mortality per day. The timing and extent of dry periods is paramount; dry springs by operating via fecundity and egg mortality, as well as snail mortality limit the number of snails available for infection when miracidium larvae hatch. Dry periods in mid-summer will cause heavy mortality of snails, including (and perhaps, in particular) those infected with *Fasciola*. An assessment of drought-induced mortality is thus crucially important in any predictive model of fluke incidence.

Heppleston (1972) using Pesigan's method (Pesigan *et al.*, 1958) estimated that the average weekly mortality of mature snails during the summer was around 17%, whereas in the winter the rate fell to about 1% (i.e. instantaneous rates of 0.17 snail per week and 0.01 snail per week respectively). Our own estimates, derived from simulation studies based on the data from 73 habitats in the North of England (Wilson, unpublished data) reveal that the mortality rate of juvenile snails is consistently higher than that of matures. Between May and June, 1978, for example, the estimated mortality of mature and juvenile snails was 0.25 snail per week and 0.98 snail per week respectively. As the year proceeded it became wetter and the mortality of mature and juvenile snails between June and October declined to 0.14 and 0.70 respectively. Overwintering mortality was lowest of all. We estimated the average overwintering mortality for all snails to be around 0.02 snail per week.

These mean values for mortality in the field give no indication of the diversity of patterns encountered. Every snail habitat examined has some individual feature marking it off from all others. Components which generate this diversity include not just the physical factors, but also largely un-quantifiable events such as the predation of snails, chiefly by mallard (*Anas platyrhyncos*) and the extent of trampling by cattle. Poaching of habitats creates large areas of mud on which the snails thrive, but at the same time makes a significant contribution to snail mortality (Wilson, unpublished data).

(d) Aggregation

Habitats exhibit spatial as well as temporal heterogeneity with the result that distribution of snails is non-random. A significant fraction of the surface area of a bog (0–50%) may consist of raised tussocks not inhabited by snails (although mats of vegetation act as refuges in times of drought). The frequency distribution of snails per quadrat gives a measure of snail distribution over the remaining habitable areas of bog. The data can be adequately described by the negative binomial distribution, the parameter R providing a measure of the aggregation (Table 9.9). Aggregation varies with the month and increases from a minimum in April to a maximum in June as habitats dry out. This could reflect migration from dry to wet areas but more likely, differential mortality. As habitats become wet again in the late summer and autumn, aggregation decreases. This most probably reflects outward migration of survivors and their progeny from areas which had remained wet.

Table 9.9 Temporal variations in the aggregated distribution of snails compared with area of habitat that was wet or under standing water. These wet areas are expressed as a proportion of total habitat area and the mean values for 74 habitats are given.

	April	May	June	July	August	September	October
k parameter	0.724	0.376	0.245	0.275	0.292	0.408	0.587
Habitat wetness	0.75	0.48	0.36	0.51	0.95	0.92	–

(e) Dispersal

Snail dispersal could be important in two respects – the recolonization of habitats where the population has become (temporarily) extinct, and in the dissemination of infected snails throughout a wide area. However, Heppleston (1972) concluded, as a result of mark-and-recapture experiments, that the snails display considerable site fidelity and the available evidence suggests that the dispersal of *L. truncatula* is a largely passive event (e.g. transport by flood water) when distances more than a metre or so are concerned (Walton, 1918; Bednarz, 1960).

Observations on ditches cleared by mechanical excavator suggest a period of 2–3 years before even limited snail populations are re-established, although this could reflect the time required for the microflora and fauna on which the snail feeds to restabilize, rather than a slow rate of dispersal. The most important instances of snail movement occur when snails are washed by heavy rainfall out of permanent habitats on to flooded fields to create temporary habitats. This could result in contamination of large areas of grass with metacercarial cysts.

9.5.2 Biology of the parasite

The population processes of the parasite (fecundity, transmission and mortality) can be treated in an identical manner to those of the snail intermediate host. The rates of these processes will be influenced by density-dependent and density-independent factors. In particular, the growth and development of the stages of *F. hepatica* between egg and metacercarial cyst will occur only during the relatively few months of the year when suitable soil surface temperatures coincide with adequate soil surface moisture on snail habitats. At any moment in time the parasite may exist in up to six discrete populations (see Fig. 9.1). The maximum time an individual resides in one of these populations may be only hours for a miracidium larva to more than 1 year for a mature fluke in a sheep.

(a) *Fecundity in adult flukes*

Egg production by mature flukes in sheep is density-dependent, ranging from an average of 25 000 day^{-1} in low infections to 8800 day^{-1} in very heavy infections (Boray, 1969) (Fig. 9.15). A similar density-dependent relationship between fluke burden and egg production presumably occurs but has not been demonstrated in cattle. Egg production in cattle averages 10 000–12 000 per fluke per day – a reflection of the smaller size of flukes from cattle (Boray, 1969).

Data from post-mortems on tracer sheep (Section 9.2) have demonstrated the heterogeneous distribution of flukes in a single flock. These findings are reinforced by observations on the distribution of *Fasciola* eggs in faecal

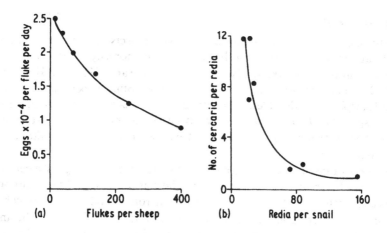

Figure 9.15 The relationship between the intensity of infection and the fecundity of the parasite. (a) Sexual reproduction of mature flukes in sheep (Boray, 1969). (b) Asexual reproduction of the intramolluscan stages (Kendall and Ollerenshaw, 1963).

samples taken from sheep or cattle (unfortunately there is no accepted formula for converting eggs per g of faeces into flukes per host).

Data from a flock of ewes on a farm in the Peak District (1975–1976) are illustrated in Fig. 9.16. The distribution is highly overdispersed. Observations on large numbers of faecal samples from cattle and sheep are summarized in Fig. 9.17. These data are grouped according to the prevalence of fascioliasis in the flock or herd sampled. When the negative binomial distribution is fitted to the data, values for the exponent k of the distribution are observed to increase with prevalence and mean eggs g^{-1}, in both sheep and cattle, suggesting that the degree of overdispersion of flukes in a flock or herd decreases as prevalence increases. The degree of overdispersion of flukes and of fluke eggs per g of faeces must be incorporated when estimates of the total parasite egg output of a flock or herd are made for epidemiological purposes.

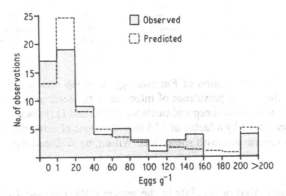

Figure 9.16   The distribution of *Fasciola* eggs in the faeces of an undosed flock of ewes, Peak District, 1975–1976. The mean eggs g^{-1} was 56.0, and prevalence was 74%. The estimated value for the k parameter of the negative binomial distribution was 0.3215. Wilson, unpublished data.

(b)   *Contamination rate*

The rate at which fluke eggs enter the habitat of *L. truncatula* is a major determinant of the rate of transmission. Contamination rate has two components, direct deposition of faeces into the habitat, and the indirect translocation of faecal material deposited on surrounding pasture. If it is assumed that in the long term, faeces are deposited or spread evenly over the whole area of pasture, then the probability of faeces entering the habitat is obtained by simply dividing the habitat area by the field area. The assumption is probably valid in the case of cattle (MacDiarmid and Watkin, 1972; Boswell and Smith, 1976) but not in the case of sheep (Hilder, 1966; Donald and Leslie, 1969, Brasher and Perkins, 1978). In general, sheep tend to avoid the wet areas where the snails are found until obliged to move there by the intensification of

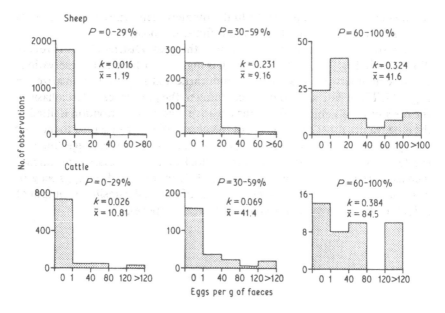

Figure 9.17 The distribution of *Fasciola* eggs in sheep and cattle faeces arranged according to the overall prevalence of infection in the flock or herd sampled. Total number of observation in sheep and cattle were 2563 and 1118 respectively. The cattle data have been scaled by a factor of 12.5 (faecal output of cattle relative to sheep) to permit direct comparison with sheep data. Wilson, unpublished data.

grazing pressure that occurs late in the season (Ollerenshaw, 1971a). This fact must also be reflected in the relative prevalence of fascioliasis in sheep and cattle (Section 9.2). Cows have approximately 1.5 times the life span of ewes, and steers graze approximately twice as long as lambs. We might therefore expect overall prevalence in sheep to be 50% or more that of cattle. Over a period of 20 years it has been very consistently 30% that of cattle. If grazing behaviour were the major reason for this difference, it would imply that sheep grazed habitats at 0.667 times the frequency of cattle.

The extent to which faeces deposited elsewhere contaminates a habitat is problematic. Rainfall and the amount of trampling by stock are key factors in faeces dispersal. The amount of faecal material remaining in a pat declines in a negatively exponential manner (Brasher and Perkins, 1978), the rate of loss varying with the season. Brasher and Perkins (1978), for example, found that 50% of the faecal material deposited by sheep in May was lost from the pats in 4–5 weeks, whereas in the relatively warmer but wetter month of August the same amount disappeared in only 2–3 weeks. The amount of rainfall is crucial (Weeda, 1967; Smith, 1978) but the original consistency of the faeces, the moisture content of the soil profile and the composition of the faunal community at or near the soil surface are each important factors in faecal decay (Castle and MacDaid, 1972; MacDiarmid and Watkin, 1972; Gronvold, 1979). The presence of stock is also important. Perkins (1978) found that faeces disappeared at three times the rate reported by Brasher and Perkins (1978) in the presence of stock and when the pasture is grazed by cattle the effect of trampling is such that an area of over $13m^2$ may be directly affected by material from a single pat (Boswell and Smith, 1976). When the faeces have been disrupted in this way it is reasonable to suppose that the fluke eggs will be spread rather thinly over the soil surface and quite quickly washed clear of faecal material in those months when rainfall is high, especially if the faeces is deposited or translocated to a wet snail habitat. Helsby (unpublished observations) estimated that 20–25 mm of rainfall over a period of 3 weeks were needed to dissipate sheep faecal pellets. In the wetter parts of the UK such conditions would generally prevail between September and April.

However, it is likely that soil will act as an efficient filter of fluke eggs so that material will only be carried on to habitats via surface run-off. This will be a quantitatively important component of total run-off when soils are at field capacity (usually October to March but in some years and locations a much briefer period, e.g. January to March).

In practical terms, what are the chances of a fluke egg reaching a snail habitat in the field? In 1978 we estimated the area of snail habitat as a percentage of field area at 17 locations in the North of England where fluke transmission occurred. The mean value was 0.38 % and the highest recorded value 2.5 %. Applying the arguments set out above the mean probability of a fluke egg reaching a habitat by direct contamination would be 0.0038 from cattle and less than 0.0038 from sheep. In the winter months this probability would be increased by an unknown factor due to contamination by surface run-off. (Hairston (1973) estimated a probability of 0.034–0.053 for an egg of *Schistosoma japonicum* reaching a snail habitat in his studies on human schistosomiasis in the Phillipines.)

(c) *Egg development and mortality*

Fasciola eggs require a surface film of moisture to survive and oxygen for development (Rowcliffe and Ollerenshaw, 1960). Little or no development occurs whilst the eggs are trapped in the faecal pat. How long eggs can remain viable whilst trapped in faeces is a matter of debate. Over and Dijkstra (1975) suggest that mortality of eggs is negligible provided that the pat remains wet either as a result of incident rainfall or capillary water drawn into the pat from the soil. *Fasciola* eggs can be routinely stored in an undeveloped state at 5 °C for approximately 8 weeks without significant loss of viability. They do, however, show a slight but definite consumption of food reserves during this period. After 8 weeks, viability declines, and those miracidia which do hatch have reduced infectivity. It therefore seems safe to assume that under field conditions in the winter months this will be the effective life span of

Table 9.10 Fluke egg mortality (data from Rowcliffe and Ollerenshaw, 1960; Over and Dijkstra, 1975; Hope-Cawdery *et al.*, 1978).

Location of eggs	Instantaneous rate of mortality/week
Faeces (wet) or water	0.005–0.007
Wet soil	0.065
Drying faeces (spring/winter)	0.608–1.289
Drying faeces (summer)	0.749–1.896

undeveloped eggs either in faeces or free on the snail habitat. Estimates of fluke egg mortality under different conditions are given in Table 9.10.

Fluke egg development is temperature-dependent and a plot of development rate (reciprocal of development time) against temperature is given in Fig. 9.18(a). The temperature cut-off below which no development occurs is 9.9 °C. Using these data in conjunction with estimates for daily maximum and minimum temperatures (see Section 9.4) a prediction can be made of the relative numbers of eggs hatching throughout the year (Fig. 9.18(b); Wilson, unpublished data). The model predicts a mass hatching of miracidia in mid to late June (using temperatures from N. England) followed by erratic but lower levels throughout the summer. Hatching has virtually ceased by the end of October. The model assumes constant egg input to habitats and incorporates

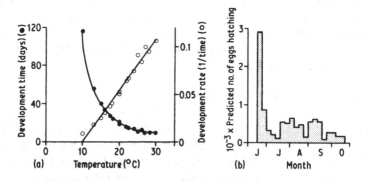

Figure 9.18 The egg of *Fasciola*. (a) The rate of development in relation to temperature. (Linear regression of development rate, *R*, on temperature, *T*. $R = 0.0539 \times T - 0.05338$; Thomas, 1979.) (b) The numbers of miracidia hatching during the summer months predicted by a simulation model, assuming constant egg input to the habitat, and incorporating the above regression, daily maximum and minimum temperatures for the Peak District 1975–1979 and drought-induced egg mortality (Wilson, unpublished data).

the effects of fluctuations in habitat wetness on egg mortality. All eggs which have undergone no development for 2 months are assumed to die. Relaxation of this restriction (see Over and Dijkstra, 1975) magnifies the initial peak of hatching. The predictions suggest that a *Fasciola* egg laid between February and approximately the end of August has a mean probability of 0.00017 of hatching into a miracidium.

(d) *The miracidium and the infection process*

The miracidium larvae are non-feeding, relying instead on endogenous energy reserves during a brief free life. As these reserves are depleted, the life expectancy and host-finding capacity of the miracidia decline. Mortality and infectivity are both functions of age and temperature (Fig. 9.19(a)–(c)) (Christensen *et al.*, 1976; Smith, unpublished work). Infectivity is also crucially dependent on the amount of water present at the soil surface. Successful infection of the host snails requires free water; a surface film of moisture is not sufficient (Wilson and Taylor, 1978). Given free water at the surface, the prevalence of infection in the snails for any particular temperature is determined by the relative densities of snails and miracidia (Fig. 9.19(d)) (Wilson and Taylor, 1978). In the field, the density of miracidia is determined by many factors, paramount among which are the contamination rate, egg mortality, temperature-dependent developmental time delays, and the proportion of habitat with standing water. The density of snails available for infection can be determined by field sampling on habitats. Similarly, the resulting density of infected snails can be found by dissection. The empirical expression relating the level of parasitization to snail and miracidial densities (Fig. 9.19(d)) can be used in conjunction with field estimates of infected snail density to estimate the approximate miracidial densities at the time of infection. (The snail data must be adjusted to take account of snail mortality between infection and sampling. An allowance must also be made for the fact that whereas a miracidium lives 24 h or less, the infection in the snail which it gives rise to will be detectable for perhaps 4 to 6 weeks). Typical values are given in Table 9.11.

(e) *The intramolluscan stages*

Three types of parasite larvae are found within the snail: sporocysts, rediae and cercariae. Their development is governed by environmental temperature and moisture conditions (Fig. 9.20) but the number of parasites that develop in each snail as opposed to the rate at which they mature is determined by the number of successful miracidial infections and by the space and nutrients available within the host (Kendall, 1949a; Kendall and Ollerenshaw, 1963; Zischke, 1967). In the field the mean parasite burden is found to be directly proportional to the size class of snail (Kendall and Ollerenshaw, 1963). It seems that the total size of the larval population is determined in part by the biomass of the infected hosts. Thus the size–class structure of the host

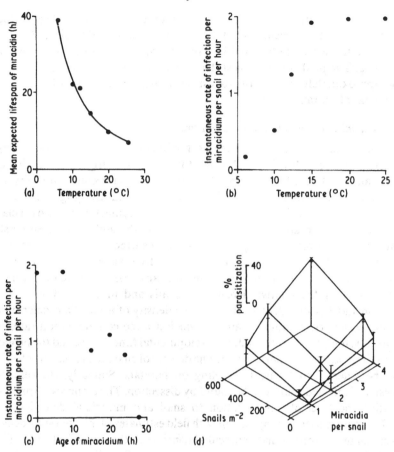

Figure 9.19 The miracidium and the infection process. (a) The life span of the miracidium of *Fasciola* at different constant temperatures. (b) The instantaneous rate of infection in relation to environmental temperature. (c) The instantaneous rate of infection in relation to miracidial age (Smith, unpublished data). (d) The relationship between miracidial density, snail density and percentage parasitization (Wilson and Taylor, 1978). Multiple regression of % snails infected (P) on miracidial (M) and snail (S) densities: $\tan h\,(P/100) = 0.244 \ln M + 0.076 \ln S - 0.282$.

population is an important constraint on the number of parasites, for it defines the carrying capacity of the redial environment. In a snail population with a constant schedule of age-specific rates of mortality and fecundity the size-class structure would eventually stabilize. However, as indicated in Section 9.5, this does not happen under field conditions. In addition the redial population is able to modify the snail biomass to its own advantage (Rondelaud and Vincent, 1973; Wilson and Denison, 1980). Quite early in parasite development

Table 9.11 Data on transmission derived from surveys on farms in the north of England, 1978–1979.

	Period	
Mean contamination rate (eggs m^{-2} habitat day^{-1})	April–June	3.625
Predicted miracidial density m^{-2} day^{-1} (incorporating developmental time delays and mortality)	June–July	3.3
Observed mean density of snails m^{-2} habitat	June–July	24.83
Predicted % parasitization (from Fig. 9.19(d))	June–July	29.08
Predicted density of infected snails (incorporating mortality of 0.14 snail per week)	Sept–Oct.	1.18
Observed mean density of infected snails m^{-2} habitat	Sept.–Oct.	0.645

the ovotestis of *L. truncatula* is partially or totally destroyed causing cessation of egg production. The nutrients thus released cause gigantism of infected snails relative to age-matched controls with an approximate doubling of biomass on which the redial population can feed. Thus the observation that infected snails are generally larger than uninfected (Smith, 1978) does not indicate that they are older.

The relationship between development rate and temperature (Fig. 9.20) can be used in conjunction with daily maximum and minimum temperatures to predict the maturation of snail infections (Nice and Wilson, 1974; Thomas, 1979). Incorporation of predictions on miracidial hatching produces the pattern illustrated in Fig. 9.20(b). The model predicts relatively more infections maturing in June and July than are observed in field collections (Fig. 9.20(c)). It must be assumed that some other factor not included in the simulation, such as the mortality of infected snails, plays a part in generating the observed variations in the density of infected snails.

An estimate of the physiological age of an infection in a snail can be obtained using three developmental criteria: the number of redia, the length of the most well-developed rediae and the proportion of germ balls recognizable as cercariae (Wilson and Draskau, 1976). The last of these is probably the most reliable indicator. If the environmental temperature regime experienced by an infection is known, then the estimate of age can be used in the model of parasite development to predict the date of infection. Results based on accumulated field observations from 1975 to 1979 are illustrated in Fig. 9.20(d). The predicted peak infection time in early July is some weeks later than the predicted peak of egg hatching (Fig. 9.18). Two caveats must be attached: the model assumes no developmental retardation due to aestivation of the snail host (see Kendall, 1949b) and we do not know what proportion of infected snails survived to the sampling time through the year. The redial death rate due to mortality of infected snails is greatest during the summer when the mean

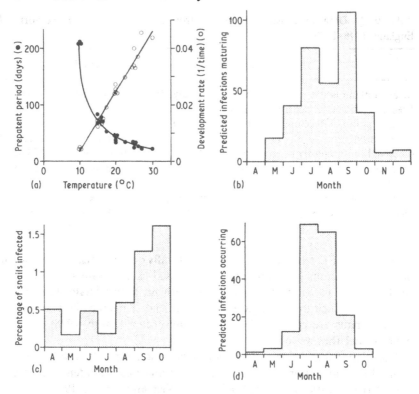

Figure 9.20 The intramolluscan stages of *Fasciola*. (a) The duration of the prepatent period in the snail host in relation to environmental temperature with moisture not limiting (Linear regression of development rate, *R*, on temperature, *T*: $R = 0.002224 \times T - 0.0197$, Thomas, 1979.) (b) The maturation of parasite infections in the snail through the year predicted by simulation model incorporating the regression in (a) above, information or miracidial hatching patterns (Fig. 9.18b) and daily maximum and minimum temperatures (Wilson, unpublished data). (c) The prevalence of snail infections in field collections 1975–1979 in the North of England. (d) The date at which snails became infected in the field predicted from a simulation incorporating the physiological age of infection, the regression in (a) above and daily maximum and minimum temperatures (Wilson, unpublished data).

expected life span of *L. truncatula* is less than half that recorded during the winter (Heppleston, 1972). There is some evidence from laboratory studies that, contrary to expectations, infected snails do not have a higher mortality than uninfected snails (Hodasi, 1972; Barrach, 1972; Wilson and Denison, 1980; but see also Kendall, 1949b, 1965; Styczynska–Jurewicz, 1965; and Sampaio–Xavier *et al.*, 1971). This remains to be confirmed in the field.

Another important aspect of fluke–snail interactions has been neglected. *L. truncatula* acts as host to a group of digeneans but double infections are seldom encountered (Wilson and Denison, 1980). The implication is that the first established infection limits the viability of subsequent infections. The population dynamics of *F. hepatica* in the field must therefore be considered in relation to the other digeneans with which it is in competition for the snail host. The prevalence of other infections such as *Cercaria cambriensis* (probably a plagiorchid of frogs) may be as high as 50 %, a fact which obviously reduces the number of snails available for *F. hepatica* and may also be a significant regulator of snail fecundity.

(f)   *Metacercarial cyst production*

The finite biomass of the snail's hepatopancreas is a constraint on the production of cercariae. Infection of snails with two or more miracidia does not result in a commensurate output of cercariae and yields only slightly greater numbers than single miracidial infections (Nice, 1979; see also Rondelaud, 1974). The relationship between the number of cercariae per redia and the intensity of infection in the snail is best described by a hyperbolic model (Thomas and Smith, unpublished) which suggests that the mean total of cercariae produced by snails of a particular size is constant whatever the redial burden (Fig. 9.15). A consequence in the field is a powerful density-dependent regulatory effect whereby multiple infections of a single snail will be wasted. It is difficult to assess the extent to which such infections occur in the field. If we assume a Poisson distribution of miracidia through a snail population, then they will only become important where the prevalence of snail infections rises above 20 % (but see Anderson, 1978). In practice mean prevalences seldom if ever rise above this level but spot estimates from single habitats may do so (Table 9.12). A single miracidial infection generally gives rise to about 40 redia

Table 9.12   Prevalence of infection in snails.

Country	Year	No. of habitats	Overall mean prevalence (%)	Highest recorded prevalence (%)	Source
Wales	1960–1966	54–79	–	15	Ollerenshaw (1971c)
Scotland	1973–1974	18	5.23	38	Ross (1977)
England	1973–1975	6	4.22	24	Smith (1978)
England	1976–1979	126	0.488	10.71	Wilson and Denison (unpublished data)
Eire	1964	1	14.56	80	Ross (1967)
Germany (DDR)	–	8	5.3	28	Holland-Moritz et al. (1977)
France	–	199	7.47	–	Rondelaud and Morel-Varielle (1975)
Czechoslovakia	1971–1973	726	0.70	4.1	Willomitzer (1974)
USSR	1965	1	16.5	24	Sosiptrov and Shumakovich (1966)

per snail at maturity. The number of mature infections in the field where the redial total greatly exceeds this figure may give a rough indication of the ratio of multiple to single infections. For our own data in the months of September and October, 1975–1979, the ratio was 1:2 at an overall prevalence of 1 % (total number of infected snails = 130). The Poisson distribution is described by a single parameter, the mean, m. The value of m can be estimated from the proportion of snails in the zero class of the frequency distribution and then used to predict the numbers of snails in the one miracidium, and two or more miracidia per snail classes. Comparison of the predicted and observed numbers of infected snails by a χ^2 test suggests a highly significant difference. Thus, the distribution of miracidia throughout snail populations in the field may be highly aggregated with important regulatory consequences for the parasite. This aspect of parasite–snail interactions would certainly repay further investigation.

The presence of standing water is an absolute requirement for cercarial shedding from the snail and dispersal (Kendall and McCullough, 1951). The stimulus for cyst production appears to be entirely physical or mechanical and dispersal distances are probably tens of centimetres at most; often no further than the shell of the infected snail. The maximum capacity for cercarial production under optimal environmental conditions is about 1000 per infected snail (Nice, 1979). Shedding, which is temperature-dependent, can continue for more than 100 days at mean daily rates up to 16 cercariae per snail. In the field, estimates for the mortality of uninfected snails suggest a mean shedding period of 27 days duration. An average shedding rate of 11 per day at optimal temperatures (Nice, 1979) would yield a total cercarial production of 300 per infected snail.

The mean density of infected snails on 17 selected habitats in September and October 1978 and 1979 was $0.645 \, m^{-2}$ (Trippick, personal communication). Using a modification of the bioassay procedure of Ross and O'Hagan (1966) (rabbits instead of guinea pigs) the corresponding density of cysts was estimated at 0.45 per 100 g of herbage. Allowing 1 kg of fresh herbage per m^2 of habitat gives seven cysts per infected snail per m^2, considerably less than predicted by laboratory results. One possible cause of the discrepancy is the availability of cysts. These are generally most abundant at the air–water interface but a considerable proportion may be on detritus etc. in pools. Another major factor is cyst mortality. Unlike fluke eggs, cysts need not be submerged in water but survival is contingent on greater than 90 % relative humidity (Boray and Enigk, 1964; Meek and Morris, 1979). It is also temperature-dependent. In Fig. 9.21 the average survival curves for meta-cercariae under winter and summer conditions in the Netherlands (Over and Dijkstra, 1975) are compared with the survival curves obtained by Ollerenshaw (1971) in the UK. Clearly metacercarial mortality varies with the season. It should be noted that the viability of the metacercariae in both these trials was tested *in vitro*. It is likely that the decline in the number of *infective* cysts will proceed at a faster rate than the number of viable cysts.

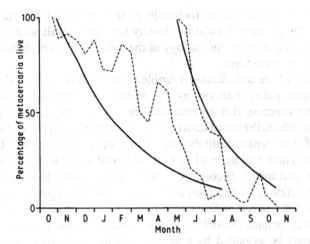

Figure 9.21 A comparison of metacercarial survival under winter and summer conditions. Data given in Over and Dijstrstra (1975) were used to estimate the average instantaneous rates of cyst mortality for winter and summer conditions in the Netherlands (μ_{winter} = 0.063 cyst per week; μ_{summer} = 0.99 cyst per week). These rates were used to construct the corresponding survival curves (dashed lines) which are superimposed in the figure on the survival curves described by Ollerenshaw (1971) for conditions in the UK.

(g) *The mortality of flukes in the primary host*

On average, only a third of the metacercariae that excyst in the gut of a primary host become established in the liver (Dixon, 1964; Boray, 1967; Berry and Dargie, 1976), but once established, in sheep at any rate, the flukes may be very long-lived indeed. The survival data presented by Durbin (1952) indicate an average instantaneous mortality rate for these established flukes in sheep of about 0.0015 fluke per week. Cattle, on the other hand, begin to reject the established flukes within 7–9 months *post infection* and manifest an enhanced resistance to further infection (Kendall and Parfitt, 1975; Kendal *et al.*, 1978). This last is a density-dependent response which regulates the mean intensity of infection in affected herds. Fluke numbers may also be regulated as the result of parasite-induced host mortality. The mortality of infected sheep, for example, is proportional to the fluke burden. The death of just a few heavily infected hosts could account for a significant proportion of the parasite population. The effectiveness of this density-dependent process increases as the distribution of the flukes becomes more overdispersed (Bradley, 1972). Some examples of the degree of overdispersion that occurs in naturally infected populations are given in Table 9.4.

(h) *The effect of farm management on the fluke life cycle*

Density-independent factors which affect the numbers of *F. hepatica* fall into two categories, microclimatic variation and farm management procedures.

The ways in which the microclimate at the surface of the snail habitats influence the parasite population density have been dealt with above so we conclude this section on the biology of the fluke with a consideration of farm management procedures.

On farms where fascioliasis *is* a problem the density of stock and the grazing management policy pursued by the farmer are important influences on transmission success. It is the total area and degree of permanence of the snail habitats which set the initial limits on the potential risk to grazing livestock but neither of these remain entirely constant on any particular farm. If stock are allowed to graze a pasture while the soil is still wet (i.e. at field capacity or above) the soil surface becomes poached (MAFF, 1970). In its deformed and compacted state it accumulates and stores water. Plainly the risk is greatest where the soil remains at field capacity for the longest periods, i.e. the North and West in Britain (MAFF, 1976). In these areas the margins of existing habitats may be extended by poaching and new habitats created in places where stock tend to congregate. Increased stocking rates and slovenly ditch or pipe maintenance exacerbate the situation. Pasture damage of this kind can be limited by housing the stock for part or all of the winter. With some exceptions sheep in Britain are usually maintained entirely out of doors on natural grazing throughout the year. Cattle on the other hand frequently are inwintered which not only alleviates the problem of poaching, but also restricts the time that stock are exposed to pasture contaminated with cysts and diminishes the pre-spring accumulation of fluke eggs (Over and Dijkstra, 1975). In some cases, cattle are permanently housed or kept in yards (King, 1978). They may be fed on cereals (e.g. barley beef) or on harvested grass (e.g. the zero grazing system). Such methods are on the increase in Britain (MAFF Annual Abstract of Statistics 1960–1979). The consequences for the transmission of *F. hepatica* are obvious.

The various methods of fascioliasis control that are available to the farmer were described in Section 9.3. In so far as they seem usually to be applied as a matter of routine, whatever the 'fluke forecast', they are mentioned again here as a powerful density-independent constraint on the parasite population.

9.6 MATHEMATICAL MODELS

In this section mathematical models are used to collate the information presented in earlier sections. There are two motives for producing such models. The first, and most common, is to gain some insight into the system in order to identify those factors which govern its dynamics. The second is the desire to mimic accurately the behaviour of the system under a wide range of conditions, with a view to assessing alternative disease management procedures.

Types of model

The structure of a model is greatly influenced by its purpose. Models used as research tools have relatively few parameters; the main interest lies in the effect of gross changes in these parameter values, or in the functional form of the relationships embodied in the model. Since these models are simple, they are expressed analytically, and their properties are frequently established using analytical rather than numerical methods. Anderson and May (1978; 1979a), May and Anderson (1978; 1979), Barbour (1978) and Bradley and May (1978) provide good examples of this approach. These workers have shown the importance of various features of parasite life cycles in stabilizing and destabilizing population equilibria. Ultimately this work may lead to a general theory of parasite dynamics allowing superficially diverse parasite–host interactions to be classified into a small number of categories.

Models developed as management aids fall into two groups: analytical models like those described above which are useful in the determination of disease *control policies* (i.e. the strategic aspects of disease control) and simulation models which are designed to reveal the optimum *control procedure* given a particular set of local circumstances and conditions (i.e. the tactical aspects of disease control). Simulation models have many parameters each of which must be estimated as accurately as possible since the performance of the models is intended to exactly mimic the course of infection observed in the field. These models are not expressed analytically; they exist only as algorithms embodied in a computer program.

Few workers have undertaken the detailed work necessary to provide models which may be used as aids to the management of fascioliasis. Gettinby (1974), Meek (1977), Hope Cawdery *et al.* (1978), Thomas (1979) and Gettinby and McLean (1979) have attempted to simulate various aspects of fascioliasis transmission but none of these models is sufficiently developed to be used as a management aid with any degree of confidence.

Although there are real differences in approach between analytical models and simulation models, there are some similarities. Both sorts of model are made up of components whose interrelationships reflect the hypothesized interrelationships between the components of the actual system and they are concerned with the dynamics of systems (even if these dynamics are investigated in the neighbourhood of equilibria). In this respect they differ from the work of Ollerenshaw and Rowlands (1959) who attempted nothing more than a convenient summary of past experience.

In our investigations of fascioliasis we have developed an analytical model and a simulation model. The structure of the analytical model is described first. It provides an overview of liver fluke transmission and reveals the way in which the equilibrium levels of prevalence and intensity of infection are determined by the various components of the system. The simulation model which follows, is concerned with only a portion of the parasite–host system but will serve to illustrate the process of constructing such a model as well as illuminating aspects of the molluscan phase of the interaction.

9.6.1 A differential equation model of fascioliasis

Anderson and May (1978) and May and Anderson (1978) developed a general theoretical framework for the investigation of the dynamics of populations of parasites and hosts. The simple mathematical model of fascioliasis presented here is a specific application of this general approach. The model is based directly on the life cycle of $F.$ $hepatica$ (Fig. 9.1). It consists of five coupled differential equations which describe the rate at which individuals are gained or lost at each of the five stages in the cycle (Table 9.13). The construction of one of these Equations is illustrated below.

$$\frac{dM(t)}{dt} = E(t-T_2)\ \exp(-T_2\mu_2)\ -\ \mu_2 M(t)\ -\ \beta_2 H_2 M(t) \quad (9.12)$$

Number of eggs T_2 weeks ago

Proportion of eggs surviving T_2 weeks

Rate of change of miracidial numbers — Miracidial hatching — Miracidial deaths — Miracidial infection

where T_2 is egg development time. The various parameters of the model are listed and defined in Table 9.14. They include instantaneous infection rates (β), stage specific rates of mortality (μ) and fecundity (λ), stage development times (T), instantaneous rates of natural and parasite-induced host mortality (b and α) and the densities of the respective host populations (H). The ways in which density-dependent and density-independent processes alter the value of these parameters have been discussed in previous sections. In incorporating the density-dependent relationships into the model it has been assumed that the distribution of parasites in both host species is adequately described by the negative binomial probability distribution.

Aspects of the behaviour of the model may be investigated by considering its equilibrium properties. This is achieved by setting the Equations defined in Table 9.13 equal to zero. This done, it may be shown that if the parasite is to persist then the following condition must be satisfied (Anderson, 1982a)

$$\frac{H_1 H_2 \beta_1 \beta_2 \lambda_1 \lambda_2 D_1 D_2 D_3}{(\mu_1 + b_1 + \alpha_1)(\mu_2 + D_2)(\mu_3 + \beta_2 H_2)(b_2)(\mu_5 + \beta_1 H_1)} > 1 \quad (9.13)$$

where $D_1 = \exp[-T(\mu_1 + b_1 + \alpha_1)]$, the proportion of flukes surviving to

Table 9.13 Five coupled differential equations describing the rates of change in the numbers of individuals at each stage in the fluke life cycle.

$$\frac{dP(t)}{dt} = \beta_1 H_1 C(t) - (\mu_1 + b_1 + \alpha_1)P(t) - \alpha_1 \frac{(k+1)}{kH_1}P^2(t) \tag{9.7}$$

$$\frac{dE(t)}{dt} = \lambda_1 P(t-T_1)D_1[1 + P(t-T_1)(1 - \exp(-0.0027)/H_1 k]^{-(k+1)}$$

$$\qquad - \mu_2 E(t) - D_2 E(t-T_2) \tag{9.8}$$

$$\frac{dM(t)}{dt} = E(t-T_2)D_2 - (\mu_3 + \beta_2 H_2)M(t) \tag{9.9}$$

$$\frac{dY(t)}{dt} = \beta_2 H_2 M(t) - b_2 Y(t) \tag{9.10}$$

$$\frac{dC(t)}{dt} = \lambda_2 Y_{(t-T_3)}D_3 - (\mu_4 + \beta_1 H_1)C \tag{9.11}$$

Where

$P(t)$ = Flukes (at time t).
$E(t)$ = Fluke eggs.
$M(t)$ = Miracidia.
$Y(t)$ = Infected snail density.
$C(t)$ = Cysts on the herbage.
H_1 = Sheep density (infected and uninfected).
H_2 = Snail density (infected and uninfected).
k = Parameter of the negative binomial distribution describing the degree of aggregation of flukes in the sheep.
D_1 = Proportion of flukes surviving T_1 weeks.
D_2 = Proportion of eggs surviving T_2 weeks.
D_3 = Proportion of infected snails surviving T_3 weeks.

maturity; $D_2 = \exp(-T_2\mu_2)$, the proportion of eggs surviving to hatch; and $D_3 = \exp(-T_3 b_2)$, the proportion of infected snails surviving prepatent period. The left side of the above relationship consists simply of parasite gains divided by parasite losses. This ratio, denoted by the symbol R and termed the *basic reproductive rate*, is a measure of an individual parasite's reproductive *potential*. The value of R reflects reproduction in the absence of density-dependent processes and differs from the effective reproductive rate per parasite (see Section 9.5) in that it remains unaltered by changes in the distribution of parasites within the host population. Nevertheless, it is sensitive to changes in climate and farm management (density-independent factors). Accordingly, the magnitude of R varies from region to region and month to month. This is illustrated by Fig. 9.22 in which seasonal and regional variations in R are compared with Froyd's (1975) map of regional variations in disease prevalence. In the calculation of R for each month in each region all of the parameters in relationship (9.13) were assumed to be constant except those directly affected by the weather. The values taken by the latter were determined by the long-term average temperatures and soil moisture deficits for each

Table 9.14 Parameter values.

Parameter (defined/week)		Summer	Winter	Estimated from data found in:
Host numbers	H_1	100		
	H_2	1000		
Reproductive rates	λ_1	17×10^4		Boray (1969), Happich and Boray (1971)
	λ_2	25	0	Nice (1979)
Natural mortality rates (parasite)	μ_1		0.003	
	μ_2	0.1	0.05	Rowcliffe and Ollerenshaw (1960)
	μ_3		7	Smith (unpublished)
	μ_5	0.1	0.025	Over and Dijkstra (1975) Ollerenshaw (1971)
Natural mortality rates (hosts)	b_1		0.013	Smith (unpublished)
	b_2	0.062		
		spring late summer	0.025	Heppleston (1972)
Parasite-induced sheep mortality rate	α_1	0.00005		Ross (1967), Boray (1969), Hawkins and Morris (1978)
Development times	T_1	10		Dixon (1964)
	T_2	Negative exponential function of temperature		Hope-Cawdery *et al.* (1978)
	T_3	Hyperbolic function of temperature		Hope-Cawdery *et al.* (1978)
Infection rates	β_1	2.5×10^{-8}		Crossland *et al.* (1977)
	β_2	0.0001	0	Wilson and Taylor (1978), Smith (Unpublished)

region (MAFF, 1976). The relationship between the prevalence of fascioliasis and the basic reproductive rate of the parasite is clear. (The *absolute* values of R given in Fig. 9.22 should be treated with caution. Since there are no field estimates of fluke egg mortality this was assumed to be the same as the mortality of the eggs *in the faeces*. As a result the value of R is probably too high by an order of magnitude. Nevertheless the relative differences in R from region to region still hold.) This relationship can be used in the assessment of alternative control strategies and will now be considered in more detail.

Control measures reduce R. As a result there is a reduction in the equilibrium number of flukes (P^*) towards which the system tends and hence there is a change in the actual prevalence and intensity of infection. The change in P^* caused by a change in control strategy can be estimated using the

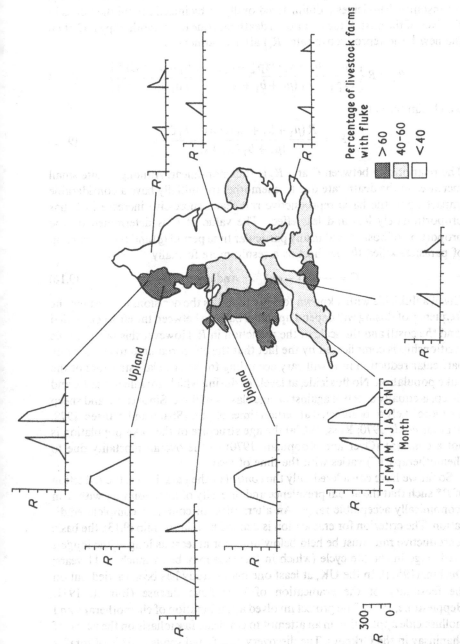

Figure 9.22 Seasonal and regional variations in *R* compared with disease prevalence. (It has been assumed that *R* < 1 when the soil moisture deficit exceeds 30mm. At this point most habitat surfaces are generally so dry that transmission ceases.) Reproduced with permission from Froyd (1975).

Percentage of livestock farms with fluke

- >60
- 40–60
- <40

equations defined in Table 9.13 but when comparing a whole set of control procedures it may be sufficient in the initial stages of the decision-making process to determine simply the relative reduction in R. Take chemotherapy, for instance. Flukicides (administered orally or by injection) kill the flukes in the liver of the host. If the additional death rate due to chemotherapy is C, then the new basic reproductive rate (R_c) after treatment is:

$$R_c = R \left\{ \frac{(\mu_1 + b_1 + \alpha_1)\exp[-T_1(\mu_1 + b_1 + \alpha_1 + C)]}{\exp[-T_1(\mu_1 + b_1 + \alpha_1)](\mu_1 + b_1 + \alpha_1 + C)} \right\} \qquad (9.14)$$

which simplifies to:

$$R_c = \frac{R(\mu_1 + b_1 + \alpha_1)\exp(-T_1 C)}{(\mu_1 + b_1 T\alpha_1 + C)} \qquad (9.15)$$

The relationship between C and R_c is thus non-linear. Although quite small increases in the death rate due to chemotherapy initially have a considerable impact upon the basic reproductive rate, each successive increase in C has proportionately less and less effect. The value of C is determined by the proportion of hosts dosed in any particular time period (g) and the proportion of parasites killed (h) per host as a result; more formally

$$C = -\ln(1 - gh) \qquad \text{Anderson (1980)} \qquad (9.16)$$

Given a flukicide with a known toxicity to flukes the decisions concerning the frequency of dosing will depend upon the balance between the effort expended (and the cost!) and the scale of the reduction in R. However this fairly simple relationship is complicated by the fact that the effort required to achieve any particular reduction in R will vary according to the age-class structure of the fluke population. No flukicide, at levels of dosing which are safe for cattle and sheep, is equally effective against all age classes of fluke. Since cattle and sheep are more likely to be infected at certain times of year (Shaka and Nansen, 1979; Armour et al., 1970; Ross, 1967a) the age structure of the fluke population is not a constant (Over and Koopman, 1970) so the overall mortality due to chemotherapy (C) varies with the time of year.

So far we have considered only the *control* of the parasite, i.e. the reduction of P^* such that the actual prevalence and intensity of infection vary within an economically acceptable range. An alternative, of course, is complete eradication. The criterion for eradication is defined by relationship (9.13), the basic reproductive rate must be held below unity for at least as long as the longest lived stage in the life cycle (which in this case may be as much as 11 years; Durbin, (1952)). In the UK, at least one major study has been carried out on the feasibility of the eradication of liver fluke disease (Burnet, 1971; Hepplestone, 1972). The project involved a combination of chemotherapy and molluscicide application in an attempt to eradicate fascioliasis on the island of Shapinsay in the Orkneys. The discovery of infected snails (0.62 % of total) 2 years after the last molluscicide application showed the eradication attempt to have been unsuccessful (Heppleston, personal communication). In addition, snail populations had returned to their pretreatment levels (see Section 9.3). The scale of the effort required was substantial but could have been assessed at the planning stage had the value of R for the region been known. Using chemotherapy alone, the death rate C required to eradicate the parasite is given by Equation (9.15), and Equation (9.16) defines the dosing regime. If molluscicides only are used, then a rearrangement of relationship (9.13) gives the threshold density of snails (H_2^*) below which the parasite fails to persist, namely:

$$H_2^* = \frac{(\mu_1 + b_1 + \alpha_1)(\mu_2 + D_2)(\mu_3)(b_2)(\mu_2 + \beta_1 H_1)}{\beta_2 [(H_1 B_1 \lambda_1 \lambda_2 D_1 D_2 D_3) - (\mu_1 + b_1 + D_1)(\mu_2 + D_2)(b_2)(\mu_5 + \beta_1 H_1)]}$$

In the case of parasites with indirect life cycles the threshold values of H are generally low (Anderson and May, 1979a; May and Anderson, 1979) and the continued maintenance of H_2 below threshold by molluscicide application alone for the required number of years would demand a prohibitive effort on most farms afflicted by fascioliasis.

9.6.2 A simulation model

In this section we consider models to be used in assisting tactical decisions. We will show that the model of the previous section is not useful in this context. An approach to developing tactical models of helminth parasite–host interactions will be introduced, and the major problems outlined. A detailed simulation model of the snail host's population dynamics will be used to illustrate the techniques.

The simple model described in the preceding section gives an overview of liver fluke transmission. It can provide answers to strategic questions such as what is the effect of increasing parasite mortality in the snail host relative to that of increasing mortality in the mammal host. Tactical models must provide answers to more detailed questions such as: is a more expensive more efficient flukicide more cost-effective than a less expensive less efficient one, and does the order of preference change given a wetter than average June or July? If the model defined in Table 9.13 is to provide answers to these questions, then at the very least all its parameters must be made explicit functions of climate.

This is not feasible. Consider, as an example, the rate of production of cercariae by infected snails. Climate certainly has a direct effect on this rate, and we can describe it reasonably accurately. Unfortunately, the size of the infected snail is equally important in determining cercarial output, and climate has a very strong effect on the size structure of the snail population. If we are to model the effect of climate on cercarial production we must model not only the direct effect, but also its interaction with the indirect effect. Similar arguments may be made concerning snail mortality, intramolluscan parasite mortality and the rate of snail infection.

It is apparent that the answers to specific questions will involve consideration of rather more parameters than those described for our simple model. Furthermore, our simple model was already so complicated as to preclude an analytical treatment of model trajectories – we discussed only the equilibrium behaviour of the system. Our specific questions, however, demand information about the model trajectories, about the numbers in each population across time. Indeed, with regular seasonal changes in transmission rates there may be no equilibrium at all. If we are to obtain answers to specific questions we are forced to consider simulation models rather than the elegant sparsely parameterized models common in the literature.

A case has been made for the use of simulation techniques in modelling fascioliasis. We will describe an approach to simulation models, placing particular emphasis on the difficulties of applying this approach to fascioliasis.

The simulation of a complex system involves many tasks, which can conveniently be grouped into four phases. The first phase is model definition. The objectives of the model are described in terms of the inputs and outputs required, and the processes which are to be included. In the second phase these processes are given separate mathematical descriptions, and in the third phase these individual models are collated to produce a population model. The fourth phase involves validating the model by comparing its predictions with independently collected data.

Problems peculiar to the simulation of fascioliasis occur during the second phase. It is necessary to find an index of environmental conditions which integrates the pattern of environmental change in the same way as the organism modelled. Any two individuals with the same index value will then be physiologically identical – despite detailed differences in their past environmental experience. Thomas (1979) provides a detailed discussion of this problem and shows how it may be resolved for *Lymnaea truncatula* and *F. hepatica*.

The third phase, in which a population model is constructed from the distinct models of aspects of parasite and host mortality, raises interesting problems. It is complicated by two aspects of heterogeneity: heterogeneity of the organisms in the various populations modelled, and heterogeneity of the habitat. Not only are the populations heterogeneous, but the nature of the heterogeneity changes with time and environment. For example, large infected snails produce more cercariae than small ones, and there are more large snails between May and July than between August and April. It is not possible to produce an average estimate of cercarial output, or any other transmission parameter which does not change with time and environment. It is therefore necessary to structure information in less aggregated units than entire populations.

Liver fluke habitats are noticeably heterogeneous, and again the nature of the heterogeneity changes with time. They are much more nearly homogeneous at the wettest and driest times of the year than at others. The seasonal changes in soil moisture conditions produce a changing patchwork of wet and dry areas on the habitat. This constant change has profound repercussions on transmission dynamics, and must be included in any predictive model.

Fortunately, the device adopted to cope with the problem of population heterogeneity is useful in dealing with habitat heterogeneity. In the simulation models we have developed, the basic data structure is the cohort, representing the largest number of individuals which are physiologically identical. These cohorts are then organized into lists, representing the populations of the transmission process. There may be many cohorts in one list. Information about the distribution of the cohort through the habitat is incorporated into the data structure representing the cohort. When each cohort is processed, this information is compared with data defining the current state of the habitat. This comparison shows whether any members of the cohort are on a piece of habitat which has changed state, i.e. become wet or become dry. This treatment is made simple by an intuitively reasonable assumption about the pattern of habitat drying. It is assumed that those areas of the habitat which become wet first become dry last, and vice versa. A sufficient, but not necessarily physical interpretation would be a circular habitat which becomes wet from the centre, but dries out from the periphery.

The major problems of simulating fascioliasis have been discussed. We have described a model in terms of the structure of population information, which facilitates solution of these problems. We will illustrate the use of this structure by means of a simulation of snail population dynamics. Choice of the snail population is easily justified. Earlier in this section we established that a snail simulation was a necessary part of a simulation model for the entire transmission process. Thomas (1979) discusses a simulation model of parasite populations given an idealized intramammalian parasite dynamics, and an idealized snail population. Meek (1977) discusses a simulation model of intramammalian dynamics (which incorporates an economic evaluation of damage) given idealized extramammalian dynamics. It is theoretically possible to combine these separate models to form a model for the entire system. We stress, however, that we are primarily concerned with illustrating the application of our model structure, rather than claiming an immediately successful simulation model of fascioliasis transmission.

We will first describe the assumptions which are built into our model, and then present the results obtained from the model. We do not have space to give a detailed step by step account of the models daily iteration, or to provide a program listing. An annotated listing is available from the authors, however. For technical reasons which we do not discuss here, the program is written in ALGOL 68.

The state of the habitat in terms of soil moisture is defined by two variables, the areas of the habitat which are above field capacity, and covered by standing water respectively, each day. A soil at field capacity will only absorb gravitational water (Bruce and Clark, 1966). We assume that snail eggs will survive only in standing water, and that snail development proceeds normally when the soil is at field capacity or wetter. Snails on soil which is below field capacity are assumed to be subjected to moisture stress. These assumptions about water relations on a habitat indicate that the model must consider three populations or lists of cohorts: snail eggs, wet snails (on ground at field capacity or wetter) and dry snails (on ground drier than field capacity). It is assumed that snails becoming wet distribute themselves evenly throughout the wet areas of the habitat, but that dry snails do not move.

Density-dependent effects on snail physiology have not been investigated but it is apparent that these must exist. They are incorporated into our model by means of a rather crude approximation. We assume that the instantaneous rate of snail mortality increases linearly with population density, and that snail fecundity is decreased proportionately with population density. It is necessary to fix both constants of proportionality. The fecundity constant is fixed by requiring fecundity to be zero when snail density is 1000 snails m^{-1}. The mortality constant is more difficult. We have no independent data, and were forced to use a range of values, and adopt the one which gave the best results. This procedure is barely satisfactory; there is no other reasonable way to proceed, but it would certainly detract from any claim that a definitive model of snail population dynamics had been produced.

The simulation model of *L. truncatula* population dynamics is driven by information about temperature and soil moisture conditions. The indices of habitat wetness used are the proportions of the habitat wet and under standing water respectively, obtained by direct observation of habitats. With a small amount of modification the predictive relationships between ln (river flow) (or soil moisture deficit) and habitat wetness (see Section 9.4) could be used instead. The index of temperature conditions required is not the same for all sub-models. Snail growth requires information about mean temperatures whilst snail egg hatching requires information about the temperature above a cut-off of $4°C$, and the proportion of time above $4°C$ (see Section 9.4). Temperature and soil moisture indices are read in on a daily basis.

A major obstacle in the application of simulation models is the validation of predictions. For this, a body of environmental and population data is needed, and it should be different from that used to estimate the model's parameters. Note that we do not satisfy this criterion, since we have estimated a mortality parameter from the data we wish to use for validation.

For our study we collected information on habitat wetness on seven farms, during 1978. We obtained spot values of the two proportions required, and obtained intermediate values by means of linear interpolation. Each value represents an average proportion for several different habitats (Fig. 9.23).

Daily maximum and minimum air temperatures used in the simulation were taken from a site close to farms 1, 2 and 3 (which are in the Peak District), but

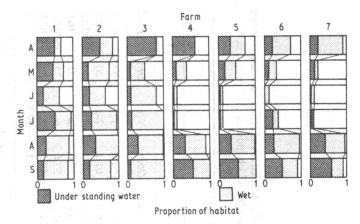

Figure 9.23 Spot values of the soil moisture indices at each of seven farms during the months April to September, 1978. Between the months October and March the proportion of habitat wet was assumed to be 1.0, and the proportion under standing water as the largest proportion observed between April and September.

which is a considerable distance from farms 4 (in the Yorkshire Dales), 5, 6 and 7 (in the Lake District). We might, therefore, expect a more reliable model performance at farms 1, 2 and 3. It will be apparent that a simulation model of this kind must have realistic estimates of the initial snail population and that these estimates must be very detailed. Such estimates are not available directly, but were obtained by starting with arbitrary population estimates and iterating the model for 3 years of duplicated data before using its results. The model, therefore, has no information about the effect of any peculiarities in soil moisture conditions in the years preceding 1978. It gives information about the snail population expected assuming that the 1978 climate is repeated endlessly.

Since the model contains information about each cohort of snails a large amount of information about the predicted snail population is available at each time interval. This information is summarized to give two population indices: the mean monthly density of snails per metre, and the mean monthly proportion of snails which are > 2 mm in length. These two indices are available for the actual snail populations at each site, for each month for which we have climate data. Observed and predicted snail densities for the months April to October are shown in Table 9.15.

It will be seen that in general terms the predicted snail densities behave as expected, rising to a maximum in August and September, and falling to a minimum at some time in May or June. Furthermore, the predicted snail population cycle is sensitive to different soil moisture conditions; quite different patterns are obtained at each of the farms. Table 9.15 also allows a more detailed examination of the results. It will be seen that farms 1, 5 and 7 show strong correlations between predicted and observed snail populations.

Table 9.15 Observed and predicted snail population densities. The table shows observed (Obs.) and predicted (Pred.) snail population densities at each farm from April 1978 to October 1978. The correlation coefficient 'r' is given as is the square 'r²' which indicates the proportion of the observed variance explained by the predictions of the model.

	Farm													
	1		2		3		4		5		6		7	
	Obs.	Pred.	Obs.	Pred.	Obs.	Pred.	Obs.	Pred.	Obs.	Pred.	Obs.	Pred.	Obs.	Pred.
April	11.5	34.1	23.0	33.2	59.0	38.8	136.6	35.0	40.0	34.8	129.6	32.4	77.8	35.6
May	26.4	53.2	28.3	35.4	28.8	32.7	156.6	32.7	24.6	30.0	61.1	24.9	20.3	29.1
June	22.1	82.2	19.8	67.7	15.0	51.0	35.4	20.6	54.1	33.6	21.8	21.3	10.9	30.8
July	11.0	75.6	33.4	58.4	12.8	39.7	15.5	9.8	49.9	14.0	89.6	26.4	31.5	16.0
Aug.	62.1	115.5	33.9	121.8	33.7	95.0	55.5	41.1	14.7	38.2	57.6	68.2	75.5	48.3
Sept.	71.8	79.5	49.0	83.8	76.3	63.4	76.3	78.0	112.0	79.2	48.5	102.4	80.0	98.0
Oct.	54.1	80.6	–	–	–	–	89.1	96.0	–	–	23.4	99.5	116.8	87.8
r	0.633		0.381		0.169		0.192		0.744		0.410		0.765	
r^2	0.401		0.145		0.029		0.036		0.554		0.168		0.585	

The percentage of variance explained lies between 40 % and 59 %. Farm 4 has a very low value of 4 % variance explained, but the observed snail density in April and May is very much greater than might reasonably be expected. These high values are quite atypical of the pattern observed at the other farms. If they are excluded, some 96 % of the variance is explained (though of course the sample size is now only 5 months). The model performs less well for farms 2, 3 and 6.

Table 9.16 gives observed and predicted proportions of snails less than 2 mm in length at each farm for the months April to October 1978. The most striking aspect of this table is the difference between predicted and observed proportions of snails below 2 mm in length. Our model always predicts more small snails than we observe in the field: the minimum observed proportion is 0, and the maximum is 0.46, whilst the range for predicted values is 0.38 to 0.87. This difference is not incompatible with a valid model and illustrates the difficulties encountered in a simulation exercise. Populations of *L. truncatula* are notoriously difficult to sample consistently. The amount of water on the habitat, the extent of vegetation cover and the tenacity of the collector all play a part. It is very much easier to find large snails than it is to find small ones.

Despite this large difference between observed and predicted proportions, there are strong correlations between observed and predicted values at farms 5 and 6 where the predicted values explain 76 % and 73 % of the variance respectively. The results are less satisfactory at the other farms.

The results of this exercise are equivocal. A snail model which incorporates a great deal of quantitative information about the effect of climate on snail biology has been constructed. Despite this the model performs indifferently well. At some sites accurate predictions of population behaviour have been obtained; at others observed and predicted populations are widely divergent.

Even if the results of the snail simulation are accepted uncritically, a snail simulation model is only part way towards a simulation model which may be used as a management aid. Such a model would consider many more lists of cohorts, at least one for each of the populations occurring in the flow chart, Fig. 9.1. The structure of this model would be a straightforward development of the structure incorporated in our snail model, and despite the extra coding, it would not be a significantly more complicated programming task to implement it.

There are, however, several problems. We do not have adequate information about density-dependent control of the snail population. The approach embodied in our snail simulation is at best reasonable supposition in the absence of real information. We do not have good estimates of fluke egg survival, and the instantaneous rate of infection of snails by miracidia. Similarly, we lack information about the instantaneous rate of infection of stock by metacercariae.

It does not seem likely that a simulation model of fascioliasis transmission which can be used to make tactical decisions is possible in the near future.

Table 9.16 Observed and predicted proportions of snails less than 2 mm in length. The observed (Obs.) and predicted (Pred.) proportions of the snail population less than 2 mm in length are compared for each farm for the period April 1978 to October 1978. The table also includes the correlation coefficient between observed and predicted values 'r', and its square 'r²', which gives the proportion of the observed variance explained by the model's predictions.

	1		2		3		4		5		6		7	
	Obs.	Pred.	Obs.	Pred.	Obs.	Pred.	Obs.	Pred.	Obs.	Pred.	Obs.	Pred.	Obs.	Pred.
April	0.013	0.410	0.065	0.378	0	0.385	0.014	0.470	0	0.459	0	0.437		0.447
May	0	0.728	0	0.540	0	0.455	0.002	0.530	0	0.519	0.007	0.562		0.551
June	0	0.868	0.011	0.843	0	0.749	0.120	0.669	0.043	0.830	0.022	0.444		0.817
July	0.138	0.699	0.139	0.586	0.444	0.412	0.295	0.541	0	0.676	0.025	0.735		0.704
Aug.	0.297	0.795	0.165	0.827	0.460	0.786	0.289	0.799	0.028	0.779	0.106	0.736		0.776
Sept.	0.204	0.641	0.264	0.665	0.219	0.498	0.170	0.738	0.032	0.757	0.116	0.775		0.812
Oct.	0.183	0.810	0.365	0.766	–	–	0.065	0.866	–	–	0.216	0.901		0.864
r	0.247		0.320		0.061		0.283		0.873		0.851			
r^2	0.061		0.102		0.004		0.08		0.762		0.725			

Nevertheless, we can reasonably claim to have given the problems of simulating fascioliasis transmission more detailed examination than they have received before. We have identified the major difficulties, and developed a model structure which we believe worthy of further development.

ACKNOWLEDGEMENTS

The authors would like to thank the following for funding the research: Agricultural Research Council, Nuffield Foundation, Shell Research Ltd (R.A.W.); Animal Health Trust (G.S.); Science Research Council (M.R.T.). They are indebted to Mrs J. Denison for data analysis and preparation of illustrations, to Ms R. Gibson for preparing the manuscript, and to Mr. M. Trippick for allowing them to use his unpublished data.

10 Epidemiological models – theory and reality

D. J. Bradley

The real world is infinitely complex. So in dealing with reality the epidemiologist must simplify. In planning a malaria control programme he will ignore the details of which days Ahmed Babu had a fever and what killed the first mosquito to emerge from a specific pool on November 10th. To that extent we all must operate with models, and as will be apparent to the reader of Albert Camus' '*La Peste*', the public health worker's model of a plague epidemic will differ from the priest's model, or that of the mayor of the town where the epidemic occurs. Thus we all work with models in order to cope with complex reality, but we usually do so unconsciously. The question to be addressed is therefore 'how far is it useful for such models to be explicit and, in particular, how important is it that they should be quantitative and mathematical?' Furthermore, do such mathematical models have decisive advantages at present over less precise intuitive and qualitative approaches in the understanding and control of infective disease? Any satisfactory answer must consider this in relation to research, teaching and operational public health work and in relation to the various diseases for which models have been proposed.

It is remarkable, especially to the mathematician entering the field from outside, how many gaps remain in our qualitative understanding of the transmission and natural history of infective disease. There is therefore always a tendency towards premature quantitative simplification to produce a spurious elegance in the analysis of messy and incompletely comprehended reality. The chief hazard of this is that it brings the whole of epidemiological modelling into disrepute, and the revulsion that the malariologists showed following Lotka's (1923) model is re-experienced with each expression of mathematical hubris in the form of an overconfident and clearly unreal (not merely unrealistic) model. No doubt the position is much the same between economic models and practical financiers, except that the epidemiologist, with a background of natural science and medicine, has a greater respect for data and the testability of hypotheses.

Indeed, a mathematical model of an epidemiological process, as it must start from an empirical account of the process modelled, has the nature of a complex hypothesis and not of deductive logic. Progress is made by testing one hypothesis and then revising it prior to further testing. The proliferation of untested hypotheses is restricted by Occam's razor and scientific custom. Where transdisciplinary issues are involved (so that a good deal has to be taken on trust by those of one discipline) confusion can be particularly counter-productive. This amounts to a plea that, given the facility with which models can be generated, their authors take responsibility for testing them and exploring their empirical validity lest they fall again into disrepute.

Malaria is remarkable because the first epidemiological model followed hard on the heels of the qualitative discovery of the transmission cycle and was applied to a specific practical end. Furthermore the model was as robust for its purpose as its author claimed, and was relatively simple and its components intuitively comprehensible. It thus reached a remarkable standard of elegance and utility by 1911. This remarkable achievement was the work of Sir Ronald Ross who combined the parasitological dexterity and persistence needed to show that mosquitoes transmitted malaria (and received the second Nobel prize for medicine for doing so) with the mathematical ability and imagination needed to model the cycle for his purposes.

The medical and public health literature of around 1900, three years after Ross's discovery of the malaria cycle, is remarkable in showing how very quickly the scientific work was fully accepted by leading workers and administrators in tropical health, yet Ross's deduction from it – that if mosquitoes transmit malaria, mosquito control could be used to stop malaria transmission – was largely rejected. The two chief grounds for this, that it was not feasible to eradicate the last mosquito from an area, and that even if it were feasible, immediate reinvasion would defeat the control programme, were strongly opposed by Ross. Although his vindication came from the field successes of Watson who controlled malaria at Klang and Port Swettenham by draining the mosquito larval habitats, Ross supported his position by constructing two, almost archetypal, models. We may doubt how far they convinced Ross's adversaries who were not primarily quantitatively rigorous men, but they probably did increase Ross's confidence in his position, and the validity of their conclusions is still accepted.

The first model that Ross put forward was a very simple equilibrium model of the entire malaria transmission cycle, using a structure based on what was known of mosquito and parasite biology at that time, and from which he showed that not every mosquito needed to be removed to stop the malaria cycle as there was a threshold level of the mosquito population below which malaria would not persist (see Chapter 5). Knowledge of mosquito biology was rudimentary at the time. Nevertheless, the conclusion has proved robust and the model is a good example of the overall cycle model that is simple, but allows of important general conclusions. Most simple models do not, or prove to be far from robust, and the problem is to know which is which! Ross's initial model was a static or equilibrium model but he later produced the important dynamic models that have been the basis of most subsequent work (Ross, 1916, 1917; Ross and Hudson, 1917). A similar equilibrium model for schistosomiasis (Hairston, 1962) was used to predict the importance of rats in maintaining the cycle of *Schistosoma japonicum* in the Philippines, though as with several other models one is left wondering whether the hypothesis or the model really came first.

Ross's second model (first chronologically: Ross, 1904) was a very simple representation of the diffusion of mosquitoes into an area rendered unsuitable for their breeding. Again it was limited by the exiguous understanding of mosquito bionomics then available, but it showed with some confidence that it was feasible to control malaria by prevention of mosquito breeding over a manageable area, provided the area of intervention exceeded the area over which malaria control was required. Here was an early example of what has often been found useful since then: a model of a very limited component of disease transmission where both realism and simplicity are attained by taking a small enough part of the cycle. Under these circumstances a precise conclusion is reached and the model's workings are sufficiently transparent to the epidemiologist for him to trust it.

In both these examples modelling was firmly a branch of epidemiology rather than mathematics and the success of the models was that each had a clear objective and this gave clear standards and criteria for what had to be represented fully and what could be ignored or simplified. I doubt if elegance and utility were so adequately combined again for 40 years. Certainly the malaria models of that intervening period contributed nothing to understanding the natural world nor to improving public health.

Ross furthermore understood what he was doing. He distinguished sharply between curve fitting to observed epidemic data followed by inductive reasoning towards determinants and processes, which he called *a posteriori* epidemiology, and his own approach. This latter, *a priori* epidemiology, involved synthesis of the known biology of transmission to build up a model and its comparison with observed data (Ross, 1916). Thus Ross's approach followed his own personal history: first determine the biological processes and then put them together to produce a quantitative model and give a sense of proportion. Not only does this approach fit our demand for realism, but also its hypothetico-deductive philosophy and improvement by falsification (observing the discrepancies between prediction and occurrence) are consistent with the Popperian theory of scientific discovery now widely accepted (Fine, 1975). The priority given by *a priori* models to biological, medical and sociological observations fits the approach of the field epidemiologist. Both have the same approach to reality.

By contrast, *a posteriori* models fit mathematical expressions to observed data and hope thereby to reach the underlying principles by induction. They have been largely relegated in transmission models to summarizing particular steps for inclusion in larger *a priori* models. For example, the use of exponential models of insect survival owes at least as much to *a posteriori* curve fitting as it does to the assumption of a constant probability of dying over time.

The family of unhappily named 'catalytic' models of Muench (1959) as applied to schistosomiasis by Hairston (1965) are again a mixture of both approaches, though owing most to *a posteriori* thinking in practice. They certainly also have a real utility in summarizing extensive data and providing a framework for comparing prevalence observations by age from different environments. Their sharp limitations have made their virtues more to do with convenience than the reality being considered in this chapter.

Underlying most of the models discussed here is the assumption that the epidemiological model must in some simplified way represent the processes involved in nature in the tradition of Ross and his *a priori* epidemiology. But several epidemiologists followed the *a posteriori* approach of fitting curves to epidemic phenomena as did Farr (1840) by assuming that the second or third ratio of successive mortality figures was constant (Fine, 1979). This form of descriptive regression method successfully predicted the course of an epidemic of rinderpest (Farr, 1866) and to that extent related to the real world. As Fine (1979) has shown, Brownlee developed Farr's approach and unfortunately followed it to the logical but fallacious conclusion that microbial infectivity falls during the course of an epidemic. Here the move to an *a priori* model, or the conclusion that Brownlee drew from it, led to much experimental work with mouse populations and to that extent affected 'reality'. Equally, one could argue that the defect was in his theory with its failure to account for multiple exposures of a single susceptible host.

Brownlee's model could be put alongside that of Hairston (1962) for schistosomiasis. In each case a simple model predicted a new component in the epidemiological process – decaying microbial infectiousness and rat reservoirs respectively – but the defect of Brownlee's conclusion was first, that it was wrong, and second, that it took many years of expensive and difficult research to prove it wrong. Perhaps the best conclusion we can draw is that the processes of the epidemiological model should be firmly based in the real world. Brownlee's problems perhaps warn against using the Muench catalytic models too much, especially in helminthic infections. They perhaps also raise doubts about the use of simple regression techniques to relate variables for incorporation in a model, though the success of such an approach in insect ecology appears established (Morris, 1963).

Returning to malaria, one sees that the next period of nearly forty years showed a steady divergence between theory and reality so that the practical malariologist, though much interested in several quantitative measures of the amount of malaria in a community and of mosquito ecology, lost all interest in formal models.

Theory and reality were brought together again in the work of Macdonald (1950, 1957) who, like Ross, was a professional public health worker with mathematical interests. Although the aspect of Ross's assumption that led him to reopen the analysis in the hope of getting a better fit to observed parasite rates in children concerned reinfection, it has been Macdonald's development of the mosquito phase of transmission that has influenced the teaching and practice of public health. Macdonald's (1952) analysis of equilibrium was notable for its clear emphasis on the role of immunity as regulator of the upper limit of infection observed. This was, however, put into the model in an explicit way rather than emerging from it, and it was the qualitative recognition of this more than any numerical expression that was of importance. So the modelling of equilibrium was of limited direct relevance. But the modelling of mosquito transmission reflected the great biological advances since Ross and that, together with the analysis being based on the basic case reproduction rate (R, see Chapter 5), rather than on incidence or prevalence, led to a simple analytically tractable and elegant formulation which is of central importance in practical malariology.

The basic reproduction rate, R, is clearly seen as a function of mosquito density, the square of its man-biting habit and the tenth power or above of the probability of survival through a day. This formulation is ideal for examining the consequences of insecticidal intervention, especially comparing larvicidal and imagicidal methods. It leads immediately to an understanding of why residual imagicides may be much more effective in malaria control even though the effects on mosquito numbers may be comparable between the two approaches. The difference between stable and unstable malaria is clearly illuminated, and the relative difficulty of malaria control in different countries becomes comprehensible.

More detailed use of the Macdonald model was less successful, showing a general limitation of models that are of manageable complexity for the epidemiologist (Najera, 1974). They are usually only applicable at one scale of analysis. Macdonald's was essentially a macro-model, and only the more recently formulated models of Dietz, Molineaux and Thomas (Molineaux and Gramiccia, 1980) have been useful in explaining small-scale detail in time, especially annual transmission cycles and the detailed consequences of different insecticidal and chemotherapeutic interventions.

The single most important insight into public health from modelling has probably been in the consequences of different insecticidal methods for transmission of mosquito-borne disease agents with an extrinsic developmental cycle in the insect. Now that a combination of environmental concern and insecticidal failure due to resistance have redirected interest to genetic control of vectors, models are crucial to the development of this area in predicting the numbers of sterile males or other genetically altered insects needing to be released and in planning the time scale of release. The exploration of interventions for the control of insects is where models and reality have frequently interacted. The optimization of spray cycles in frequency and timing during the year has been modelled for agricultural and medical pest insects. Both modelling and field activity have been more successful in vector control than in disease control predictions. This is partly because the vector population is viewed as a whole, while disease transmission is often very heterogeneously aggregated in space and time over the vector population. With the increase of interest in the micro-distribution of disease in space and human behavioural aspects of transmission, the data required for better modelling of disease consequences of vector control are becoming available.

While malaria models have had great application to the real world, in schistosomiasis by contrast there has been little, if any, clear and usable input to practical public health, in spite of numerous research studies and publications over the last two decades. This is due to two reasons: the absence of epidemiological data of a fundamental, almost qualitative, type prevents useful modelling, and the lack of field testing means that epidemiologists, with good cause, lack confidence in the various model predictions. The models produced so far have, however, clarified thinking and stimulated important research, though its outcome has often been beneficial in ways that are separate from model building.

The earliest contribution (Hairston, 1962) of a model of schistosomiasis basically dealt with the magnitudes of multiplication and loss rates at each stage in the *Schistosoma japonicum* life cycle required to maintain endemic equilibrium. Its contribution, apart from the pioneering nature of the work, was to indicate that the importance of rats as reservoirs of the worms had been underestimated. Thus, as with malaria, a simple model had epidemiological predictive value, though whether the modelling process was really the first thing to hint that the rats needed study is not clear.

Subsequent models by Hairston (1965) developed this approach in relation to all three major schistosome species and gave an intellectual coherence to the quantitative epidemiological data then accumulating, though the models themselves had little effect upon practical control procedures. In his subsequent independent work on schistosomiasis, Macdonald (1965) incorporated the dioecious nature of the adult worms, as had Hairston (1962), but placed great emphasis upon its consequences at low levels of infection, where the concept of 'breakpoint' – a level of infection in the human population below which the helminth population would proceed to extinction in spite of continuingly favourable circumstances for transmission – emerged from his analysis (Macdonald, 1965). Here is a concept of great relevance to practical public health. If true, it would be as important as Ross's threshold concept in malaria because it would imply that at some level of human schistosomiasis, short of extinction, control efforts could cease in the knowledge that the remaining worms would die out. The problems raised by the breakpoint illustrate three major barriers between theory and reality: lack of data in construction of the model and so numerical uncertainty about its conclusions, a less robust structure than hoped, and lack of a field test of its conclusions. To prepare a sound model requires both a clear qualitative empirical understanding of what regulates schistosome populations, the longevity of the worms and extent of human acquired immunity, and also numerical data on adult worm load. In the absence of these fundamental data, Macdonald had to make assumptions not only about the numerical values, but also about the regulators of the worm population, as discussed fully by Barbour in Chapter 6. We are left with uncertainty over the numerical levels of the breakpoint. When it is further found that the breakpoint concept is dependent on the distribution of worms between human hosts and is not robust to change from the assumed Poisson distribution to the more realistic aggregated distributions (May, 1977; Bradley and May, 1978), the theoretical basis for the breakpoint is shaken.

Empirical test of the concept depends on substantial field control programmes relying heavily on chemotherapy. Only recently have such been feasible because earlier schistosomicides were too toxic. Now the situation after several years of intensive control in St. Lucia allows of such a test of the breakpoint concept and results are awaited. Earliest indications (Jordan, personal communication) suggest that it is lower than the levels attained there, and therefore probably of little help as a practical public health concept (see also the hookworm and *Ascaris* examples discussed in Chapter 3). The earlier work on *Schistosoma haematobium* in the Cameroons (Duke and Moore, 1976) gave no support to the existence of a practically accessible breakpoint.

Here then was an example of the hazards which surround any attempt at an overall transmission model. But it is necessary to start somewhere. Rather, it points towards a second generation of such models which can explore parts or components of the cycle with special emphasis on empirical data, validity of assumptions, and most of all the robustness of that part of the model to changes in the less secure assumptions involved. Such exploration will both improve model quality and retain the confidence of the field epidemiologist. As will be clear from this chapter, the latter is of great importance to the future of the subject. Until an adequate body of accepted theory exists – and this will depend on field testing – the credibility of most modelling depends on the extent to which the models are comprehensible and 'transparent' to the epidemiologist.

The history of schistosomiasis models also shows how models help change reality: the wish of such epidemiologists as Macdonald and Hairston to test models played a large part in the motivation leading to the major control project in St. Lucia, and influenced two others in Africa. The same was true of malaria, where the project in Nigeria at Kankiya was intended to test the Macdonald model, and the Garki project was developed along with a renewed attempt at operational modelling, with notable success. Although the schistosomiasis projects were subsequently little affected by modelling, the design was considerably affected by such thinking and, in the author's view, greatly benefitted from this, even if it was not always at a conscious level. So although the cost and difficulty have meant that few models have received thorough testing in the real world, the attempts to do so have encouraged large-scale control attempts and much improved their design and conduct.

Work on mathematical models of epidemiological processes has been peculiarly subject to the hazards of disproportionate growth. A likely approach is begun to a particular disease or situation by experienced workers and is taken up by many with adequate understanding of only one of the disciplines involved. Finally the research leads into a blind alley and is abandoned. These cycles of disillusionment and rediscovery are at least less harmful than the similar activities of economic model builders outside health, whose untested theories are widely applied at great cost to the community before being abandoned (if then!), whereas epidemiological models are rarely allowed to influence the real world so much. In both areas, untested models combined with sweeping policy conclusions and a lack of common sense and experience have led to trouble.

It is this tendency to over-sweeping generalization which is the chief bar to steady progress. Hubris seems to be the chief vice of the model builder without, and even with, field experience. It induces justified scepticism and is counterproductive. It serves only to convince the determinedly non-numerate public health worker that models are a seductive alternative to understanding.

Among the more directly transmitted viral and bacterial infections there is a rather separate literature on transmission based on mass-action and Reed–Frost models. These have been useful in explaining the regular cycles of such infections as measles (Soper, 1929; Yorke and London, 1973; Fine and Clarkson, 1982; Anderson and May, 1982a) and have given encouragement to the prospects of stopping transmission by high levels of child immunization. How far they have influenced public health action otherwise is more doubtful, though the teaching of epidemiology using those models, especially at John Hopkins School of Public Health in the 1930s, has clearly inspired several of the most active field epidemiologists, including Langmuir. The strategy of smallpox vaccination for eradication, however, owes nothing to modelling and much to the intelligent exploitation of serendipity.

It may be useful to consider the reasons for this limited practical output from models of direct infections, though opinions on this are likely to vary, and the author's tropical viewpoint may bias his perception of the issues. There is no doubt that far more theoretical work has been done on the direct infections. They are much more tractable mathematically and, prior to the introduction of computers, the only type of model that could be handled readily on a variety of scales and from both deterministic and stochastic aspects. Yet I would suggest that it is the simplicity of the transmission process that may limit the utility of the models so far devised.

It is possible to gain a good understanding of the broad epidemiological processes by reflection and intuition in the case of organisms with a relatively simple life cycle. Or is this again an example of hubris this time on the part of the practical epidemiologist?

Public health action is a blunt instrument: there are relatively few options available for tackling a disease in the community and where there are apparently multiple approaches many are likely to be variants on changing human behaviour, in which the cultural problems are likely to exceed the subtle policy options. In other words the choice between chemotherapy, environmental control and vaccination is likely to depend on issues of feasibility and broad policy rather than the results of subtle analysis.

The one major concept that must depend on the analysis of infection spread is that of herd immunity, and in particular the point at which transmission dies out. It was early realized that a contagious disease, even in the absence of subclinical infections, will die out before every susceptible has been infected, for an infection with a limited infective duration in the individuals. Any rigorous formulation of such a theory of herd immunity depends on some model of the infectious process and a threshold theorem such as results from the Kermack–McKendrick or Reed–Frost formulations of transmission. Further progress beyond the concept has been more limited because of the difficulty of setting a level at which the infection would in fact die out but methods to help solve this problem are slowly evolving (see Chapter 1 and Anderson and May, 1982a). In the case of smallpox, particularly, it was found that the 'herd immunity' approach of aiming at a very high vaccination coverage was relatively unsuccessful in attempts to deliberately stop transmission. The effective alternative of case finding and vaccination of all visitors and contacts was arrived at by serendipity (adequate vaccine stocks failed to arrive in Nigeria and the new strategy was used as a temporary expedient, with unexpectedly successful results).

If it be true, as the past suggests, that models have most to offer to the real world in the case of infections whose transmission cycle is too complicated to be intuitively understood quantitively, it is probably also the case that reality can offer most to models of simpler systems.

To test a model of malaria or schistosomiasis in a useful way is very expensive. The Garki project on malaria cost $6 million. Even then, if such a project is used to develop a model it really needs another project to test its overall predictive value. A simpler cycle is less greedy of data not only because there are less components and variables involved, but also because the logistic problem of co-ordinating the measurements of these variables in space and time is very much simpler. The directly transmitted infections and the soil-transmitted helminths are thus more attractive in some ways than schistosomiasis and sleeping sickness for data to interact with modelling (Anderson and May, 1982b). In part this seems clear, and there is a real opportunity for development of this area (see Chapters 1 and 3). But two qualifications are necessary. For some of these infections the human behavioural component is both large and intractable. For the geohelminths the interaction of transient defaecation behaviour (which may be hard to record!) with a long-term environmental persistence of the worm eggs or larvae may pose difficult problems of analysis, though that is not a reason against their study. Similarly, venereal disease transmission also depends on relatively private activities and it may reasonably be postulated that if one knew who slept with whom, it would be feasible to take the necessary public health action without much help from a mathematical model! This mild scepticism over useful outcomes is not a reason for abandoning such studies but suggests that for a fruitful development of the subject, objectives need to be clear and systems selected with some care (Yorke *et al.*, 1978). The successes being obtained in fitting models with data in the case of measles show the increased feasibility of studying rather publicly transmitted infections; indeed the relation between school reopening and epidemic spread becomes sharper with the improved data now analysed (Fine and Clarkson, 1982), and a rather simple model fits the data relatively well (Anderson and May, 1982a).

A predictive model, to be useful in the real world, needs to indicate the best type of intervention and its frequency and degree of application. This often involves comparing unlike variables: the use of insecticides or drugs or some environmental change for vector-borne diseases; treatment or immunization for viral and some bacterial infections. Relative costs are clearly of major significance. An economic component is therefore an important component of such models and this links them to the very extensive economic modelling experience where practical relevance can be combined with sophistication and precision. But, of course, the biological and social data underlying the model will still limit its reliability. Even when only a single intervention is being considered, such as residual insecticide spraying, the economic component is essential to optimize the conclusions because the relative costs of labour and insecticide will determine the outcome.

In this type of optimization model, especially as applied to tuberculosis, there is a combination of realism and relevance which is very attractive. The models were well developed 10 years ago and it is surprising that they do not dominate practical action today. Several reasons exist, though their relative weight is unclear. Predominant are the crude nature of most available data and of feasible action in most developing countries. The actual prevalence of active cases may be uncertain along with their relative infectiousness. The options open to the public health administrator are also very limited, and subtle differences in intervention policies may be irrelevant where the gap between policy and implementation is great. Much greater doubts exist over the available interventions: in particular, the available studies give efficacies for the protection afforded by BCG that range from 80% to 0%! No model, nor any reality, can be robust, to variance of that order. There are, furthermore, differences in the time course of benefits to those already ill between immunization and case finding followed by chemotherapy. Where there is little operational choice between alternatives, an optimization model can have limited utility, though it may serve to broaden perception of the available options.

It is the central preoccupation of this chapter that theory and reality must remain closely in touch. Yet in the physical sciences theory has often far outrun experimental work with beneficial results for the development of the subject as a whole. In one sense this may be true of epidemiology and that is where theory points to neglected topics for study, to aspects of the transmission cycle which will repay field investigation. But in other respects the physical sciences are not a good analogy and a subject like economics has much more in common with epidemiological modelling. In these areas the number of variables is excessively great and one is not dealing with a few fundamental properties of the physical world but with the need to select from a vast array of biological and sociological variables those most relevant to understanding epidemiological processes. This needs both mathematical insight and epidemiological experience.

The time scales of theoretical and practical work are so different that, apart from retrospective analyses of data, the attempt to keep them congruent is peculiarly difficult. Whereas the average biological experiment takes hours or up to weeks, a major epidemiological study will take a decade. The Garki malaria project formally began to be set up from May 1969 and the report of the whole project was published in 1980. The St. Lucia schistosomiasis project was conceived in the lifetime of G. Macdonald, who died in 1967, and the fieldwork is due to be concluded in 1981. Indeed, it has been suggested that the intervention period of chemotherapy in Garki was too short. There can be no doubt, therefore, that experimental epidemiology of human disease requires patience and perseverance in the field over a prolonged period. Furthermore, much of the actual work has to be administrative and logistic, combined with much local political acumen, while much of the scientific work is of a relatively tedious nature if completely reliable results are to be obtained. These virtues stand in some contrast to those of the mathematical modeller whose time scales of thought and work, preferred environment and gifts are likely to be of a quite different type.

The most enduring advances have been made by those few men, Ross, Macdonald, Frost, who have combined attributes of both types. The work of teams has only succeeded where the mathematicians have immersed themselves in the field work and the epidemiologists have become fully numerate and familiar with modelling. For more workers to emerge who will combine both approaches will depend heavily on the way in which epidemiologists are educated. The right balance of theory and field work are seen in the education of some ecologists but there is a real danger that the medical component may be neglected. This too would separate theory from reality and lose a necessary group of insights as well as making much of the field work unfeasible. In particular, it is important that the epidemiological modeller be immersed in the day-to-day operations if new insights are to be gained, in the same way that the experimental biologist both designs and carries out his own experiments.

How are the difficulties of joining theory with reality to be best overcome? It is clear from the history of the subject that this depends on the same individual carrying out both activities, probably with assistance from more specialized workers. The crucial integration occurs in one mind. This has immediate implications for education of communicable disease epidemiologists. Such education needs to convey an adequate understanding of epidemiological models. This is an advantage in all ways, in that the greatest contribution of models so far is in education. Without any theoretical framework the teaching of malariology, in particular, requires the learning of a vast number of specific situations whereas with a model framework the general principles and interrelations of the various components can be set out in a few hours. This is a major, I would say the chief, contribution of models to reality so far.

There is a useful analogy between epidemiological and physical models. A child learns most from a model or toy if not only does it behave like the real thing (whether car, yacht or toy crane) but also if he can take it to pieces and reassemble it. Much of the educational value of epidemiological models to reality results when the epidemiologist can take the model apart, inspect the components, and fit them together in various ways. The limited mathematical expertise of most epidemiologists places marked limitations on their ability to do this with any but the simplest models – this has clear implications for their education, but it also places almost intolerable limits on what models are useful, and there is bound to be a period in which the few who work at the interface between the disciplines of epidemiology and mathematics have a heavy burden of interpretation.

Attempts to bridge the gap by means of computer models for self-instruction have both great advantages and risks. Very recently several malaria models have been written in a form compatible with more readily available microcomputers, so making it possible for postgraduate students to explore the consequences of various control interventions upon the prevalence, incidence and intensity of infection. The Garki malaria model is now available for several types of computer and microcomputer, so that the student can study the effects of varying chemotherapy and spraying with insecticides in a realistic way, against a background of seasonally varying transmission. This makes familiarity with such models a practical part of the education of the field epidemiologist. The hazard is that the student can too easily accept the model structure and assumptions, consequently believing too readily the output of the model. It needs to be balanced by teaching and practical work in the selection of variables for inclusion in model structure; without such critical analysis the way will be encouraged for a spurious confidence based on a full understanding of the outcome from manipulating quite inadequate models.

It may be helpful to attempt some ordering of the models available and likely to be generated in the near future, in relation to their uses rather than their mathematical structure. We lay emphasis on goals and objectives rather than the difference between deterministic and stochastic models since the choice between them, when not forced by tractability, will depend on the sort of problem being tackled.

The earliest, and in many ways most helpful, models so far have been rather simple macromodels of whole life cycles. They have often been developed before the computer era and greatly over-simplify reality, but they have been of decisive value in understanding complex reality and hence in teaching it (Macdonald on malaria), in formulating new and important questions or drawing attention to parts of the life cycle that are important but neglected (Hairston, 1962, on schistosomiasis). Such models can predict the broad consequences of different interventions and inform public health policy rather than give precise numerical values. If such simplified models are to be relied on, however, the sensitivity of the model to changes in different components needs full exploration.

Such total cycle models can be made of more specific predictive value by increasing their complexity. Today this usually implies a switch to a computer model and moves towards realism. This may either affect the whole cycle, or may more simply explore one step in transmission with great detail. A much less ambitious aim of such segment models may be to help summarize data, to estimate parameters, or to empirically relate two adjacent steps in transmission or steps in the life cycle (see Chapter 7).

I tend to the view that prediction is the all-important aim and test of models. It is possible to describe data mathematically (Von Euler's elephant comes to mind), but the test is to make predictions of the consequences of intervention, natural environmental change or other happenings. Furthermore, the model needs to outrun the ability of the experienced field worker if it is to be of real value – but these are long-term goals, as with weather-forecasting, and more modest steps forward are of real value.

The discussion of the real world has centred on medical and health issues, on human disease. This is historically appropriate as most modelling of infections has been directed to human disease, and adequate data and opportunities for testing are so costly that only human disease has provided the appropriate opportunities. However, wildlife disease and infections of domestic stock should not be neglected and veterinary situations in particular could be much more fully exploited (see Chapters 8 and 9). Some animal diseases are economically important enough to justify such effort. The removal of many human value problems (is a child worth more than a young adult!) makes optimization models using economic measures both more valid and more feasible, while the replication of similarly managed herds makes for useful application of conclusions.

Can any general conclusions be drawn from this critical review of the application of epidemiological models? A few may be proposed.

Firstly, the utility of quantitative models is limited by their selection of variables. This truism may be rephrased as stating that the selection of variables for inclusion has limited the values of models far more than the mathematical handling of those variables. Progress in useful modelling can only come from extremely close co-operation between the epidemiologist or biologist and the mathematician. Indeed progress has largely come where the key investigator has combined these two functions in himself even though he seeks advice from many others.

All models have proved less robust than their authors hoped, and often claimed. Each model has been proposed as covering a range of situations and tolerating considerable variation in parameter values and sometimes in the assumptions made. The clearest example is the Macdonald schistosomiasis model where the main qualitative advance, the concept of the breakpoint, was considered very robust but has since been shown to depend heavily on the degree of parasite aggregation within hosts, while its application in the real world depends on just how low a community worm burden is needed before a breakpoint is attained. It may be so low as to be operationally almost irrelevant (see Chapter 3).

In general, simpler models have contributed more to reality than complex ones. The simplicity in the case of analytical models lies in their mathematical structure and in the case of computer models in the flow diagram: the actual computation procedures in the computer-based model may be very lengthy.

The reason for the utility of simpler models lies in their use in teaching and research, as models have so far contributed most to the real world in two ways. The first is in teaching, in providing a picture of how a complex transmission cycle operates, that can form a basis for teaching epidemiologists. The Macdonald malaria model is the best example of this. Secondly, the contribution to research of models is in sharpening the questions to be asked and provoking precise thought on the epidemiologist's part. He can explore an idea rapidly and at low cost before designing a hypothesis for slow field testing at great expense.

It follows that the useful model is also as explicit in its processes as possible. If the epidemiologist can interpret into reality each step in the model's computations or each component of the model so that he gains insight and retains confidence in the model, then epidemiological modelling can contribute greatly to improving health in the real world. For real progress, the mathematical modeller as well as the epidemiologist must have mud on his boots.

REFERENCES

Aitken, M. M., Jones, P. W., Hall, G. A. and Hughes, D. L. (1976). The effect of fascioliasis on susceptibility of cattle to *Salmonella dublin*. *British Veterinary Journal*, **132**, 119–20.

Alonge, D. O. and Fasanmi, E. F. (1979) A survey of abattoir data in Northern Nigeria. *Tropical Animal Health and Production* **11**, 57–62.

Ambroise–Thomas, P. (1974) La réaction d'immunofluorescence dans l'étude séroimmunologique du paludisme. *Bulletin of World Health Organization*, **50**, 267–76.

Ambroise–Thomas, P., Wernsdorfer, W. H., Grab, B., Cullen, J. R. and Bertagna, P. (1974) Longitudinal sero-epidemiological studies on malaria in Tunisia. WHO/MAL/74.834, unpublished document of the World Health Organization.

Ames, W. R. and Robins, M. (1943) Age and sex as factors in the development of the typhoid carrier state and a method for estimating carrier prevalence. *American Journal of Public Health*, **33**, 221–30.

Anderson, J., Fuglsang, H., Hamilton, P. J. S. and Marshall, T. F. de C. (1974) Studies on onchocerciasis in the United Cameroon Republic II. Comparison of onchocerciasis in rain-forest and Sudan–Savanna. *Transactions of the Royal Society of Tropical Medicine and Hygiene*, **68**, 209–22.

Anderson, R. M. (1974) Population dynamics of the cestode *Caryophyllaeus laticeps* (Pallas, 1781) in the bream (*Abramis brama* L.). *Journal of Animal Ecology*, **43**, 305–21.

Anderson, R. M. (1976) Some simple models of the population dynamics of eucaryotic parasites. *Lecture Notes in Biomathematics*, **11**, 16–57.

Anderson, R. M. (1978) Population dynamics of snail infection by miracidia. *Parasitology*, **77**, 201–24.

Anderson, R. M. (1979) The persistence of direct life-cycle infectious diseases within populations of hosts, in *Some Mathematical Questions in Biology Lectures on Mathematics in the Life Sciences*, **12**, pp. 1–68.

Anderson, R. M. (1980) The dynamics and control of direct life-cycle helminth parasites. *Lecture Notes in Biomathematics*, **39**, 278–322.

Anderson, R. M. (1981a) Infectious disease agents and cyclic fluctuations in host abundance, in *The Mathematical Theory of the Dynamics of Biological Populations* (ed. R. W. Hiorns and D. Cooke), Academic Press, London, pp. 47–80.

Anderson, R. M. (1981b) Population Ecology of Infectious Disease Agents, in *Theoretical Ecology* (ed. R. M. May), Blackwell Scientific Publications, Oxford, pp. 318–355.

Anderson, R. M. (1982a) Reproductive Strategies in Trematode Species, in *Reproductive Biology of Invertebrates*. Vol. VI (ed. K. G. Adiyodi and R. G. Adiyodi), John Wiley, New York, in press.

Anderson, R. M. (1982b) Epidemiology of infectious disease agents, in *Modern Parasitology* (ed. F. E. G. Cox), Blackwell Scientific Publications, Oxford, in press.

Anderson, R . M., Jackson, H. C., May, R. M. and Smith, A. M. (1981) Population dynamics of fox rabies in Europe. *Nature (London)*, **289**, 765–71.

Anderson, R. M. and May, R. M. (1978) Regulation and stability of host-parasite population interactions. I. Regulatory processes. *Journal of Animal Ecology*, **47**, 219–47.

Anderson, R. M. and May, R. M. (1979a) Population biology of infectious diseases: I. *Nature (London)*, **280**, 361–7.

Anderson, R. M. and May, R. M. (1979b) Prevalence of schistosome infections within molluscan populations: observed patterns and theoretical predictions *Parasitology*, **79**, 63–94.

Anderson, R. M. and May, R. M. (1980) The population dynamics of microparasites within invertebrate hosts. *Philosophical Transactions of the Royal Society London Series B* **291**, 451–524.

Anderson, R. M. and May, R. M. (1982a) Directly transmitted infectious diseases: control by vaccination. *Science*, **215**, 1053–60.

Anderson, R. M. and May, R. M. (1982b) The population dynamics and control of human helminth infections: control by chemotherapy. *Nature* (London), in press.

Andral, L. and Toma, B. (1977) Epidemiology of fox rabies. *Advances in Virus Research*, **21**, 1–36.

Andrews, J. M. (1942) Hookworm disease control in Georgia. *Journal of Medical Association, State of Alabama*, **11**, 4–8.

Anon. (1976) The invisible worm. *The Lancet*, **61**, 552–4.

Anon. (1980) Seven year study finds tuberculosis vaccine ineffective (from NY Times News Service). *Tropical Medicine and Hygiene News*, **29**, 11–12.

Arfaa, F. and Ghadirian, E. (1977) Epidemiology and mass-treatment of ascariasis in six rural communities in Central Iran. *American Journal of Tropical Medicine and Hygiene*, **26**, 866–71.

Armour, J. (1975) The epidemiology and control of bovine fascioliasis. *Veterinary Record*, **96**, 198–201.

Armour, J. and Dargie, J. D. (1975) Mechanisms of acquired immunity to *Fasciola hepatica*, in *Facts and Reflections. II. Lelystad Workshop on Fascioliasis* (Ed H. J. Over and J. Armour).

Armour, J., Jennings, F. W. and Reid, J. F. S. (1970) Studies on ovine fascioliasis. II. The relationship between the availability of metacercariae of *Fasciola hepatica* on pastures and the development of clinical disease. *Veterinary Record*, **86**, 274–7.

Armstrong, A. C. (1978) A digest of drainage statistics. *Field Drainage Experimental Unit, Technical Report* 78/7. Land Drainage Service, ADAS.

Armstrong, J. C. (1978) Susceptibility to vivax malaria in Ethiopia. *Transactions of the Royal Society of Tropical Medicine and Hygiene*, **72**, 342–4.

Aron, J. L. (1982) Malaria epidemiology and detectability. *Transactions of the Royal Society of Tropical Medicine and Hygiene*, in press.

Augustine, D. L. (1923) Investigations on the control of hookworm disease. XVI. Variation in length of life of hookworm larvae from the stools of different individuals. *American Journal of Hygienes*, **3**, 127–36.

Azurin, J. C. and Alvero, M. (1974) Field evaluation of environmental sanitation measures against cholera. *Bulletin of World Health Organization*, **51**, 19–26.

Bacon, P. J. and MacDonald, D. W. (1980) To control rabies: vaccinate foxes. *New Scientist*, **87**, 640–5.

Baer, G. M. (1975) *The Natural History of Rabies*, Vols. I and II. Academic Press, New York.

Bailey, N. T. J. (1957) *The Mathematical Theory of Epidemics*. Griffin, London.

Bailey, N. T. J. (1973) Estimation of parameters from epidemic models, in *Mathematical Theory of the Dynamics of Biological Populations* (ed. M. S. Bartlett and R. W. Hiorns), Academic Press, London, pp. 253–67.

Bailey, N. T. J. (1975) *The Mathematical Theory of Infectious Diseases and its Application*, Griffin, London.

Bailey, N. T. J. (1979) Introduction to the modelling of venereal disease. *Journal of Mathematical Biology*, **8**, 301–22.

Bain, O. (1969) Morphologie des stades larvaires d'*Onchocerca volvulus* chez *Simulium damnosum* et redescription de la microfilaire. Annales de parasitologie humaine et comparée, **44**, 69–81.

Barbour, A. D. (1978a) Macdonald's model and the transmission of bilharzia. *Transactions of the Royal Society of Tropical Medicine and Hygiene*, **72**, 6–15.

Barbour, A. D. (1978b) A stochastic model for the transmission of bilharzia. *Mathematical Biosciences*, **38**, 303–312.

Barrach, A. (1972) Effect of temperature and infection with *Fasciola hepatica* larvae on *Galba truncatula*. Thesis, Freien University, Berlin.

Bartlett, M. S. (1955) *Stochastic Processes*. Cambridge University Press, Cambridge.

Bartlett, M. S. (1956) Deterministic and stochastic models for recurrent epidemics. *Proceedings of the 3rd Berkeley Symposium on Mathematical Statistics and Probability* **4**, 81–109.

Bartlett, M. S. (1957) Measles periodicity and community size. *Journal of the Royal Statistical Society Series A*, **120**, 48–70.

Bartlett M. S. (1960) The critical community size for measles in the United States. *Journal of the Royal Statistical Society Series B*, **123**, 37–44.

Barua, D. and Burrows, W. (eds) (1974) *Cholera*, Saunders, London.

Basson, P. A., McCully, R. M., Kruger, S. P., van Niekerk, J. W., Young, E. and deVos, V. (1970) Parasitic and other diseases of the African buffalo in the Kruger National Park. *Onderstepoort Journal of Veterinary Research*, **37** (1), 11–28.

Beale, G. H., Carter, R. and Walliker, D. (1978) Genetics in *Rodent Malaria*, (ed. R. Killick–Kendrick and W. Peters), Academic Press, London and New York, pp. 213–45.

Becker, N. (1976) Estimation for an epidemic model. *Biometrics* **32**, 769–77.

Becker, N. (1977a) Estimation for discrete time branching processes with application to epidemics. *Biometrics*, **33**, 515–22.

Becker, N. (1977b) On a general epidemic model. *Theoretical Population Biology*, **12**, 23–36.

Becker, N. (1979) The uses of epidemic models. *Biometrics*, **35**, 295–305.

Beddington, J. R. and May, R. M. (1977) Harvesting natural populations in a randomly fluctuating environment. *Science*, **197**, 463–465.

Bednarz, S. (1960) On the biology and ecology of *Galba truncatula* and cercariae of *Fasciola hepatica* in the basin of the river Barycz. *Acta Parasitologica Polonica*, **8**, 279–88.

Bekessy, A., Molineaux, L. and Storey, J. (1976) Estimation of incidence and recovery rates of *Plasmodium falciparum* parasitemia from longitudinal data. *Bulletin of World Health Organization*, **54**, 685–91.

Bell, G. I., Perelson, A. S. and Pimbley, G. H., Jr. (eds) (1978) *Theoretical Immunology*, Marcel Dekker, New York and Basel.

Benenson, A. S. (ed) (1975) *Control of Communicable Diseases in Man* (12th edn). American Public Health Association, Washington, D.C.

Berger, J. (1976) Model of rabies control. *Lecture Notes in Biomathematics*, **11**, 74–88.

Berry, C. I. and Dargie, J. D. (1976) The role of host nutrition in the pathogenesis of ovine fascioliasis. *Veterinary Parasitology*, **2**, 317–32.

Binford, C. H. and Connor, D. H. (eds) (1978) *Pathology of Tropical and Extraordinary Diseases, An Atlas*, Vol. 2. Armed Forces Institute of Pathology, Washington DC.

Birdsell, J. B. (1972) *Human Evolution*. Rand McNally and Company, Chicago.

Black, F. L. (1966) Measles endemicity in insular populations: critical community size and its evolutionary implication. *Journal of Theoretical Biology*, **11**, 207–211.

Black, N. M. and Froyd, G. (1972). The possible influence of liver fluke infestation on milk quality. *Veterinary Record*, **90**, 71–2..

Blamire, R. V., Crowley, A. J. and Goodhand, R. H. (1970) A review of some animal diseases encountered at meat inspection 1960–1968. *Veterinary Record*, **87**, 234–8.

Blamire, R. V., Goodhand, R. H. and Taylor, K. C. (1980) A review of some animal diseases encountered at meat inspections in England and Wales, 1969–1978. *Veterinary Record*, **106**, 195–199.

Blancou, J. (1979) Prophylaxie medicale de la rage chez le renard. *Recueil de Médicine Vétérinaire* **155**, 733–41.

Bliss, C. A. and Fisher, R. A. (1953) Fitting the negative binomial distribution to biological data and a note on the efficient fitting of the negative binomial. *Biometrics*, **9**, 176–200.

Bloom, B. R. (1979) Games parasites play: how parasites evade immune surveillance. *Nature (London)*, **279**, 21–6.

Bogel, K., Moegle, H., Knorpp, F., Arata, A., Dietz, K. and Dietheln, P. (1976) Characteristics of the spread of a wildlife rabies epidemic in Europe. *Bulletin of World Health Organization*, **54**, 433–47.

Boray, J. C. (1967) Studies on experimental infections with *Fasciola hepatica* with particular reference to acute fascioliasis in sheep. *Annals of Tropical Medicine and Parasitology*, **61**, 439–50.

Boray, J. C. (1969) Studies on experimental infections with *Fasciola hepatica* with particular reference to fascioliasis in sheep. *Advances in Parasitology*, **7**, 95–210.

Boray, J. C. (1977) Fascioliasis in Australia. *Bulletin de l'office international des epizoites*, **87**, 675–91.

Boray, J. C. and Enigk, K. (1964) Laboratory studies on the survival and infectivity of *Fasciola hepatica* and *Fasciola gigantica* metacercariae. *Zeitschrift für Tropenmedizin und Parasitologie*, **15**, 324–31.

Boreham, P. F. L. and Garrett–Jones, C. (1973) Prevalence of mixed blood meals and double feeding in a malaria vector (*Anopheles sacharovi* Favre). *Bulletin of World Health Organization*, **48**, 605–14.

Boswell, C. C. and Smith, A. (1976) The use of fluorescent pigment to record the distribution by cattle of traces of faeces from dung pats. *Journal of the British Grassland Society*, **31**, 135–6.

Boyd, M. F. (1949a) Epidemiology of malaria: factors related to the intermediate host, in *Malariology* (ed. M. F. Boyd), W. B. Saunders, Philadelphia, pp. 551–607.

Boyd, M. F. (1949b) Epidemiology: factors related to the definitive host, in *Malariology* (ed. M. F. Boyd), W. B. Saunders, Philadelphia, pp. 608–97.

Bradley, D. J. (1972) Regulation of parasite populations: a general theory of the epidemiology and control of parasitic infections. *Transactions of the Royal Society of Tropical Medicine and Hygiene*, **66**, 697–708.

Bradley, D. J. (1977) Human pest and disease problems: contrasts between developing and developed countries, in *Origins of Pest, Parasite, Disease and Weed Problems* (ed. J. M. Cherrett and G. R. Sagar), Blackwell, Oxford, pp. 329–45.

Bradley, D. J. and McCullough, F. S. (1973) Egg output stability and the epidemiology of *Schistosoma haematobium*. Part II. An analysis of the epidemiology of endemic *S. haematobium*. *Transactions of the Royal Society of Tropical Medicine and Hygiene*, **67**, 491–500.

Bradley, D. J. and May, R. M. (1978) Consequences of helminth aggregation for the dynamics of schistosomiasis. *Transactions of the Royal Society of Tropical Medicine and Hygiene*, **72**, 262–273.

Brasher, S. and Perkins, D. F. (1978) Production Ecology of British Moors and Montane Grasslands, in *Ecological Studies 27*, (ed. O. W. Heal and D. F. Perkins) Springer–Verlag, Berlin, Ch. 19.

Bromel, J. and Zettl, K. (1974) Beitrag zur altersbestimmung beim Rotfuchs (*Vulpes vulpes* L., 1758). *Zeitschrift für Jagdwissenschaft*, **20**, 96–104.

Brown, H. W. and Cort, W. W. (1927) The egg production of *Ascaris lubricoides*. *Journal of Parasitology*, **14**, 88–90.

Brown, I. N. (1969) Immunological aspects of malaria infection. *Advances in Immunology*, **11**, 267–349.

Brown, K. N. (1977) Antigenic variation in malaria, in *Immunity to Blood Parasites of Animals and Man* (ed. L. H. Miller, J. A. Pino and J. J. McKelvey, Jr.) Plenum Press, New York, pp. 5–25.

Brownlee, J. (1906) Statistical studies in immunity: the theory of an epidemic. *Proceedings of the Royal Society, Edinburgh*, **26**, 484–521.

Bruce, J. P. and Clark, R. H. (1966) *Introduction to Hydrometeorology*. Pergamon Press, Oxford.

Bruce–Chwatt, L. J. (1979) Man against malaria: conquest or defeat. *Transactions of the Royal Society of Tropical Medicine and Hygiene*, **73**, 605–17.

Bruce–Chwatt, L. J. (1980) *Essential Malaria*. Heinemann Medical Publication, London.

Bruce–Chwatt, L. J., Garrett–Jones, C. and Weitz, B. (1966) Ten years' study (1955–64) of host selection by anopheline mosquitoes. *Bulletin of World Health Organization* **35**, 405–39.

Brumpt, E. (1949) The human parasites of the genus *Plasmodium*, in *Malariology* (ed. M. F. Boyd), W. B. Saunders, Philadelphia, pp. 65–121.

Burnet, G. F. (1971) The Shapinsay Project. *Agriculture*, **78**, 470–1.

Burridge, M. J. and Schwabe, C. W. (1977) An epidemiological analysis of factors influencing the increase in *Taenia ovis* prevalence during the New Zealand *Echinococcus granulosus* control programme. *Australian Veterinary Journal*, **53**, 374–9.

Bytchenko, B. (1966) Geographical distribution of tetanus in the world: A review of the problem. *Bulletin of World Health Organization*, **34**, 71–104.

Bytchenko, B. (1967) Tetanus as a world problem. *Proceedings of International Conference on Tetanus*, Vol. 1, pp. 21–41.

Bytchenko, B. (1975) Factors determining mortality due to tetanus. *Proceedings of 4th International Conference on Tetanus*, Vol. 1, pp. 43–66.

Camus, A. (1960) *The Plague*, Penguin Books, Hamondsworth, (first published, 1947, as *La Peste*).

Carter, R. and Chen, D. H. (1976) Malaria transmission blocked by immunization with gametes of the malaria parasite. *Nature, (London)* **263**, 57–60.

Castle, M. E. and MacDaid, E. (1972) The decomposition of cattle dung and its effect on pasture. *Journal of the British Grassland Society*, **27**, 133–7.

Chambers, P. G. (1978) Hydatid disease in slaughter cattle in Rhodesia. *Tropical Animal Health and Production*, **10**, 74.

Chandler, A. C. (1929) *Hookworm Disease*. Macmillan, London.

Chappell, L. H. and Pike, A. W. (1976) Loss of *Hymenolepis diminuta* from the rat. *International Journal for Parasitology*, **6**, 333–9.

Cheever, A. W. (1977) A quantitative post-mortem study of schistosomiasis mansoni in man. *American Journal of Tropical Medicine and Hygiene*, **17**, 38–64.

Chen, D. H., Tigelaar, R. E. and Weinbaum, F. I. (1977) Immunity to sporozoite-induced malaria infection in mice I. The effect of immunization of T- and B-cell-deficient mice. *Journal of Immunology*, **118**, 1322–7.

Chen, E. R. (1971) Recent studies on endemic ascariasis in Taiwan. *Formosan Science*, **25**, 27–50.

Cheng, T. C. (1973) *General Parasitology*. Academic Press, New York.

Cheong, W. H. (1968) *Abstr. Pap. Sem. Med. Ent. As. Reg. SEAMEC, Bangkok, 15–17 January 1968* (cited in Slooff and Verdrager, 1972).

Chowdhury, A. B., Schad, G. A. and Schiller, E. L. (1968) The prevalence of intestinal helminths in religious groups of a rural community near Calcutta. *American Journal of Epidemiology*, **87**, 313–7.

Chowdhury, A. B. and Schiller, E. L. (1968) A survey of parasitic infections in a rural community near Calcutta. *American Journal of Epidemiology*, **87**, 299–312.

Christensen, N. O., Nansen, P. and Frandsen, F. (1976) The influence of temperature on the infectivity of *Fasciola hepatica* miracidia to *Lymnaea truncatula*. *Journal of Parasitology*, **62**, 698–701.

Christie, A. B. (1974) *Infectious Diseases: Epidemiology and Clinical Practice*. Churchill Livingstone, London.

Christophers, S. R. (1949) Endemic and epidemic prevalence, in *Malariology* (ed. M. F. Boyd), W. B. Saunders, Philadelphia, pp. 698–721.

Chu, G. S. T., Palmier, J. R. and Sullivan, J. T. (1977) Beetle-eating: a Malaysia folk medical practice and its public health implications. *Tropical and Geographical Medicine*, **29**, 422–7.

CIBA Foundation Symposium No. 49 (1977) *Health and Disease in Tribal Societies*. Elsevier, Amsterdam.

Ciuca, M., Ballif, L. and Chelarescu–Vieru, M. (1934) Contribution à l'étude de l'immunité dans l'infection paludéenne intentionellement provoquée par inoculation de sang virulent. *Hommage à la Mémoire du Professeur Cantacuzene*. Paris, Masson et Cie.

Clark, R. H. P. and Choudhury, M. A. (1941) Observations on *A. leucosphyrus* in

Digboi area, Upper Assam. *Journal of Malaria Institute in India*, **4**, 103–7.

Clarke, B. (1976) The ecological genetics of host-parasite relationships. *Symposium of the British Society for Parasitology*, **14**, 87–103.

Clegg, J. A. and Smith, M. A. (1978) Prospects for the development of dead vaccines against helminths. *Advances in Parasitology*, **16**, 165–218.

Cohen, J. E. (1973) Heterologous immunity in human malaria. *Quarterly Review of Biology*, **48**, 467–89.

Cohen, J. E. (1977) Mathematical models of schistosomiasis. *Annual Review of Ecology and Systematics*, **8**, 209–33.

Cohen, J. E. (1979) Malaria, a moving target. *New York Times*, Sunday, July 1, op-ed, p. 21.

Cohen, S. (1979) Review lecture. Immunity to malaria. *Proceedings of the Royal Society of London, Series B*, **203**, 323–45.

Cohen, S. and Sadun, E. H. (1976) *Immunology of Parasitic Infections*. Blackwell Scientific Publications, Oxford.

Cole, H. H. and Ronning, M. (1974) *Animal Agriculture*. W. H. Freeman & Co, San Francisco.

Coleman, D. A. (1978) Regulation and Stability of |Rat Tapeworm Populations: an Experimental Study and Matrix Model. PhD Thesis, University of Bristol.

Colless, D. H. (1952) Observations on periodicity of natural infections in anopheline mosquitoes of Borneo. *Medical Journal of Malaya*, **6**, 234–40.

Constable, G. M. (1975) The problem of V. D. modelling. *Bulletin of the Institute of International. Statistics*, **106**(2), 256–63.

Conway, G. R., Glass, N. R. and Wilcox, J. C. (1970) Fitting non-linear models to biological data by Marquart's algorithm. *Ecology*, **51**, 503–8.

Cooke, K. L. and Yorke, J. A. (1973) Some equations modelling growth processes and gonorrhea epidemics. *Mathematical Biosciences*, **16**, 75–101.

Cornille–Brögger, R., Mathews, H. M., Storey, J., Ashkar, T. S., Brögger, S. and Molineaux, L. (1978) Changing patterns in the humoral immune response to malaria before, during, and after the application of control measures: a longitudinal study in the West African savanna. *Bulletin of World Health Organization*, **56**, 579–600.

Coutinho, F. A. B., Griffin, M. and Thomas, J. D. (1981), A model of schistosomiasis incorporating the searching capacity of the miracidium, *Parasitology*, **82**, 111–120.

Cox, F. E. G. (1975) Factors affecting infections of mammals with intraerythrocytic protozoa. *Symposia of the Society for Experimental Biology*, **29**, 429–51.

Cox, F. E. G. (1978a) Specific and nonspecific immunisation against parasite infections. *Nature (London)*, **273**, 623–6.

Cox, F. E. G. (1978b) Heterologous immunity between piroplasms and malaria parasites: the simultaneous elimination of *Plasmodium vinckei* and *Babesia microti* from the blood of doubly infected mice. *Parasitology*, **76**, 55–60.

Cox, F. E. G. (1980) Monoclonal antibodies and immunity to malaria. *Nature (London)*, **284**, 304–5.

Crewe, B. and Owen, R. (1978) 750,000 eggs a day – £750,000 a year. *New Scientist*, **80**, 344–6.

Crofton, H. D. (1971) A quantitative approach to parasitism. *Parasitology*, **62**, 179–94.

Croll, N. A., Anderson, R. M., Gyorkos, T. W. and Ghadirian, E. (1981). The population biology and control of *Ascaris lumbricoides* in a rural community in Iran. *Transactions of the Royal Society of Tropical Medicine and Hygiene*, **76**, 187–197.

Cross, J. H., Gunawan, S., Gaba, A., Watten, R. H. and Sulianti, J. (1970) Survey for human intestinal and blood parasites in Bojolali, Central Java, Indonesia. *South East Asian Journal of Tropical Medicine and Public Health*, **1**, 354–60.

Crossland, N. O. (1976) The effect of the molluscicide *N*-tritylmorpholine on transmission of *Fasciola hepatica*. *The Veterinary Record*, **98**, 45–8.

Crossland, N. O., Bennet, M. S. and Hope–Cawdery, M. J. (1969) Preliminary observations on the control of *Fasciola hepatica* with the molluscicide *N*-tritylmorpholine. *The Veterinary Record*, **84**, 182–4.

Crossland, N. O., Johnstone, A., Beaumont, G. and Bennet, M. S. (1977) The effect of chronic fascioliasis on the productivity of lowland sheep. *British Veterinary Journal*, **133**, 518–25.

Cruikshank, R., Standerd, K. and Russell, H. B. L. (1976) *Epidemiology and Community Health in Warm Climate Countries*. Churchill–Livingstone, New York.

Cvjetanović, B. (1973) Typhoid fever and its prevention. *Public Health Review*, **2**, 229–46.

Cvjetanović, B. (1974) Cost-effectiveness and cost-benefit aspects of preventive measures against communicable diseases. *Ciba Foundation Symposium*, **23**, 187–203.

Cvjetanović, B., Grab, B. and Uemura K. (1971) Epidemiological model of typhoid fever and its use in the planning and evaluation of antityphoid immunization and sanitation programmes. *Bulletin of World Health Organization*, **45**, 53–75.

Cvjetanović, B., Grab, B., Uemura, K. and Bytchenko, B. (1972) Epidemiological model of tetanus and its use in the planning of immunization programmes. *International Epidemiological Journal*, **1**, 125–37.

Cvjetanović, B., Grab, B. and Uemura, K. (1978) Dynamics of acute bacterial diseases, epidemiological models and their application in public health. *Bulletin of World Health Organization, Supplement No. 1*, **56**, 1–143.

Cvjetanović, B. and Uemura, K. (1965) The present status of field and laboratory studies of typhoid and paratyphoid vaccines, with special reference to studies sponsored by the World Health Organization. *Bulletin of World Health Organization*, **32**, 29–36.

Dada, B. J. O. (1978) Prevalence of hydatid disease in food animals reported at meat inspection in Nigeria, 1971–1975. *Journal of Helminthology*, **52**, 70–2.

Dajani, Y. F. (1978) Prevalence of hydatid disease in Syria and Jordan: preliminary results. *Transactions of the Royal Society of Tropical Medicine and Hygiene*, **72(3)**, 320–1.

Dalton, P. R. and Pole, D. (1978) Water contact patterns in relation to *Schistosoma haematobium* infection. *Bulletin of World Health Organization*, **56**, 417–26.

Dar, F. K. and Taguri, S. (1978) Human hydatid disease in eastern Libya. *Transactions of the Royal Society of Tropical Medicine and Hygiene*, **72(3)**, 313–4.

Dargie, J. D. (1975) Factors affecting the pathogenesis of fascioliasis in ruminants, In *Facts and Reflections II. Lelystad Workshop on Fascioliasis* (ed. H. J. Over and J. Armour).

Dargie, J. D., Berry, C. I. and Parkins, J. J. (1979) The pathophysiology of ovine fascioliasis: studies on the feed intake and digestibility, body weight and nitrogen balance of sheep given rations of hay or hay plus a pelleted supplement. *Research in Veterinary Science*, **26**, 289–95.

Darrow, W. W. (1975) Changes in sexual behaviour and venereal disease. *Clinical Obstetrics and Gynecology*, **18**, 255–67.

Davis, D. E. and Wood, J. E. (1959) Ecology of foxes and rabies control. *Public Health Reports*, **74**, 115–8.

Deans, J. A., Dennis, E. D. and Cohen, S. (1978) Antigenic analysis of sequential erythrocytic stages of *Plasmodium knowlesi*. *Parasitology*, **77**, 333–44.

Delgado y Garnica, R. and Martinez–Murry, R. (1970) L'irregularité de la ponte d'*Ascaris lumbricoides*. *Annals of Parasitologie*, **45**, 223–6.

Dietz, K. (1974) Transmission and control of arbovirus diseases, in *Epidemiology* (ed. D. Ludwig and K. L. Cooke). Proceedings of the Society for Industrial and Applied Mathematics, Philadelphia, pp. 104–21.

Dietz, K. (1976) The incidence of infectious diseases under the influence of seasonal fluctuations. *Lecture Notes in Biomathematics*, **11**, 1–15.

Dietz, K. (1980) Models for vector–borne parasitic diseases. *Lecture Notes in Biomathematics*, **39**, 264–77.

Dietz, K., Molineaux, L. and Thomas, A. (1974) A malaria model tested in the African savannah. *Bulletin of World Health Organization*, **50**, 347–57.

Disko, R. and Weber, L. (1979) The attraction of miracidia of *Schistosoma mansoni* to the snail *Biomphalaria glabrata*. Technical report, Inst. f. Med. Mikrobiologie d. Techn. Univ. München.

Dixon, K. E. (1964) The relative suitability of sheep and cattle as hosts for the liver fluke *Fasciola hepatica*. *Journal of Helminthology*, **28**, 203–12.

Dogiel, V. A. (1962) *General Parasitology*. Oliver and Boyd, Edinburgh and London.

Donald, A. D. and Leslie, R. T. (1969) Population studies on the infective stage of some nematode parasites of sheep II. The distribution of faecal deposits on fields grazed by sheep. *Parasitology*, **59**, 141–57.

Doyle, J. J. (1972) Evidence of an acquired resistance in calves to a single experimental infection with *Fasciola hepatica*. *Research in Veterinary Science*, **13**, 456–9.

Doyle, J. J. (1973) The relationship between the duration of a primary infection and the subsequent development of an acquired resistance to experimental infections with *Fasciola hepatica* in calves. *Research in Veterinary Science*, **14**, 97–103.

Dubreuil, M., Andral, L., Aubert, M. F. and Blancou, J. (1979) Oral vaccination of foxes against rabies. An experimental study. *Annals of Veterinary Research*, **10**, 9–21.

Duke, B. O. L. (1957) The reappearance, rate of increase, and distribution of the microfilariae of *Onchocerca volvulus* following treatment with diethylcarbamazine. *Transactions of the Royal Society of Tropical Medicine and Hygiene*, **51**, 37–44.

Duke, B. O. L. (1962a) Studies on factors influencing the transmission of onchocerciasis I. The survival rate of *Simulium damnosum* under laboratory conditions and the effect upon it of *Onchocerca volvulus*. *Annals of Tropical Medicine and Parasitology*, **56**, 130–5.

Duke, B. O. L. (1962b) Studies on factors influencing the transmission of onchocerciasis. II. The intake of *Onchocerca volvulus* microfilariae by *Simulium damnosum* and the survival of the parasites in the fly under laboratory conditions. *Annals of Tropical Medicine and Parasitology*, **56**, 255–63.

Duke, B. O. L. (1968) The effects of drugs on *Onchocerca volvulus*. I. Methods of assessment, population dynamics of the parasite and the effects of diethylcarbamazine. *Bulletin of World Health Organization*, **39**, 137–46.

Duke, B. O. L. (1973) Studies on factors influencing the transmission of onchocerciasis. VIII. The escape of infective *Onchocerca volvulus* larvae from feeding 'forest' *Simulium damnosum*. *Annals of Tropical Medicine and Parasitology*, **67**, 95–9.

Duke, B. O. L. (1975) The differential dispersal of nulliparous and parous *Simulium damnosum*. *Zeitschrift für Tropenmedizin Parasitologie*, **26**, 88–97.

Duke, B. O. L. and Lewis, D. J. (1964) Studies on factors influencing the transmission of onchocerciasis. III. Observations of the effect of the peritrophic membrane in limiting the development of *Onchocerca volvulus* microfilariae in *Simulium damnosum*. *Annals of Tropical Medicine and Parasitology*, **58**, 83–8.

Duke, B. O. L. and Moore, P. J. (1976) The use of molluscicide, in conjunction with chemotherapy, to control *Schistosoma haematobium* at the Barombi Lake foci in cameroon. *Tropenmedizin und Parasitologie*, **27**, 297–313.

Dungal, N. (1946) Echinococcosis in Iceland. *American Journal of Medical Science*, **212**, 12–17.

Durbin, C. G. (1952) The longevity of the liverfluke, *Fasciola* sp. in sheep. *Proceedings of the Helminthological Society*, Washington, **19**, 120.

Earle, W. C., Pérez, M., Del Rio, J. and Arzola, C. (1939) Observations on the course of naturally acquired malaria in Puerto Rico. *Puerto Rico Journal of Public Health and Tropical Medicine*, **14**, 391–406.

Eckmann, L. (ed) (1967). *Principles of Tetanus* (*Proceedings of the International Conference on Tetanus*, Bern, July 15–19, 1966), Hans Huber, Bern.

Edwards, C. M. (1968) Liver fluke in sheep. Field trials in Wales on control by planning in advance. *The Veterinary Record*, **80**, 718–28.

Edwards, C. M., al-Saigh, M. N. R., Williams, G. H. and Chamberlain, A. G. (1976) Effects of liverfluke on wool production in Welsh Mountain sheep. *Veterinary Record*, **98**, 372.

Elderkin, R. H., Berkowitz, D. P., Farris, F. A., Gunn, C. F., Hickernell, F. J., Kass, S. N., Mansfield, F. I. and Taranto, R. G. (1977) On the steady state of an age dependent model for malaria, in *Nonlinear Systems and Applications*, (ed. V. Lakshmikantham), Academic Press, New York, pp. 491–512.

Englund, J. (1970) Some aspects of reproduction and mortality rates in Swedish foxes. *Viltrevy*, **8**, 1–82.

Euzeby, J. and Jolivet, G. (1972) Les maladies animales. Leur incidence sur l'économie agricole. Les maladies parasitaires, in *Regards sur la France*, 229–50.

Evans, D. G. and Pratt, J. H. (1978) A critical analysis of condemnation data for cattle, pigs and sheep 1969 to 1975. *British Veterinary Journal*, **134**, 476–92.

Eyles, D. E., Wharton, R. H., Cheong, W. H. and Warren, M. (1964). Studies on malaria and *Anopheles balabacensis* in Cambodia. *Bulletin of World Health Organization*, **30**, 7–21.

Farr, W. (1840a) Progress of epidemics. *Second report of the Registrar General of England and Wales*, 16–20.

Farr, W. (1840b) Progress of epidemics. *Second report of the Registrar General of England and Wales*, 90–98.

Farr, W. (1866) On the cattle plague. Letter to the editor of the *Daily News* (London), February 19.

FAO/UNEP/WHO Report (1976) *Consultation on Field control of Taeniasis and Echinococcosis*, Nairobi, Kenya.

Feldman, F. M. (1957) How much control of tuberculosis 1937–1957–1977? *American Journal of Public Health*, **10**, 1235–41.

Feldman, F. M. (1973) Resource allocation model for Public Health Planning. *Bulletin of World Health Organization*, Supplement Vol. 48.

Fenner, F. and White, D. O. (1970) *Medical Virology*, Academic Press, New York.

Fine, P. E. M. (1975a) Ross' *a priori* pathometry – a perspective. *Proceedings of the Royal Society of Medicine*, **68**, 547–51.

Fine, P. E. M. (1975b) Superinfection – a problem in formulating a problem. *Tropical Diseases Bulletin*, **72**, 475–88.

Fine, P. E. M. (1979) John Brownlee and the measurement of infectiousness: an historical study in epidemic theory. *Journal of the Royal Statistical Society Series, A*, **142**, 347–362.

Fine, P. E. M. and Clarkson, J. A. (1982) Measles in England and Wales I. An analysis of factors underlying seasonal patterns. *International Journal of Epidemiology*, **11**, 5–14.

Fisher, R. A. (1930) *The Genetical Theory of Natural Selection*, Clarendon Press, Oxford.

Fleming, A. F., Storey, J., Molineaux, L., Iroko, E. A. and Attai, E. D. E. (1979) Abnormal haemoglobins in the Sudan savanna of Nigeria. I. Prevalence of haemoglobins and relationships between sickle cell trait, malaria and survival. *Annals of Tropical Medicine and Parasitology*, **73**, 161–72.

Foreyt, W. J. and Todd, A. C. (1976) Liver flukes in cattle. *Veterinary Medicine and the Small Animal Clinician*, **71**, 816–22.

Frame, A. D., Bendezu, P, Mercado, H., Otiniano, H., Frame, S. H. and Flores, W. (1979) Increase in bovine fascioliasis in Puerto Rico as determined by slaughter house surveys. *Journal of Agriculture of the University of Puerto Rico*, **63**, 27–30.

Freeman, R. R., Trejdosiewicz, A. J. and Cross, G. A. M. (1980) Protective monoclonal antibodies recognising stage-specific merozoite antigens of a rodent malaria parasite. *Nature (London)*, **284**, 366–8.

Friend, M. (1968) History and epidemiology of rabies in wildlife in New York. *Fisheries Game Journal, New York*, **15**, 71–97.

Frost, W. H. (1937) How much control of tuberculosis? *American Journal of Public Health*, **27**, 759–60.

Froyd, G. (1965) Bovine cysticercosis and human taeniasis in Kenya. *Annals of Tropical Medicine and Parasitology*, **59**, 169–180.

Froyd, G. (1975) Liver fluke in Great Britain. *The Veterinary Record*, **97**, 492–5.

Galbraith, N. S., Forbes, P. and Mayon–White, R. T. (1980) Changing patterns of communicable disease in England and Wales: Part II – disappearing and declining diseases. *British Medical Journal*, **281**, 489–92.

Garrett–Jones, C. (1964) The human blood-index of malaria vectors in relation to epidemiological assessment. *Bulletin of World Health Organization*, **30**, 241–61.

Garrett–Jones, C. and Shidrawi, G. R. (1969) Malaria vectorial capacity of a population of *Anopheles gambiae. Bulletin of World Health Organization,* **40,** 531–45.

Geeraerts, J. (1971) Distribution and expansion in the distribution of cattle fascioliasis in the Belgian province of East Flanders. *Second International Liverfluke Colloquium, Wageningen,* 2–6 Oct. 1967.

Gemmell, M. A. (1960) Advances in knowledge on the distribution and importance of hydatid disease as world health and economic problems during the decade 1950– 1959. *Helminthological Abstracts,* **29**(4), 355–63.

Gemmell, M. A. (1967) Species specificity and cross-protective functional antigens of the tapeworm embryo. *Nature (London),* **213,** 500–1.

Gemmell, M. A. (1977) Taeniidae: modification to the lifespan of the egg and the regulation of tapeworm populations. *Experimental Parasitology,* **41,** 314–28.

Gemmell, M. A. (1979) Hydatidosis control – a global view. *Australian Veterinary Journal,* **55,** 118–25.

Gettinby, G. (1974) Assessment of the effectiveness of control techniques for liver fluke infection, in *Ecological Stability* (ed. M. B. Usher and M. H. Williamson), Chapman and Hall, London, pp. 89–97.

Gettinby, G. and McLean, S. (1982) A matrix formulation of the life cycle of the liver fluke. *Proceedings of the Royal Irish Academy, B* (in press).

Ghadirian, E. and Arfaa, F. (1972) Human infection with *Hymenolepis diminuta* in villages of Minab, Southern Iran. *International Journal for Parasitology,* **2,** 481–2.

Ghazal, A. M. and Avery, R. A. (1974) Population dynamics of *Hymenolepis nana* in mice: fecundity and the 'crowding effect'. *Parasitology,* **69,** 403–15.

Ghestem, A., Morel–Vareille, C., Rondelaud, D. and Vilks, A. (1974) Premiers documents phytosociologiques des biotopes à *Lymnaea truncatula* dans le nord – ouest du Limousin. *Bulletin Société d'histoire Naturelle de Toulouse,* **110,** 235–240.

Giglioli, G. (1972) Changes in the pattern of mortality following the eradication of hyperendemic malaria from a highly susceptible community. *Bulletin of World Health Organization,* **46,** 181–202.

Gottlieb, S. (1967) Long-term immunity of diptheria and tetanus: a mathematical model. *American Journal of Epidemiology,* **85,** 207–19.

Gough, K. J. (1977). The estimation of latent and infectious periods *Biometrika,* **64,** 559–65.

Greenberg, M., Pellitteri, O. and Barton, J. (1957) Frequency of defects in infants whose mothers had Rubella during pregnancy. *Journal of the American Medical Association,* **165,** 675–8.

Greenwood, M. (1931) On the statistical measure of infectiousness. *Journal of Hygiene. Cambridge,* **31,** 336–51.

Greer, N. R. (1976). Characterisation of a habitat for *Lymnaea truncatula,* the dwarf pond snail and intermediate host in the life cycle of *Fasciola hepatica.* Undergraduate project, University of York.

Gregory, G. G. (1977) The prevalence of tapeworms in dogs during the hydatid limitation program in Tasmania. *Australian Veterinary Journal,* **53,** 88–90.

Griffiths, D. A. (1973) The effect of measles vaccination on the incidence of measles in the community. *Journal of Royal Statistical Society Series, A,* **136,** 441–8.

Griffiths, D. A. (1974) A catalytic model of infection for measles. *Applied Statistics,* **23,** 330–9.

Griffiths, R. B. (1979) Veterinary aspects, in *The Relevance of Parasitology to Human*

Welfare Today (B. S. P. Symposium No. 16) (ed. A. E. R. Taylor and R. Muller), Blackwell Scientific Publications, Oxford.

Grindle, R. J. (1978) Economic losses resulting from bovine cysticercosis with special reference to Botswana and Kenya. *Tropical Animal Health and Production*, **10**, 127–40.

Gronvold, J. (1979). On the possible role of earthworms in the transmission of *Ostertogia ostertagi* 3rd stage larvae from faeces to soil. *Journal of Parasitology*, **65**, 831–2.

Grossman, Z. (1980) Oscillatory phenomena in a model of infectious diseases. *Theoretical Population Biology*, **18**, 204–43.

Grossman, Z., Gumowski. I. and Dietz, K. (1977) The incidence of infectious diseases under the influence of seasonal fluctuations – analytical approach, in *Nonlinear Systems and Applications*, Academic Press, New York, pp. 525–46.

Gurney, W. S. C., Blythe, S. P. and Nisbet, R. M. (1980) Nicholson's blowflies revisited. *Nature (London)*, **287**, 17–21.

Hairston, N. G. (1962) Population ecology and epidemiological problems. *Proceedings of the CIBA Foundation Symposium on Bilharziasis*, J. and A. Churchill, London, pp. 36–80.

Hairston, N. G. (1965) On the mathematical analysis of schistosome populations. *Bulletin of World Health Organization*, **33**, 45–62.

Hairston, N. G. (1973) The dynamics of transmission, in *Epidemiology and Control of Schistosomiasis* (ed. N. Ansari), University Park Press, Baltimore.

Hamer, W. H. (1906) Epidemic disease in England. *Lancet*, **1**, 733–9.

Happich, F. A. and Boray, J. C. (1971) The quantitative diagnosis of *Fasciola hepatica* infection in sheep, in *Second International Liver Fluke Colloquium*, 2–6 Oct. 1967, Wageningen, pp. 63–4.

Harris, S. (1977) Distribution, habitat utilization and age structure of a suburban fox (*Vulpes vulpes*) population. *Mammal Review*, **7**, 25–39.

Harrison, G. (1978) *Mosquitoes, Malaria and Man.*, Clarke, Irwin and Co., New York.

Hawkins, C. D. and Morris, R. S. (1978) Depression of productivity in sheep infected with *Fasciola hepatica*. *Veterinary Parasitology*, **4**, 341–51.

Hayden, G. F., Modlin, J. F. and Witte, J.J. (1977) Current status of Rubella in the United States 1969–75. *Journal of Infectious Diseases*, **185**, 337–40.

Heath, D. D. and Lawrence, S. B. (1978) The effect of mebendazole and praziquantel on the cysts of *Echinococcus granulosus*, *Taenia hydatigena* and *T. ovis* in sheep. *New Zealand Veterinary Journal*, **26**, 11–15.

Heppleston, P. B. (1972) Life history and population fluctuations of *Lymnaea truncatula* (Mull.), the snail vector of fascioliasis. *Journal of Applied Ecology*, **9**, 235–48.

Hesselberg, C. A. and Andreassen, J. (1975) Some influences of population density on *Hymenolepis diminuta* in rats. *Parasitology*, **71**, 517–23.

Hethcote, H. W. (1974) Asymptotic behaviour and stability in epidemic models. In *Lecture Notes in Biomathematics*, **2**, 83–92.

Hethcote, H. W. (1976) Qualitative analyses of communicable disease models. *Mathematical Biosciences*, **28**, 335–56.

Heyneman, D. (1958) Effect of temperature on rate of development and viability of the cestode, *Hymenolepis nana* in its intermediate host. *Experimental Parasitology*, **7**, 374–82.

Hien, N. T. (1968) The genus *Anopheles* in the Republic of Vietnam N. M. P., Saigon, Vietnam (cited in Slooff) and Verdrager, 1972).

Hilder, E. J. (1966) Distribution of excreta by sheep at pasture. *Proceedings of the 10th International Grassland Congress, Helsinki*, 977–981.

Hill, R. B. (1926) The estimation of the number of hookworm harboured by the use of the dilution egg count method. *American Journal of Hygienes*, **6**, 19–41.

Hoagland, K. E. and Schad, G. A. (1978) *Nector americanus* and *Ancylostoma duodenale*: life history parameters and epidemiological implications of two sympatric hookworms of humans. *Experimental Parasitology*, **44**, 36–49.

Hodasi, J. K. M. (1972) The effects of *Fasciola hepatica* on *Lymnaea truncatula*. *Parasitology*, **65**, 359–69.

Holland–Moritz, Von W., Nickel, S. and Hiepe, Th. (1977) Untersuchungen zür Epizooliologie der Fasziolose der Jungrinder. *Monatshefte für Veterinärmedizin*, **23**, 889–93.

Honer, M. R. and Vink L. A. (1963) Contributions to the epidemiology of *Fasciola hepatica* in the Netherlands. II. Studies on cattle fascioliasis. *Zeitschrift für Parasitenkunde*, **23**, 106–20.

Hope–Cawdery, M. J. (1976) The effects of fascioliasis on ewe fertility. *British Veterinary Journal*, **132**, 568–75.

Hope–Cawdery, M. J. and Moran, M. A. (1971) A method for estimating the level of infection of fascioliasis to which sheep are exposed. *British Veterinary Iournal*, **127**, 118–24.

Hope–Cawdery, M. J., Strickland, K. L., Conway, A. and Crowe, P. J. (1977) Production effects of liver fluke in cattle. I. The effects of infection on liveweight gain, feed intake and food conversion efficiency in beef cattle. *British Veterinary Journal*, **133**, 145–59.

Hope–Cawdery, M. J., Gettinby, G. and Grainger, J. N. R. (1978) Mathematical models for predicting the prevalence of liver fluke disease and its control from biological and meteorological data. *World Meteorological Organisation, Technical Note No. 159. Weather and parasitic animal disease*, 21–38.

Horak, I. G. and Louw, J. P. (1977) Parasites of domestic and wild animals in South Africa. IV. Helminths in sheep or irrigated pasture on the transvaal highveld. *Onderstepoort Journal of Veterinary Research*, **44(4)**, 261–70.

Hornick, R. and Woodward, T. E. (1967) Appraisal of typhoid vaccine in experimentally infected human subjects. *Transactions of the American Clinical Medicine Association*, **78**, 70–8.

Howard, R. J. and Mitchell, G. F. (1979) Accelerated clearance of uninfected red cells from *Plasmodium berghei*-infected mouse blood in normal mice. *Australian Journal of Experimental Biology and Medicine*, **57**, 455–57.

Hsieh, H. C. (1970) Studies on endemic hookworm. I. Survey and longitudinal observations in Taiwan. *Japan Journal of Parasitology*, **19**, 508–22.

Insler, G. D. and Roberts, L. S. (1976) *Hymenolepis diminuta*: lack of pathogenicity in the healthy rat host. *Experimental Parasitology*, **39**, 351–57.

Islam, N. and Rashid, H. (1977) Hydatid cysts in bovines, caprines and ovines in Dacca, Bangladesh. *Annals of Tropical Medicine and Parasitology*, **71**, 239–41.

Johnston, D. H. and Beauregard, M. (1969) Rabies epidemiology in Ontario. *Bulletin of Wildlife Disease Association*, **5**, 357–70.

Jordan, P. (1977) Schistosomiasis – research to control. *American Journal of Tropical Medicine and Hygiene*, **26**, 877–86.

Jordan, P. and Webbe, G. (1969) *Human Schistosomiasis*. William Heinemann, London.

Kaplan, C. (ed) (1977) *Rabies: the Facts*. Oxford University Press, Oxford.

Karim, M. A. (1979) A survey of bovine cysticercosis in Northern Iraq. *Tropical Animal Health and Production*, **11**, 239–40.

Karlin, S. and Taylor, H. M. (1975) *A First Course in Stochastic Processes* (2nd edn.), Academic Press, New York.

Kauker, E. and Zettl, K. (1963) The epidemiology of sylvan rabies in central Europe and the possibilities of combating it. *Veterinär-medizinische Nachrichten*, **2/3**, 96–116.

Kendall, S. B. (1949a) Nutritional factors affecting the rate of development of *Fasciola hepatica* in *Lymnaea truncatula*. *Journal of Helminthology*, **23**, 179–90.

Kendall, S. B. (1949b) Bionomics of *Lymnaea truncatula* and the parthenitae of *Fasciola hepatica* under drought conditions. *Journal of Helminthology*, **23**, 57–68.

Kendall, S. B. (1965) Relationships between the species of *Fasciola* and their molluscan host. *Advances in Parasitology*, **3**, 59–98.

Kendall, S. B. and McCullough, F. S. (1951) The emergence of the cercariae of *Fasciola hepatica* from the snail *Lymnaea truncatula*. *Journal of Helminthology*, **25**, 77–92.

Kendall, S. B. and Ollerenshaw, C. B. (1963) Effect of nutrition on the growth of *Fasciola hepatica*. *Proceedings of the Nutrition Society*, **22**, 41–6.

Kendall, S. B. and Parfitt, J. W. (1975) Chemotherapy of infection with *Fasciola hepatica* in cattle. *The Veterinary Record*, **97**, 9–12.

Kendall, S. B., Sinclair, I. J., Everett, G. and Parfitt, J. W. (1978) Resistance to *Fasciola hepatica* in cattle. I. Parasitological and serological observations. *Journal of Comparative Pathology*, **88**, 112–15.

Kermack, W. O. and McKendrick, A. G. (1927) A contribution to the mathematical theory of epidemics. *Proceedings of the Royal Society of London Series A*, **115**, 700–21.

Kermack, W. O. and McKendrick, A. G. (1932) A contribution to the mathematical theory of epidemics. Part II. The problem of endemicity. *Proceedings of the Royal Society of London Series A*, **138**, 55–83.

Kermack, W. O. and McKendrick, A. G. (1933) A contribution to the mathematical theory of epidemics, Part III. Further studies of the problem of endemicity. *Proceedings of the Royal Society of London Series A*, **141**, 92–122.

Kern, P., Dietrich, M. and Volkmer, K. (1979) Chemotherapy of echinococcosis with mebendazole. *Tropenmedizin und Parasitologie*, **30**, 65–72.

Keymer, A. E. (1980a) The influence of *Hymenolepis diminuta* on the survival and fecundity of the intermediate host. *Tribolium confusum*. *Parasitology*, **81**, 405–21.

Keymer, A. E. (1980b) *The Population Dynamics of the Rat Tapeworm, Hymenolepis diminuta*. Unpublished PhD Thesis, University of London.

Keymer, A. E. (1981) Population dynamics of *Hymenolepis diminuta* in the intermediate host. *Journal of Animal Ecology*, **50**, 941–50.

Keymer, A. E. (1982) The dynamics of infection of *Tribolium confusum* by *Hymenolepis diminuta*: the influence of exposure time and host density. *Parasitology*, **84**, 157–66.

Keymer, A. E. and Anderson, R. M. (1979) The dynamics of infection of *Tribolium confusum* by *Hymenolepis diminuta*: the influence of infective-stage density and spatial distribution. *Parasitology*, **79**, 195–207.

Khan, A. Q. and Talibi, S. A. (1972) Epidemiological assessment of malaria transmission in an endemic area of East Pakistan and the significance of congenital immunity. *Bulletin of World Health Organization*, **46**, 783–92.

King, J. O. L. (1978) *An Introduction to Animal Husbandry*, Blackwell Scientific Publications, Oxford.

Klob, H. H. and Hewson, R. (1980) A study of fox populations in Scotland from 1971 to 1976. *Journal of Applied Ecology*, **17**, 7–19.

Kloetzel, K. and da Silva, J. R. (1967) *Schistosomiasis mansoni* acquired in adulthood: behaviour of egg counts and the intradermal test. *American Journal of Tropical Medicine and Hygiene*, **16**, 167–9.

Knox, E. G. (1980) Strategy for rubella vaccination. *International Journal of Epidemiology*, **9**, 13–23.

Koino, S. (1922) In *Medicine in the Tropics* (ed. A. W. Woodruff, 1974).

Krafsur, E. S. and Armstrong, J. C. (1978) An integrated view of entomological and parasitological observations on falciparum malaria in Gambela, Western Ethiopia lowlands. *Transactions of the Royal Society of Tropical Medicine and Hygiene*, **72**, 348–56.

Krause, R. A. and Massie, L. B. (1975) Predictive systems: modern approaches to disease control. *Annual Review of Phytopathology*, **13**, 31–47.

Krebs, C. J. (1972) *Ecology. The Experimental Analysis of Distribution and Abundance*, Harper and Row, New York.

Krupp, I. M. (1962) Effects of crowding and of superinfection on habitat selection and egg production in *Ancylostoma caninum*. *Journal of Parasitology*, **47**, 957–61.

Kulasiri, C. (1954) Some cestodes of the rat, *Rattus rattus* Linaeus, of Ceylon and their epidemiological significance for man. *Parasitology*, **44**, 349–52.

Lajmanovich, A. and Yorke, J. A. (1976) A deterministic model for gonorrhea in a nonhomogeneous population. *Mathematical Biosciences*, **28**, 221–36.

Langreth, S. G. and Reese, R. T. (1979) Antigenicity of the infected erythrocyte and merozoite surfaces in falciparum malaria. *Journal of Experimental Medicine*, **150**, 1241–54.

Lechat, M. F. (1971) An epidemiometric approach for planning and evaluating leprosy control activities. *International Journal of Leprosy*, **39**, 603–7.

Lewis, T. (1975a) The loss of immunity in age-prevalence models for bilharzia in man. *Mathematical Biosciences*, **23**, 205–18.

Lewis, T. (1975b) A model for the parasitic disease bilharzia. *Advances in Applied Probability* **7**, 673–704.

Lewis, T. (1976) Threshold results in the study of schistosomiasis. *Mathematical Biosciences*, **30**, 205–11.

Leyton, M. K. (1968) Stochastic models in populations of helminthic parasites in the definitive host. II. Sexual mating functions. *Mathematical Biosciences*, **3**, 413–9.

Li, S. Y. and Hsu, H. F. (1951) On the frequency distribution of parasitic helminths in their naturally infected hosts. *Journal of Parasitology*, **37**, 32–41.

Lloyd, H. G. (1976) Wildlife rabies in Europe and the British situation. *Transactions of the Royal Society of Tropical Medicine and Hygiene*, **70**, 175–203.

Lloyd, H. G. (1980) *The Red Fox*, Batsford, London.

Lloyd, H. G., Jensen, B., van Haaften, J. L., Nuwold, F. J., Wandeler, A., Bogel, N.

and Arata, A. A. (1976) Annual turnover of fox populations in Europe. *Zentralblatt Veterinärmedizin* **B23**, 580–9.

London, W. P. and Yorke, J. A. (1973) Recurrent outbreaks of measles, chickenpox and mumps. I. Seasonal variation in contact rates. *American Journal of Epidemiology*, **98**, 453–68.

Lotka, A. J. (1923) Contributions to the analysis of malaria epidemiology. *American Journal of Hygiene*, 3, (*Suppl.* I), 1–21.

Lysenko, A. J., Beljaev, A. E. and Rybalka, V. M. (1977) Population studies of *Plasmodium vivax*. 1. The theory of polymorphism of sporozoites and epidemiological phenomena of tertian malaria. *Bulletin of World Health Organization*, **55**, 541–9.

McArthur, J. (1947) The transmission of malaria in Borneo. *Transactions of the Royal Society of Tropical Medicine and Hygiene*, **40**, 537–58.

McArthur, R. H. and Wilson, E. O. (1967) *The Theory of Island biogeography*, University Press, Princeton.

McConnell, J. D. and Green, R. J. (1979) The control of hydatid disease in Tasmania. *Australian Veterinary Journal*, **55**, 140–5.

MacDiarmid, B. N. and Watkin, B. R. (1972) Distribution and rate of decay of dung patches and their influence on grazing behaviour. *Journal of the British Grassland Society*, **27**, 48–54.

Macdonald, D. W. (1980) *Rabies and Wildlife: a Biologists Perspective*, Oxford University Press, Oxford.

Macdonald, G. (1950) The analysis of infection rates in diseases in which super-infection occurs. *Tropical Diseases Bulletin*, **47**, 907–15.

Macdonald, G. (1952) The analysis of equilibrium in malaria. *Tropical Diseases Bulletin*, **49**, 813–28.

Macdonald, G. (1957) *The Epidemiology and Control of Malaria*, Oxford University Press, London.

Macdonald, G. (1965) The dynamics of helminth infections, with special reference to schistosomes. *Transactions of the Royal Society of Tropical Medicine and Hygiene*, **59**, 489–506.

Macdonald, G. (1973) *Dynamics of Tropical Disease* (collected papers, ed. L. J. Bruce–Chwatt and V. J. Glanville), Oxford University Press, London.

McGregor, I. A. (1974) Mechanisms of acquired immunity and epidemiological patterns of antibody responses in malaria in man. *Bulletin of World Health Organization*, **50**, 259–66.

MacInnes, C. D. & Johnston, D. H. (1975). Rabies control: experiments in behavioural engineering. *Ontario Fish and Wildlife Reviews*, **14**: 17–20.

McKeown, T. (1979) *The Role of Medicine: Dream, Mirage or Nemesis*, Princeton University Press, Princeton.

McMillan, B., Kelly, A. and Walker, J. C. (1971) Prevalence of *Hymenolepis diminuta* infection in man in the New Guinea Highlands. *Tropical and Geographical Medicine*, **23**, 390–2.

McNamee, R. (1978) Manchester–Sheffield Research Report 72/RM/1.

McNeill, W. H. (1976) *Plagues and People*, Blackwell Scientific Publishers, Oxford.

May, R. M. (1976) Models for single populations, in *Theoretical Ecology: Principles and Applications* (ed. R. M. May) Blackwell Scientific Publications, Oxford, pp. 4–25.

May, R. M. (1977a) Thresholds and break points in ecosystems with a multiplicity of stable slates. *Nature, (London)* **269**, 471–7.

May, R. M. (1977b) Togetherness among schistosomes: its effects on the dynamics of the infection. *Mathematical Biosciences*, **35**, 301–43.

May, R. M. and Anderson, R. M. (1978) Regulation and stability of host-parasite population interactions. II. Destabilising processes. *Journal of Animal Ecology*, **47**, 249–67.

May, R. M. and Anderson, R. M. (1979) Population biology of infectious diseases: II. *Nature* (London), **280**, 455–61.

Maynard–Smith, J. (1978) *Models in Ecology*, Cambridge University Press, Cambridge.

Meek, A. H. (1977) Economically Optimal Control Strategies for Ovine Fascioliasis. PhD Thesis, University of Melbourne, Australia.

Meek, A. H. and Morris, R. S. (1979) The longevity of *Fasciola hepatica* metacercariae encysted on herbage. *Australian Veterinary Journal*, **55**, 58–60.

Mello, D. A. (1974) A note on egg production of *Ascaris lumbricoides*. *Journal of Parasitology*, **60**, 380–1.

Mendis, K. N. and Targett, G. A. T. (1979) Immunisation against gametes and asexual erythrocytic stages of a rodent malaria parasite. *Nature (London)*, **277**, 389–91.

Merselis, J. G. (1964) Quantitative bacteriology of the typhoid carrier state. *American Journal of Tropical Medicine*, **13**, 425–9.

Meuwissen, J. H. E. Th. (1974) The indirect haemagglutination test for malaria and its application to epidemiological surveillance. *Bulletin of World Health Organization*, **50**, 277–86.

Miller, D. L. (1964) Frequency of complications of measles, 1963. *British Medical Journal*, **2**, 75–8.

Miller, M. J. (1958) Observations on the natural history of malaria in the semi-resistant West African. *Transactions of the Royal Society of Tropical Medicine and Hygiene*, **52**, 152–68.

Miller, T. A. (1978) Industrial development and field use of the canine hookworm vaccine. *Advances in Parasitology*, **16**, 333–42.

Ministry of Agriculture, Fisheries and Food (1970) Modern farming and the soil. *Agricultural Advisory Council*, HMSO.

Ministry of Agriculture, Fisheries and Food (1976) The agricultural climate of England and Wales. *Technical Bulletin No. 35*, HMSO.

Ministry of Agriculture, Fisheries and Food (1976–1977) Farm incomes in England and Wales, 1976–1977; *Ministry of Agriculture, Fisheries and Food*, HMSO.

Ministry of Agriculture, Fisheries and Food (1960–1979). Annual Abstract of Statistics 1960–1979. *Central Statistical Office*, HMSO.

Moegle, H. Knorpp, F., Bogel, K., Arata, A. A., Dietz, N. and Dethelm, P. (1974) Zur Epidemiologie der Wildliertollarut. *Zentralblatt Veterinärmedizin*, **B21**, 647–59.

Molineaux, L. (1975) Dynamics of transmission. Unpublished Working Paper: *Expert Committee on Epidemiology of Onchocerciasis* (ONCHO/WP/75.23).

Molineaux, L., Dietz, K. and Thomas, A. (1978) Further epidemiological evaluation of a malaria model. *Bulletin of World Health Organization*, **56**, 565–71.

Molineaux, L. and Gramiccia, G. (1980) *The Garki Project*, World Health Organization, Geneva.

Molineaux, L., Shidrawi, G. R., Clarke, J. L., Boulzaguet, J. R. and Ashkar, T. S.

(1979) Assessment of insecticidal impact on the malaria mosquito's vectorial capacity, from data on the man-biting rate and age-composition. *Bulletin of World Health Organisation*, **57**, 265–74.

Molineaux, L., Storey, J., Cohen, J. E. and Thomas, A. (1982) A longitudinal study of human malaria in the West African savanna in the absence of control measures: relationships between *P. falciparum* and *P. Malariae*. *American Journal of Tropical and Medical Hygiene*, **29**, 725–37.

Mollison, D. (1977) Spatial contact models for ecological and epidemic spread. *Journal of Royal Statistical Society Series B*, **39**, 283–326.

Morris, R. F. (ed.) (1963) The dynamics of epidemic spruce budworm populations. *Memoirs of Entomological Society, in Canada*, **31**.

Muench, H. (1959) *Catalytic Models in Epidemiology*, Harvard University Press, Cambridge, Mass.

Muller, R. (1975) *Worms and Disease, a Manual of Medical Helminthology*, William Heinemann Medical Books Ltd., London.

Murdoch, W. W. and Oaten, A. (1975) Predation and population stability. *Advances in Ecological Research*, **9**, 1–131.

Nagano, Y. and Davenport, F. (eds) (1971) *Rabies*, University Park Press, Baltimore.

Nájera, J. A. (1974) A critical review of the field application of a mathematical model of malaria eradication. *Bulletin of World Health Organization*, **50**, 449–57.

Nansen, P. and Midtgaard, N. (1977) Fascioliasis in sheep in South-western Jutland. *Nordisk Veterinaermedicin*, **29**, 257–62.

Nardin, E. H., Nussenzweig, R. S., McGregor, I. A. and Bryan, J. H. (1979) Antibodies to sporozoites: their frequent occurrence in individuals living in an area of hyperendemic malaria. *Science*, **206**, 597–9.

Nåsell, I. and Hirsch, W. M. (1973) The transmission dynamics of schistosomiasis. *Communications in Pure and Applied Mathematics*, **26**, 395–453.

Nawalinski, T., Schad, G. A. and Chowdhury, A. B. (1978a) Population biology of hookworms in children in rural west Bengal. I. General parasitological observations. *American Journal of Tropical Medicine and Hygiene*, **27**, 1152–61.

Nawalinski, T., Schad, G. A. and Chowdhury, A. D. (1978b) Population biology of hookworms in children in rural west Bengal. II. Acquisition and loss of hookworms. *American Journal of Tropical Medicine and Hygiene*, **27**, 1162–73.

Nelson, G. S. and Saoud, M. F. A. (1966) The daily egg output of *Schistosoma mansoni* in rhesus monkeys. *Transactions of the Royal Society of Tropical Medicine and Hygiene*, **60**, 429.

Nice, N. G. (1979) Aspects of the Biology of *Fasciola hepatica* and its Intermediate Snail Host, *Lymnaea truncatula*. PhD Thesis, University of York.

Nice, N. G. and Wilson, R. A. (1974) A study of the effect of temperature on the growth of *Fasciola hepatica* and *Lymnaea truncatula*. *Parasitology*, **68**, 47–56.

Nikolitsch, M. (1965) Rabies – aspects of the history of the disease and its mode of transmission. *Blue Book for the Veterinary Profession*, **10**, 7–12.

Nold, A. (1982) Heterogeneity in disease transmission modelling. *Mathematical Biosciences*, **52**, 227–40.

Nollen, P. M. (1975) Studies on the reproductive system of *Hymenolepis diminuta* using autoradiography and transplantation. *Journal of Parasitology*, **61**, 100–4.

Nussenzweig, R. S. (1977) Immunoprophylaxis of malaria: sporozoite-induced immunity, in *Immunity to Blood Parasites of Animals and Man*, (ed. L. H. Miller, J.

A. Pino and J. J. McKelvey, Jr.) Plenum Press, New York, pp. 75–87.

Oakley, G. A. Owen, B. and Knapp, N. H. H. (1979) Production effects of subclinical liver fluke infection in growing dairy heifers. *Veterinary Record*, **104**, 503–7.

Obiamiwe, B. A. (1977) The pattern of parasitic infection in human gut at the Specialist Hospital, Benin City, Nigeria. *Annals of Tropical Medicine and Parasitology*, **71**, 35–43.

Ollerenshaw, C. B. (1966) The approach to forecasting the incidence of fascioliasis over England and Wales 1958–1962. *Agricultural Meteorology*, **3**, 35–63.

Ollerenshaw, C. B. (1971a) The influence of climate on the life cycle of *Fasciola hepatica* in Britain with some observations on the relationship between climate and the incidence of fascioliasis in the Netherlands. *Symposium – Parasitological Department of the Centraal Diergeneestundig Institut at Lelystad.*

Ollerenshaw, C. B. (1971b) Some observations on the epidemiology of fascioliasis in relation to the timing of molluscicide applications in the control of the disease. *The Veterinary Record*, **88**, 152–64.

Ollerenshaw, C. B. (1971c) Some observations on the epidemiology and control of fascioliasis in Wales. *Second International Liverfluke Colloquium*, Wageningen, 2–6 Oct. 1967.

Ollerenshaw, C. B. (1974) Forecasting liver fluke disease. *Symposia of the British Society for Parasitology*, **12**.

Ollerenshaw, C. B. and Rowcliffe, S. A. (1961) A survey and appraisal of the methods used by farmers to control fascioliasis. *The Veterinary Record*, **73**, 1113–21.

Ollerenshaw, C. B. and Rowlands, W. T. (1959) A method of forecasting the incidence of fascioliasis in Anglesey. *The Veterinary Record*, **71**, 591–8.

Over, H. J. (1962) A method of determining the liver fluke environment by means of the vegetation type. *Bulletin de l'office international des epizoites*, **58**, 297–304.

Over, H. J. and Dijkstra, J. (1975) Infection rhythm in fascioliasis, *In Facts and Reflections II. (Lelystad Workshop on Fascioliasis)*, (ed. H. J. Over and J. Armour).

Over, H. J. and Koopman, J. J. (1970) Field trials with 'Frescon' in the Netherlands. *The Control of Fascioliasis* (Proceedings of the symposium held 23–25 Feb. 1970). Shellstar Ltd.

Pampiglione, S. and Ricciardi, M. L. (1972) Geographic distribution of *Strongyloides fulleborni* in humans in tropical Africa. *Parasitologia*, **14**, 329–38.

Parker, R. L. and Wilsnack, R. E. (1966) Pathogenesis of skunk rabies virus. *American Journal of Veterinary Research*, **27**, 33–43.

Pawlowski, Z. S. (1978) Ascariasis. *Clinics in Gastroenterology*, **7**, 157–78.

Pawlowski, Z. S. and Schultz, M. G. (1972) Taeniasis and cysticercosis (*Taenia saginata*). *Advances in Parasitology*, **10**, 269–347.

Payne, F. K. (1924) Investigations on the control of hookworm disease XXXI. The relation of the physiological age of hookworm larvae to their ability to infect the human host. *American Journal of Hygiene*, **3**, 584–97.

Pearson, A. J. A. (1970) Frescon – application methods for control of *Lymnaea truncatula*, in *The Control of Fascioliasis* (Proceedings of the symposium 23–25 Feb. 1970), Shellstar Ltd.

Penman, H. L. (1948) Natural evaporation from open water, bare soil and grass. *Proceedings of the Royal Society, London Series A*, **193**, 120–45.

Pennycuik, L. (1971) Frequency distributions of parasites in a population of three-spined sticklebacks, *Gasterosteus aculeatus* L., with particular reference to the negative binomial distribution. *Parasitology*, **63**, 389–406.

Perkins, D. F. (1978) Production ecology of British moors and montane grasslands. *Ecological Studies 27* (ed. O. W. Heal and D. F. Perkins), Springer-Verlag, Berlin, ch. 20.

Pesigan, T. P., Farooq, M., Hairston, N. G., Jauregui, J. J., Garcia, E. G., Santos, A. T., Santos, B. C. and Besa, A. A. (1958a) Studies on *Schistosoma japonicum* infection in the Philippines. 1. General considerations and epidemiology. *Bulletin of World Health Organization*, **18**, 345–455.

Pesigan, T. P., Hairston, N. G., Jauregui, J. J., Garcia, E. G., Santos, A. T., Santos, B. C. and Besa, A. A. (1958b) Studies on *Schistosoma japonicum* infection in the Philippines. 2. The molluscan host. *Bulletin of World Health Organization*, **18**, 481–578.

Peters, B. G. and Clapham, P. A. (1942) Infestation with liver fluke among 73,000 cattle slaughtered in Great Britain during June 1942. *Journal of Helminthology*, **20**, 115–38.

Peters, W. (1974) Recent advances in antimalarial chemotherapy and drug resistance. *Advances in Parasitology*, **12**, 69–114.

Peters, W. (1978) Medical aspects – comments and discussion II, in *The Relevance of Parasitology to Human Welfare Today* (ed. A. E. R. Taylor and R. Muller), Blackwell Scientific Publications, Oxford.

Peters, W. and Standfast, H. A. (1960) Studies on the epidemiology of malaria in New Guinea. II. Holoendemic malaria, the entomological picture. *Transactions of the Royal Society of Tropical Medicine and Hygeine*, **54**, 249–60.

Philippon, B. and Bain, O. (1972) Transmission de l'onchocercose humaine en zone de savane d'Afrique occidentale, passage de microfilaires *d'Onchocerca volvulus* Leuck. dans l'hémocèle de la femelle de *Simulium damnosum* Th., *Cahiers ORSTOM Series Entomologiste Médecire Parasitologie*, **10**, 251–61.

Pickering, J. (1980) Sex Ratio, Social Behaviour and Ecology in *Polistes* (Hymenoptera, Vespidae), *Pachysomoides* (Hymenoptera, Ichneumonidae) and *Plasmodium* (Protozoa, Haemospovidia) *PhD Thesis*, Department of Biology, Harvard university, 362 pp.

Polydorou, K. (1977) The anti-echinococcosis campaign in Cyprus. *Tropical Animal Health and Production*, **9**, 141–6.

Preston, E. M. (1973) Computer simulated dynamics of a rabies-controlled fox population. *Journal of Wildlife Management*, **36**, 237–48.

Price, P. W. (1980) *Evolutionary Biology of Parasites*, Princeton University Press, Princeton.

Pringle, G. and Avery–Jones, S. (1966) Observations on the early course of untreated falciparum malaria in semi-immune African children following a short period of protection. *Bulletin of World Health Organisation*, **34**, 269–72.

Prost, A., Hervouet, J. P. and Thylefors, B. (1979) Les niveaux d'endémicité dans l'onchocercose, *Bulletin de l'Organisation Mondiale de la Santé*, **57**, 655–62.

Pull, J. H. and Grab, B. (1974) A simple epidemiological model for evaluating the malaria inoculation rate and the risk of infection in infants. *Bulletin of World Health Organisation*, **51**, 507–16.

Pullan, N. B., Sewell, M. M. H. and Hammond, J. A. (1970) Studies on the pathogenicity of massive infections of *Fasciola hepatica* in lambs. *British Veterinary Journal*, **126**, 543–58.

Rahman, A., Ahmed, M. U. and Mia, A. S. (1975) Diseases of goats diagnosed in slaughterhouses in Bangladesh. *Tropical Animal Health and Production*, **7**, 164.

Rajendram, S. and Jayewickreme, S. H. (1951a) Malaria in Ceylon, Part I, the control and prevention of epidemic malaria by the residual spraying of houses with DDT. *Indian Journal of Malariology*, **5**, 1–73.

Rajendram, S. and Jayewickreme, S. H. (1951b) Malaria in Ceylon, Part II, the control of endemic malaria at Anuradhapura by the residual spraying of houses with DDT. *Indian Journal of Malariology*, **5**, 75–124.

Ratliff, C. R. and Donaldson, L. (1965) A human case of *Hymenolepiasis diminuta* in Alabama. *Journal of Parasitology*, **51**, 808.

Rau, M. E. (1979) The frequency distribution of *Hymenolepis diminuta* cysticercoids in natural sympatric populations of *Tenebrio moliter* and *Tenebrio obscurus*. *International Journal for Parasitology*, **9**, 85–7.

Rees, G. (1967) Pathogenesis of adult cestodes. *Helminthological Abstracts*, **36**, 1–23.

Registrar General (1940–1979) *Annual Review of the Registrar General of England and Wales*. HMSO (for 1974–1979 morbidity records were taken from *the Office of Population Census and Surveys. Infectious disease quarterly monitor*. HMSO)

Reuss, U. (1973) *Fascioliasis Symposium Proceedings*, Tecklenburg, 3–4 Oct 1973 A. I. P., Bonn-Bad Godesberg.

Revelle, C., Lynn, W. R. and Feldman, F. (1967) Mathematical models for the economic allocation of tuberculosis control programs. *American Review of Respiratory Diseases*, **96**, 893–909.

Reynolds, G. H. and Chan, Y. K. (1975) A control model for gonorrhea. *Bulletin Institutions of International Statistics*, **106–2**, 264–79.

Ribbeck, R. and Witzel, G. (1979) Okonomische Verluste infolge Fasziolose bei Rind und Schaf. *Monatshefte für Veterinärmedizin*, **34**, 56–61.

Rieckmann, K. H., Carson, P. E. Beaudoin, R. L., Cassells, J. S. and Sell, K. W. (1974) Sporozoite induced immunity in man against an Ethiopian strain of *Plasmodium falciparum*. *Transactions of the Royal Society of Tropical Medicine and Hygiene*, **68**, 258–9.

Roberts, J. M. D., Neumann, E., Göckel, C. W. and Highton, R. B. (1967) Onchocerciasis in Kenya, 9, 11 and 18 years after elimination of the vector. *Bulletin of World Health Organization*, **37**, 195–212.

Roberts, L. S. (1961) The influence of population density on patterns and physiology of growth in *Hymenolepis diminuta* (Cestoda: Cyclophyllidea) in the definitive host. *Experimental Parasitology*, **11**, 332–71.

Roden, A. T. and Heath, W. C. C. (1977) Effects of vaccination against measles on the incidence of the disease and on the immunity of the child population in England and Wales. *Health Trends*, **9**, 69–72.

Rondelaud, D. (1974) L'évolution des rédies de *Fasciola hepatica* L. chez *Galba truncatula* Müller en Limousin. *Revue de Medicine Veterinaire*, **125**, 237–50.

Rondelaud, D. and Vincent, M. (1973) The effect of parasitisation on the growth of *Galba truncatula* in Limousin. *Comptes Rendues des Séances de la Societé de Biologié*, **167**, 736–8.

Rondelaud, D. and Morel–Vareille, C. (1975) Distribution estivale et survie des

Limnées tronquées, *Lymnaea truncatula* (Muller) saines ou infestees par *Fasciola hepatica* L. *Annales de Parasitologie, Humaine et Comparee*, **50**, 603–16.

Ross. J. G. (1965) Experimental infections of cattle with *Fasciola hepatica*: a comparison of low and high infection rates. *Nature (London)*, **208**, 907.

Ross, J. G. (1966) An abattoir survey of cattle liver infections with *Fasciola hepatica*. *British Veterinary Journal*, **122**, 489–94.

Ross, J. G. (1967a) An epidemiological study of fascioliasis in sheep. *Veterinary Record*, **80**, 214–17.

Ross, J. G. (1967b) A further season of epidemiological studies of *Fasciola hepatica* in sheep. *Veterinary Record*, **80**, 368–371.

Ross, J. G. (1970) The economics of *Fasciola hepatica* infections in cattle. *British Veterinary Journal*, **126**, 23–5.

Ross, J. G. (1977) A five year study of the epidemiology of fascioliasis in the North, East and West of Scotland. *British Veterinary Journal*, **133**, 263–72.

Ross, J. G. and O'Hagan, J. (1966) A biological technique to assess numbers of *Fasciola hepatica* cercariae on pastures. *Journal of Helminthology*, **40**, 375–8.

Ross, R. (1904) On the logical basis of the sanitary policy of mosquito reduction. *Proceedings of the Congress, Arts, Science, St. Louis, USA*, **6**, 89. (Also (1905) *British Medical Journal*, **1**, 1025–9.)

Ross, R. (1911) *The prevention of malaria* (2nd ed.), Murray, London.

Ross, R. (1915) Some *a priori* pathometric equations. *British Medical Journal*, **1**, 546–7.

Ross, R. (1916) An application of the theory of probabilities to the study of *a priori* pathometry. I. *Proceedings of the Royal Society of London Series A*, **92**, 204–30.

Ross, R. (1917) An application of the theory of probabilities to the study of *a priori* pathometry. II. *Proceedings of the Royal Society of London Series A*, **93**, 212–25.

Ross, R. and Hudson, H. P. (1917) An application of the theory of probabilities to the study of *a priori* pathometry. III. *Proceedings of the Royal Society of London Series A*, **93**, 225–40.

Rowcliffe, S. A. and Ollerenshaw, C. B. (1960) Observations on the binomics of the egg of *Fasciola hepatica*. *Annals of Tropical Medicine and Parasitology*, **54**, 172–81.

Rowland, M. G. M., Cole, T. J. and Whitehead, R. G. (1977) A quantitative study into the role of infection in determining nutritional status in Gambian village children. *British Journal of Nutrition*, **37**, 441–50.

Sadun, E. H. and Vajrasthira, S. (1953) Studies on intestinal parasitic infections in Cholburi province (Thailand). *American Journal of Tropical Medicine and Hygiene*, **2**, 286–97.

Sahba, G. H. Arfaa, F. and Bijan, H. (1967) Intestinal helminthiasis in the rural area of Khuzestan, south-west Iran. *Annals of Tropical Medicine and Parasitology*, **61**, 352–7.

Sampaio–Xavier, M. de L., Martinez Fernandez, A. R. and Mattos dos Santos, M. A. (1971) The susceptibility to *Fasciola hepatica* of some fresh-water snails in Portugal and Spain. *Second International Liverfluke Colloquium* Wageningen 2–6 Oct. 1967.

Scanlon, J. E. and Sandhinand, U. (1965) The distribution and biology of *Anopheles balabacensis* in Thailand (Diptera: Culicidae). *Journal of Medical Entomology*, **2**, 61–9.

Scanlon, J. E., Peyton, E. L. and Gould, D. J. (1967) The *Anopheles (cellia) leucosphyrus* donitz 1901 group in Thailand. *Proceedings of the Annual Conference in California of Mosquito Control Association,* **35**, 78–83.

Schad, G. A. (1971) The ecology of interacting populations of man and hookworms in rural west Bengal. *Report of the Johns Hopkins Center for Medical Research and Training,* 1969–1970, 5–24.

Schad, G. A., Tonascia, J. A., Chowdhury, A. B. and Thomas, J. (1982) The ecology of interacting populations of man and hookworms in rural west Bengal. I. The frequency distribution of faecal egg counts, in preparation.

Schaefer, M. B. (1954) Some aspects of the dynamics of populations important to the management of commercial fish populations. *Inter-American Tropical Tuna Commission Bulletin,* **1**, 26–56.

Schantz, P. M. and Schwabe, C. (1969) Worldwide status of hydatid disease control. *Journal of the American Veterinary Medical Association,* **155**(12), 2104–21.

Schiefer, B. A., Ward, R. A. and Eldridge, B. F. (1977) *Plasmodium cynomologi*: effects of malaria infection on laboratory flight performance of *Anopheles stephensi* mosquitoes *Experimental Parasitology,* **41**, 397–404.

Scott, J. A. and Barlow, C. H. (1938) Limitations in the control of helminth parasites in Egypt by means of treatment and sanitation. *American Journal of Hygiene,* **27**, 619.

Scrimshaw, N. S., Taylor, C. E. and Gordon, J. E. (1968) Interactions of nutrition and infection. *World Health Organization Monographic Series,* **57**, 329 pp.

Segal, H. E., Wilkinson, R. N., Thiemanun, W., Gresso, W. E. and Gould, D. J. (1974) Longitudinal malaria studies in rural north-east Thailand: demographic and temporal variables of infection. *Bulletin of World Health Organisation,* **50**, 505–12.

Sergent, E. and Poncet, A. (1956) Etude expérimentale du paludisme des rongeurs à *P. berghei*, IV. Resistance acquisé. *Archives Institut Pasteur d'Algérie,* **34**, 1–51.

Shaka, S. and Nansen, P. (1979) Epidemiology of fascioliasis in Denmark. Studies on the seasonal availability of metacercariae and the parasite stages overwintering on pasture. *Veterinary Parasitology,* **5**, 145–54.

Sikes, K (1962) Pathogenesis of Rabies in Wildlife, I. *American Journal of Veterinary Research,* **13**, 1041–7.

Sinclair, K. B. (1962) Observations on the clinical pathology of ovine fascioliasis. *British Veterinary Journal,* **118**, 37–53.

Sinclair, K. B. (1972) The pathogenicity of *Fasciola hepatica* in pregnant sheep. *British Veterinary Journal,* **128**, 249–59.

Slooff, R. and Verdrager, J. (1972) *Anopheles balabacensis* Baisas 1936 and malaria transmission in south-eastern areas of Asia. WHO/MAL/72.765, unpublished document of the World Health Organization.

Smalley, M. E. and Sinden, R. E. (1977) *Plasmodium falciparum* gametocytes: their longevity and infectivity. *Parasitology,* **74**, 1–8.

Smart, C. W. and Giles, R. H. (1973) A computer model of wildlife rabies epizootics and an analysis of incidence patterns. *Wildlife Diseases,* **61**, 1–89.

Smillie, W. G. (1924) Control of hookworm disease in South Alabama. *Southern Medical Journal,* **17**, 494–9.

Smith, C. E. G. (1970) Prospects for the control of infectious diseases. *Proceedings of the Royal Society of Medicine,* **63**, 1181–90.

Smith, G. (1978) A Field and Laboratory Study of the Epidemiology of Fascioliasis. D Phil Thesis, University of York.

Smith, G. (1981) Copulation and oviposition in *Lymnaea truncatula* (Muller). *Journal of Molluscan Studies*, **47**, 108–11.

Smith, G. (1982) Climate, soil and regional variations in the prevalence of fascioliasis. *Welsh Soils Discussion Group Report* (in press).

Smith G. and Wilson, R. A. (1980) Seasonal variations in the microclimate of *Lymnaea truncatula* habitats. *Journal of Applied Ecology*, **17**, 329–42.

Smithers, S. R. and Terry, R. J. (1969) Immunity in schistosomiasis. *Annals of New York Academy of Sciences*, **160**, 826–40.

Smyth, J. D. (1977) Strain differences in *Echinococcus granulosus*, with special reference to the status of equine hydatidosis in the United Kingdom. *Transactions of the Royal Society of Tropical Medicine and Hygiene*, **71**, 93–100.

Smyth, J. D. and Smyth, M. M. (1964) Natural and experimental hosts of *Echinococcus granulosus* and *E. multilocularis*, with comments on the genetics of speciation in the genus *Echinococcus*. *Parasitology*, **54**, 493–514.

Soper, H. E. (1929) Interpretation of periodicity in disease-prevalence. *Journal of Royal Statistical Society*, **92**, 34–73.

Sosiptrov, G. V. and Shumakovich, E. E. (1966) Population dynamics and density of the mollusc, *Galba truncatula* and its infestation with larvae of *Fasciola hepatica* in Moscow Province conditions. *Mater. Knof. obshch. gel'mint.*, **1**, 253–6.

Steele, J. H. (1973) The epidemiology and control of rabies. *Scandinavian Journal of Infectious Diseases*, **5**, 299–312.

Stoll, N. R. (1923) Investigations on the control of hookworm disease. XVIII. On the relation between the number of eggs found in human faeces and the number of hookworms in the host. *American Journal of Hygiene*, **3**, 103–17.

Stoll, N. R. (1938) Tapeworm studies. VII. Variation in pasture infestation with *M. expansa*. *Journal of Parasitology*, **24**, 527–45.

Stoll, N. R. (1947) This wormy world. *Journal of Parasitology*, **33**, 1–18.

Sturrock, R. F. (1967) Hookworm studies in Tanganyika (Tanzania): The results of a series of surveys on a group of primary school children and observations on the survival of hookworm infective larvae exposed to simulated field conditions. *East African Medical Journal*, **44**, 142–9.

Sturrock, R. F. (1973) Field studies on the population dynamics of *Biomphalaria glabrata*, intermediate host of *Schistosoma mansoni*, on the West Indian islands of St. Lucia. *International Journal of Parasitology*, **3**, 175–94.

Sturrock, R. F. and Webbe, G. (1971) The application of catalytic models to schistosomiasis in snails. *Journal of Helminthology*, **45**, 189–200.

Styczynska–Jurewicz, E. (1965) Adaptation of eggs and larvae of *Fasciola hepatica* to the conditions of astatic habitats of *Galba truncatula*. *Acta Parasitologica*, **13**, 151–68.

Sullivan, A. V. (1977) Some diseases of animals communicable to man. *Environmental Health*, **85(7)**, 151–7.

Sutherland, I. and Fayers, P. M. (1971) Effects of measles vaccination on incidence of measles in the community. *British Medical Journal*, **1**, 698–702.

Sykes, A. R. Coop, R. L. and Rushton, B. (1980) Chronic subclinical fascioliasis in sheep: effects on food intake, food utilisation and blood constituents. *Research in Veterinary Science*, **28**, 63–70.

Taliaferro, W. H. (1949) Immunity to the malaria infections, in *Malariology* (ed. M. F. Boyd), W. B. Saunders, Philadelphia, pp. 935–65.

Tallis, G. M. and Leyton, M. K. (1969) Stochastic models of populations of helminthic parasites in the definitive host: I. *Mathematical Biosciences*, **4**, 39–48.

Taylor, D. W. and Siddiqui, W. A. (1978) Effect of falciparum malaria infection on the *in vitro* mitogen responses of spleen and peripheral blood lymphocytes from owl monkeys. *American Journal of Tropical Medicine and Hygiene*, **27**, 738–42.

Thomas, M. R. (1979) Towards a Mathematical Model for the Transmission of Fascioliasis. D. Phil. Thesis, University of York.

Thompson, R. C. A. and Smyth, J. D. (1974) Potential danger of hydatid disease of horse dog origin. *British Medical Journal*, **iii**, 807.

Thylefors, B., Philippon, B. and Prost, A. (1978) Transmission potentials of *Onchocerca volvulus* and the associated intensity of onchocerciasis in a Sudan-savanna area. *Tropenmedizin und Parasitologie*, **29**, 346–54.

Tierkel, E. S. (1959) Rabies *Advances in Veterinary Sciences*, **5**, 183–226.

Upatham, E. S. and Sturrock, R. F. (1973) Field investigations on the effect of other aquatic animals on the infection of *Biomphalaria glabrata* by *Schistosoma mansoni* miracidia. *Journal of Parasitology*, **59**, 448–53.

Urquhart, G. M., Doyle, J. and Jennings, F. W. (1970) Studies on ovine fascioliasis. III. The comparative use of molluscicide and an anthelmintic in the control of the disease. *The Veterinary Record*, **86**, 338–45.

Van Haaften, J. (1970) Fox ecology studies in the Netherlands. *Transactions of the International Congress of Game Biologists*, **9**, 539–43.

Varley, G C., Gradwell, G. R. and Hassell, M. P. (1973) *Insect population ecology: an analytical approach.* Blackwell Scientific Publications, Oxford.

Vink, L. A. (1971) The practical diagnosis of fascioliasis in sheep and cattle. *Second International Liverfluke Colloquium*, Wageningen, 2–6 Oct., 1967.

Voge, M. and Turner, J. A. (1956) Effect of temperature on larval development of the cestode, *Hymenolepis diminuta. Experimental Parasitology*, **5**, 580–6.

von Bonsdorff, K. (1977) *Diphyllobothriasis in Man*, Academic Press, New York.

Waaler, H. T. (1968) A dynamic model for the epidemiology of tuberculosis. *American Review of Respiratory Diseases*, **98**, 591–600.

Waaler, H. T., Gesser, A. and Anderson, S. (1962) The use of mathematical models in the study of the epidemiology of tuberculosis. *American Journal of Public Health*, **52**, 1002–13.

Waaler, H. T. and Piot, M. A. (1969) The use of an epidemiological model for estimating the effectiveness of tuberculosis control measures. Sensitivity of the effectiveness of tuberculosis control measures to the coverage of the population. *Bulletin of World Health Organization*, **41**, 75–93.

Walsh, J. F., Davies, J. B. and Le Berre, R. (1979) Entomological aspects of the first five years of the Onchocerciasis Control Programme in the Volta River Basin. *Tropenmedizin und Parasitologie*, **30**, 328–44.

Walters, T. M. H. (1977) Hydatid disease in Wales. *Transactions of the Royal Society of Tropical Medicine and Hygiene*, **71(2)**, 105–8.

Walton, C. L. (1918) Liver rot of sheep, and bionomics of *Lymnaea truncatula* in the Aberystwyth area. *Parasitology*, **10**, 232–66.

Wandeler, A. (1976) Fox ecology in Central Europe in relation to rabies control.

Proceedings of the Symposium on Advances in Rabies Research, 1976, *United States Department of Health, Education and Welfare*, Atlanta, pp. 6–21.

Wandeler, A., Wachendorfer, J., Forster, U., Krekel, H., Schale, W., Muller, J. and Steck, F. (1974) Rabies in wild carnivores in Central Europe. I. Epidemiological studies. *Zeitschrift für Tropenmedizin und Parasitologie*, **B21**, 735–56.

Warren, K. S. (1973) Regulation of the prevalence and intensity of schistosomiasis in man: immunology or ecology? *Journal of Infectious Diseases*, **127**, 595–609.

Warren, K. S. (1981) The control of helminths: non-replicating infectious agents of man. Annual Review of Public Health, **2**, 101–115.

Warren, K. S., Mahmoud, A. A. F., Muruka, J. F., Whittacker, L. R., Ouma, J. H. and Arap Siongok, T. K. (1979) Schistosomiasis haematobia in Coast Province, Kenya: relationship between egg output and morbidity. *American Journal of Tropical Medicine and Hygiene*, **28**, 864–70.

Warren, K. S. and Mahmoud, A. A. F. (1976) Targeted mass treatment: a new approach to the control of schistosomiasis. *Transactions of the Association of American Physicians*, **89**, 195–204.

Watson, K. C. (1967) Intravascular *Salmonella typhi* as a manifestation of the carrier state. *Lancet*, **ii**, 332–4.

Webbe, G. (1962) The transmission of *Schistosoma haematobium* in an area of Lake Province, Tanganyika. *Bulletin of World Health Organization*, **27**, 59–85.

Webbe, G. (1967) The hatching and activation of taeniid ova in relation to the development of cysticercosis in man. *Zeitschrift für Tropenmedizin und Parasitologia*, **18**, 354–69.

Weeda, W. C. (1967) The effect of cattle dung patches on pasture growth, botanical composition and pasture utilisation. *New Zealand Journal of Agriculture*, **10**, 150–9.

Weinbaum, F. I., Evans, C. B. and Tigelaar, R. E. (1976) Immunity to *Plasmodium berghei yoelii* in mice. I. The course of infection in T-cell and B-cell deficient mice. *Journal of Immunology*, **117**, 1999–2005.

Weinbaum, F. I., Weintraub, J., Nkrumah, F. K., Evans, C. B., Tigelaar, R. E. and Rosenberg, Y. J. (1978) Immunity to *Plasmodium berghei yoelii* in mice, II. Specific and nonspecific cellular and humoral responses during the course of infection. *Journal of Immunology*, **121**, 629–636.

Wellde, B. T., Diggs, C. L. and Anderson, S. (1979) Immunization of *Aotus trivirgatus* against *Plasmodium falciparum* with irradiated blood forms. *Bulletin of World Health Organization*, **57**, (*Suppl*. 1), 153–7.

Whitehead, R. G. (1977) Some quantitative considerations of importance to the improvement of the nutritional status of rural children. *Proceedings of the Royal Society of London (Biol.)*, **199**, 49–60.

Whittle, P. (1955) The outcome of a stochastic epidemic – a note on Bailey's paper. *Biometrika*, **42**, 154–62.

WHO (1967) Control of ascariasis. *World Health Organization Technical Report Series*, **379**, 47 pp.

WHO (1970) Principles and practice of cholera control. (Public Health papers, No. 40), WHO, Geneva.

WHO (1980) *Rabies Bulletin Europe*, **1**, 1980.

Wickwire, K. (1977) Mathematical models for the control of pests and infectious diseases: a survey. *Theoretical Population Biology*, **11**, 181–238.

Williams, H. H. and McVicar, A. (1968) Sperm transfer in Tetraphyllidea (platyhelminths: cestoda). *Nytt Magasin for Zoologi*, **16**, 61–71.

Willomitzer, J. (1974) Examination of some Lymnaeidae for the developmental stages of *Fasciola hepatica*. *Acta Veterinaria, Brno*, **43**, 381–5.

Wilson, E. G. and Burke, M. H. (1942) The epidemic curve. *Proceedings of the National Academy of Science U.S.A.*, **28**, 361–7.

Wilson, R. A. and Draskau, T. (1976) The stimulation of daughter redia production during the larval development of *Fasciola hepatica*. *Parasitology*, **72**, 245–57.

Wilson, R. A. and Taylor, S. L. (1978) The effect of variations in host and parasite density on the level of parasitisation of *Lymnaea truncatula* by *Fasciola hepatica*. *Parasitology*, **76**, 91–8.

Wilson, R. A. and Denison, J. (1980) The parasitic castration and gigantism of *Lymnaea truncatula* infected with the larval stages of *Fasciola hepatica*. *Zeitschrift für Parasitenkunde*, **61**, 109–19.

Wilson, R. J. M. (1980) Serotyping *Plasmodium falciparum* malaria with S-antigens. *Nature (London)*, **284**, 451–2.

Winkler, W. G. (1975) Fox rabies, in *The Natural History of Rabies*, (ed. G. M. Baer), Academic Press, New York, pp. 3–22:

Winkler, W. G. and Baer, G. M. (1976) Rabies immunisation of red foxes (*Vulpes fulva*) with vaccine in sausage baits. *American Journal of Epidemiology*, **103**, 408–15.

Winkler, W. G., McLean, R. G. and Cowart, J. C. (1975) Vaccination of foxes against rabies using ingested baits. *Journal of Wildlife Diseases*, **11**, 382–8.

Witenberg, G. G. (1964) Cestodiases, in *Zoonoses* (ed. J. van Hoeden), Elsevier Pub. Co., Amsterdam.

Woodruff, A. W. (1974) *Medicine in the Tropics*, Churchill–Livingstone, London.

Yanagisawa, R. and Mizuno, T. (1963) On the infection mode of hookworm. *Medical Culture*, **5**(1), 112–18.

Yekutiel, P. (1960) Problems of epidemiology in malaria eradication. *Bulletin of World Health Organization*, **22**, 669–83.

Yorke, J. A., Hethcote, H. W. and Nold, A. (1978) Dynamics and control of the transmission of gonorrhea. *Sexually Transmitted Diseases*, **5**, 51–6.

Yorke, J. A. and London, W. P. (1973) Recurrent outbreaks of measles, chickenpox and mumps. II. Systematic differences in contact rates and stochastic effects. *American Journal of Epidemiology*, **98**, 469–82

Yorke, J. A. Nathanson, N., Pianigiani, G. and Martin, J. (1979) Seasonality and the requirements for perpetuation and eradication of viruses in populations. *American Journal of Epidemiology*, **109**, 103–23.

Yoshida, N., Nussenzweig, R. S., Potocnjak, P., Nussenzweig, V. and Aikawa, M. (1980) Hybridoma produces protective antibodies directed against the sporozoite stage of malaria parasite *Science*, **207**, 71–3.

Zahar, A. R. (1974) Review of the ecology of malaria vectors in the WHO Eastern Mediterranean region. *Bulletin of World Health Organisation*, **50**, 427–40.

Zimen, E. (ed.) (1980) *The Red Fox*, Kluwer Boston, Hingham, Mass.

Zischke, J. A. (1967) Redial populations of *Echinostoma revolutum* developing in snails of different sizes. *Journal of Parasitology*, **53**, 1200–4.

Zuckerman, A. (1974) Functional aspects of immunity in malarial rats, in *Basic Research on Malaria*, (ed. J. B. Bateman), Technical Report ERO-5-74, US Army European Research Office, London, pp. 87–102.

Index

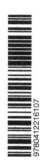